Mastering Single Best Answer Questions for the Part 2 MRCOG Examination

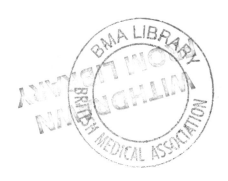

Mastering Single Best Answer Questions
for the Part 2 MRCOG Examination

Mastering Single Best Answer Questions for the Part 2 MRCOG Examination

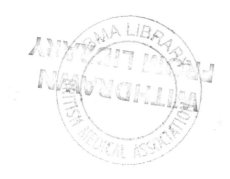

An Evidence-Based Approach

Adel Elkady FRCOG
Boulak El Dakror Hospital, Giza, Egypt

Bashir Dawlatly FRCOG
Whipps Cross Hospital, London, UK

Mustafa H. Ahmed MD MRCOG
Southend University Hospital, Southend, UK

Editor: **Alexandra E. Rees FRCOG**
University Hospital of Wales, Cardiff, UK

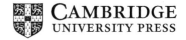

CAMBRIDGE
UNIVERSITY PRESS

University Printing House, Cambridge CB2 8BS, United Kingdom

One Liberty Plaza, 20th Floor, New York, NY 10006, USA

477 Williamstown Road, Port Melbourne, VIC 3207, Australia

4843/24, 2nd Floor, Ansari Road, Daryaganj, Delhi – 110002, India

79 Anson Road, #06–04/06, Singapore 079906

Cambridge University Press is part of the University of Cambridge.

It furthers the University's mission by disseminating knowledge in the pursuit of
education, learning, and research at the highest international levels of excellence.

www.cambridge.org
Information on this title: www.cambridge.org/9781316621561
DOI: 10.1017/9781316756447

First published 2017

Printed in the United Kingdom by Clays, St Ives plc

A catalogue record for this publication is available from the British Library.

ISBN 978-1-316-62156-1 Paperback

Cambridge University Press has no responsibility for the persistence or accuracy
of URLs for external or third-party Internet Web sites referred to in this publication
and does not guarantee that any content on such Web sites is, or will remain,
accurate or appropriate.

....

Every effort has been made in preparing this book to provide accurate and up-to-date
information, which is in accord with accepted standards and practice at the time of
publication. Although case histories are drawn from actual cases, every effort has been
made to disguise the identities of the individuals involved. Nevertheless, the authors,
editors and publishers can make no warranties that the information contained herein is
totally free from error, not least because clinical standards are constantly changing through
research and regulation. The authors, editors and publishers therefore disclaim all liability
for direct or consequential damages resulting from the use of material contained in this
book. Readers are strongly advised to pay careful attention to information provided by the
manufacturer of any drugs or equipment that they plan to use.

I dedicate my involvement in this work to the memories of my teachers and mentors (AbdElslam ElMenebawy, Gamal Samy and Haidar Fahmy), who helped and educated me when I was just crawling in this fascinating specialty and inspired me to become a Member of our Royal College.

Adel Elkady

I dedicate this book to my family, Marmar, Nic and Bells, for their support and patience during its preparation.

Bashir Dawlatly

I dedicate my contribution to my parents, brothers and sisters; to Dr. Hassan A Abdulla and all my teachers; to Hassan, Kareem, Aseel and Talya; to my wife.

Mustafa H. Ahmed

Contents

Mock examinations can be found online at www.cambridge.org/9781316621561

Contributors

YOUSSEF ABO ELWAN MD, MRCOG
Professor of Obstetrics and Gynaecology, Zagazig University, Zagazig, Egypt

MUSTAFA HASSAN AHMED MD, MRCOG
Obstetrics and Gynaecology Fellow, Southend University Hospital, Southend, UK

WAFAA BASTA MRCOG
Consultant, Mataria Hospital, Cairo, Egypt

BASHIR DAWLATLY FRCOG
Consultant Obstetrician and Gynaecologist, Whipps Cross University Hospital, London, UK

MAGDY EL SHEIKH FRCOG, FRCS
Consultant Obstetrician and Gynaecologist, Dr Soliman Fakeeh Hospital, Jeddah, Saudi Arabia

AHMED ELBOHOTY MD, MRCOG
Assistant Professor of Obstetrics and Gynaecology, Faculty of Medicine, Ain Shams University, Cairo, Egypt

ADEL ELKADY DGO, FRCOG, FICS
Consultant Obstetrician and Gynaecologist, Police Force Hospital, Egypt and Honorary Consulate Boulak El Da Kror Hospital, Giza, Egypt

IRENE GAFSON MBBS, BMEDSCI, MRCOG, FHEA, PGCPCE
Senior Registrar in Obstetrics and Gynaecology and Clinical Teaching Fellow, Whipps Cross Hospital, London, UK

BISMEEN JADOON MBBS, MRCOG, DFFP, DCLHCM
Reproductive and Maternal Health Unit, WHO Eastern Mediterranean Regional Office, Cairo, Egypt

AHMED M KHALIL MBBCH, MSC, MD, MRCOG
Lecturer, Benha University Faculty of Medicine, Banha, Egypt

TAMARA KUBBA MBBS, PGCME, MRCOG
Clinical Research Fellow, University College London Hospital, London, UK

RADWA MANSOUR MD, MRCOG
Lecturer in Obstetrics and Gynaecology, Ain Shams University, Cairo, Egypt

ROSHNI R PATEL FRCOG, MSC, PHD
Consultant in Maternal Medicine and High-Risk Obstetrics, Chelsea and Westminster Healthcare National Health Service Foundation Trust, London, UK and MBRRACE assessor.

ALEXANDRA REES MBCHB, FRCOG
Honorary Consultant, University Hospital of Wales, Cardiff, UK

AMY SHACALUGA MBBCH, MRCOG
Senior Registrar, Department of Obstetrics and Gynaecology, University Hospital of Wales, Cardiff, UK.

NAHED SHALTOOT MBBCH, MRCOG, DFFP, MSC, PGC
Consultant Obstetrics and Gynaecologist, Home Minimal Invasive and Robotic Surgery, Bedford Hospital National Health Service Trust, Bedford, UK

AKANKSHA SOOD MS, DNB, MRCOG, FACOG
Senior Clinical Fellow in Obstetrics and Gynaecology, St. Mary's Hospital, Central Manchester University Hospitals National Health Service Foundation Trust, Manchester, UK

Editor's Preface

Achieving membership of the Royal College of Obstetricians and Gynaecologists (RCOG) is an essential step along the path to a career in obstetrics and gynaecology. Passing the MRCOG examination is a key stepping stone towards this goal.

Until 2015, the examination was in two parts and contained a variety of different question types, including extended matched questions (EMQs), multiple choice questions (MCQs), short essay questions and true/false questions. The examination is now in three parts and success in Part 2 is required before progression to the Part 3 objective structured clinical examination (OSCE) or clinical assessment.

The Part 2 written examination consists of both single best answer (SBA) questions and EMQs. The examination is designed to be taken during years 3 to 5 of core training, and the questions cover the whole syllabus as described on the RCOG website; SBA questions make up 40% of the total marks and EMQs 60%.

This text book is designed to assist the candidates in their revision for the Part 2 examination. It comprises 26 chapters, which cover all areas of the Part 2 syllabus. The layout is clear and easy to follow with explanations and references to assist in understanding the answers to the questions. Evidence-based explanations are included for most of the answers to indicate the level of evidence for the answers.

I was delighted when Dr Adel Elkady asked me to edit this textbook. He is experienced in running membership courses both in the UK and abroad and has previously written an excellent best-selling book on mastering short answer questions.

As a Part 2 examiner, a member of the MCQ and then the SBA committees of the RCOG, and from my involvement in assisting on Part 2 courses, I feel I am well placed to add my expertise and experience to this textbook.

Single best answer questions require careful reading and the candidate should be able to produce the correct answer without reading the five answers offered (the so-called 'cover test'). Although incorrect answers are not penalised, the format does not lend itself to guessing the correct answer and a well-designed SBA question will reward the well-prepared candidate who has a thorough knowledge of the subject. Unlike MCQs, which test recall of medical knowledge, SBAs test the candidate's ability to apply clinical knowledge.

There is no pass mark in any Part 2 examination. A process of 'standard setting' is undertaken to ensure that every examination tests candidates to the same level. This is a laborious exercise involving some 20 or so senior consultants who assess the questions individually and consider whether a good trainee who is preparing for the examination would know the correct answer.

Medical knowledge is continually changing and new evidence and guidelines are produced, which are then incorporated in and tested by the MRCOG examination. It is essential therefore to use up-to-date textbooks, and current RCOG and the National Institute for Health and Care Excellence (NICE) guidelines when preparing for the examination.

Alexandra Rees FRCOG MBChB
Honorary Consultant, University Hospital of Wales, Cardiff, UK
Faculty Lead for Quality, Post-Graduate Medical Education Department
University Hospital of Wales, Cardiff, UK

Foreword

Passing the MRCOG Part 2 examination determines whether one could proceed to Part 3. The Part 2 examination consists of single best answer (SBAs) questions (40% of the marks) and extended matching questions (EMQs) (60% of the marks). Unlike the true/false multiple choice questions (MCQs) in the past, which test one's ability to recollect facts, the SBAs test one's ability to apply clinical knowledge. The candidate should have adequate knowledge in the subject of obstetrics and gynaecology and practise to answer SBAs to pass the Part 2 examination. Practice makes one perfect. The book *Mastering Single Best Answer Questions for the Part 2 MRCOG Examination, An Evidence-Based Approach* authored by Adel Elkady, Bashir Dawlatly and Mustafa Ahmed, and edited by Alex Rees, is one of the best books available for improving your knowledge and practising to get maximum marks in the SBAs section of the paper. Many candidates in the past have benefitted from Adel Elkady's best-selling book on short answer questions (SAQs) for the MRCOG Part 2 examination – before the SAQs were omitted. I am sure this book will enjoy the same popularity as Adel's previous book.

This book has 26 chapters covering the span of obstetrics and gynaecology ('blue printing') needed for the examination. The number of questions in each area varies on the breadth and depth of the knowledge tested in the examination; for example, gynaecological oncology: 46, infections in obstetrics and gynaecology: 40, urogynaecology: 29, conception and assisted reproduction: 24, obstetric medicine: 25, saving mothers' lives: 34, and labour ward practice: 24 questions. It also covers subjects of importance such as adolescent health and teenage pregnancy. There are 501 questions (205 pages). Each question stem has five options and evidence-based answers are given with suitable references. This should encourage further learning by the candidate. Sample answer sheets are provided to practise 50 questions in 70 minutes.

I would strongly recommend *Mastering Single Best Answer Questions for the Part 2 MRCOG Examination, An Evidence-Based Approach* published by Cambridge University Press as essential reading for those who appear for the Part 2 MRCOG examination.

Best wishes to all candidates for the examination.

Sir Sabaratnam Arulkumaran PhD DSc FRCS FRCOG
Professor Emeritus of Obstetrics & Gynaecology
St George's, University of London, London, UK
Past President of RCOG, BMA, FIGO

Authors' Introduction

Dear Colleagues

We, the editor and authors, trust that you will find this book a valuable tool to help you prepare and pass the Part 2 of the Membership examination.

This book is a follow-up from the principal author's previous very successful short answer question book *Mastering Short Answer Questions for the Part 2 MRCOG Examination with Evidence-Based Answers*. It was extremely helpful to use Dr Elkady's experience of writing books for the Part 2 examination. The RCOG has now replaced the short answer questions with the new single best answer (SBA) questions, so it was felt that another well-referenced, evidence-based question book was required to fill the gap.

Becoming a member of the RCOG is an important step in the career progress of an obstetrician and gynaecologist. Passing the Part 2 MRCOG examination entitles you to attempt the Part 3 clinical assessment, which is the last leg of this long process to achieve membership.

In order to pass Part 2, you need clinical experience, extensive up-to-date evidence-based knowledge, familiarity with UK practices and a good examination technique to achieve a satisfactory score. We trust that our book adequately covers these essentials.

This book comprises 26 chapters covering the RCOG syllabus and is divided into chapters to help you with your reading and preparation in a systematic fashion.

The questions for each chapter are collated, followed by the correct answer. The answers are well referenced, evidence based and with detailed explanations, which will also help you as a revision exercise, particularly on some topics where you may have some difficulty finding up-to-date sources; for example, Chapter 4, Labour Ward Management, and Chapter 12, Paediatric and Adolescent Medicine.

To achieve the maximum benefit from this book, supposing you have already done your revision, you should try to answer the questions before looking at the answers. After you have written down your answers on a separate sheet, cross check against the correct answer and read the explanation. You may still have to review other sources (recent textbooks, Green Top guidelines, *The Obstetrician and Gynaecologist* journal or the NICE guidelines) so that you eventually have full knowledge of the topic and are ready to answer any questions across the syllabus.

After your first review as suggested here, keep reviewing and answering the questions until you achieve at least an 80%–90% correct answer response.

To assist your revision further, we have included a mock examination that is as close as possible to the real examination. You should only attempt this after having done all your homework to avoid disappointment if you do so before you are fully prepared. The mock examination papers, answer sheets and correct answers can be found at www.cambridge.org/9781316621561.

Sometimes there is no absolute right or wrong answer, therefore you may find the occasional discrepancy in an answer that may not match with other sources or references.

You will find out all you need to know about the Part 2 written examination at the college website, using the link [https://www.rcog.org.uk/en/careers-training/mrcog-exams/part-2-mrcog/]

The editor and the authors are senior Members/Fellows of the RCOG and are experienced examiners, or very successful organizers of the written and OSCE courses. The contributors, most of them being sub-specialists, have been carefully chosen to offer you the best and most useful questions, answers and explanations. In addition, some of the contributors are new members of the RCOG and can offer you the added advantage of the perspective of fresh graduates who have been through the process just before you, having done their revision adequately and passed the examination.

The authors would like to acknowledge the help and support offered by Paul Fogarty and thank him for suggesting Alexandra Rees as an editor.

We would also like to acknowledge the support of Dr Mohamed Hamed, an MRCOG trainee, on whom we tested a random sample of the questions to get feedback from the perspective of a trainee.

Medical knowledge is constantly changing and newer evidence is always emerging. While we have taken due care that the medical information given is both accurate and up to date according to the best available evidence, readers are strongly advised to confirm for themselves that the information given complies with standard practices.

Last but not least, we wish you good luck with your endeavours to become a member of this internationally accredited elite club, the RCOG.

Adel Elkady

Bashir Dawlatly

Mustafa H. Ahmed

Chapter 1

Early Pregnancy

QUESTIONS

1.

A woman who is nine weeks pregnant comes to the early pregnancy assessment unit complaining of severe nausea and occasional vomiting. She is not keen on drug therapy.

What is your advice?

A. Drink decaffeinated coffee.
B. Drink ginger syrup.
C. Drink herbal tea.
D. Take a long break from work.
E. Take up yoga.

2.

A 33-year-old woman, gravida 3, para 2, comes to the emergency department complaining of excessive vomiting for the last three days. She is otherwise asymptomatic with a normal past medical history. She is admitted and her thyroid function tests showed a low thyroid stimulating hormone (TSH) level with raised free thyroxine (T4).

What is the most important feature to differentiate transient hyperthyroidism of hyperemesis gravidarum (THHG) from hyperthyroidism?

A. Absence of current clinical signs and symptoms of hyperthyroidism.
B. Absence of a history of hyperthyroidism.
C. Absent enlarged thyroid gland.
D. Negative thyroid receptor antibodies titre.
E. Normal TSH and T4 in a repeat thyroid function test.

3.

A primigravida who is 10 weeks pregnant is complaining of slight vaginal bleeding and the occasional abdominal colic. Ultrasound showed a live singleton pregnancy corresponding to her last menstrual period. She is worried about losing this pregnancy and asks for any medication to help keep the pregnancy. She has read something about progesterone treatment.

How will you counsel her?

A. She can start oral progesterone therapy.
B. She can start a combination of oral and vaginal progesterone, as it is more effective than single therapy.
C. She should start a combination therapy if she gets severe colic.
D. There is no strong evidence to recommend the use of any progesterone therapy.
E. Vaginal progesterone is more effective to treat threatened miscarriage.

4.

A 20-year-old woman who was nine weeks into her first pregnancy has just had a complete miscarriage. She is distressed and very tearful. You have explained that miscarriage does not affect her future fertility. Her partner is worried her anxiety may persist and be a possible cause of a delayed pregnancy.

What else will you tell them?

A. Her anxiety will go away when she misses her next period.
B. Her anxiety will persist until she achieves another pregnancy.
C. Her anxiety will continue until she has a healthy baby.
D. Her anxiety will most likely disappear in around four months when she gets over it.
E. She should be referred to a phychiatrist.

5.

A woman who is 11^{+3} weeks pregnant complained of abdominal colic and an attack of brisk vaginal bleeding. A repeat ultrasound confirmed fetal demise. You diagnosed inevitable miscarriage. She is considering expectant management.

How will you counsel her?

A. Arrange for expectant management in a hospital setting as she is under a higher risk of bleeding.
B. Agree that expectant management is her best option.
C. Explain that she is at a higher risk of bleeding
D. Recommend surgical management as she is at a higher risk of bleeding.
E. Wait for 14 days before you recommend other options.

6.

A woman who is 11 weeks pregnant with confirmed miscarriage was very hesitant in deciding on medical or surgical management. She was still keen on avoiding the anaesthetic and surgical risks, if possible.

What will you tell her about her chances of not having surgery if she opts for medical management?

A. It avoids the need for surgery in over 30% of women.
B. It avoids the need for surgery in over 40% of women.
C. It avoids the need for surgery in over 50% of women.
D. It avoids the need for surgery in over 60% of women.
E. It avoids the need for surgery in over 70% of women.

7.

A 20-year-old woman comes to the early pregnancy assessment unit with 7^{+6} weeks amenorrhea and mild to moderate vaginal bleeding with the occasional abdominal pain. She has a positive pregnancy test but refuses a transvaginal ultrasound scan.

How will you handle the situation?

A. Ask the consultant to talk to her.
B. Ask her to sign a form that she refused medical advice.
C. Refer her to the radiology departmental for a scan in the earliest available appointment.
D. Respect her wishes but explain the limitations of a transabdominal (TAS) versus a transvaginal scan (TVS).
E. Send her back to her general practitioner.

8.

A woman who is eight weeks pregnant complains of vaginal bleeding. An ultrasound scan showed a crown rump length of 7 mm but no visible fetal heart. You advised her to come for a follow-up scan after seven days. She expressed her concern that waiting that long may harm the pregnancy or her health.

How will you counter her concern?

A. Assure her that waiting for a repeat scan will have no detrimental effect on the outcome of the pregnancy or her health.
B. Ask the midwife to talk to her and explain the unit's regulations.
C. Explain that a serum human chorionic gonadotropin (beta-hCG/BhCG) measurement will confirm the diagnosis of fetal demise.
D. Give her a leaflet explaining the unit's procedures.
E. Offer her termination of the pregnancy as this is most likely an unviable pregnancy.

9.

The community midwife calls you about an eight-week pregnant woman who is complaining of vaginal bleeding and abdominal colic. A repeat scan confirmed fetal demise. She opted for expectant management. Her bleeding and abdominal pains have resolved. The woman wants to know how to confirm that miscarriage is complete.

What is your advice?

A. No need for any further follow-up as she is no longer symptomatic.
B. Return for advice if the bleeding starts again.
C. Repeat a pregnancy test after one week.
D. Repeat a pregnancy test after two weeks.
E. Repeat a pregnancy test after three weeks.

10.

A woman who is 11 weeks pregnant is diagnosed with incomplete miscarriage. She opts for medical management.

What will you offer her?

A. Oral mifepristone and 800 mcg misoprostol in one setting.
B. Oral mifepristone and then 800 mcg misoprostol when she starts having contractions.

C. Oral 800 mcg misoprostol.
D. Vaginal 600 mcg misoprostol.
E. Vaginal 800 mcg misoprostol.

11.

A pregnant woman is diagnosed with miscarriage based on absent cardiac pulsation in repeat scans. She opted for surgical management as her work commitments would not allow for a long wait and she feels she may not be able to cope with bleeding and pain if she opts for medical management. She was undecided, however, about an outpatient setting manual vacuum aspirating (MVA) under a local anaesthetic or a hospital evacuation curettage (EVA) under a general anaesthetic.

How will you counsel her?

A. Arrange for a meeting with an experienced counsellor.
B. Ask the consultant to come and talk to her.
C. Explain that the median waiting time, the number of women requiring a blood transfusion, and the mean blood loss were all lower in an outpatient setting.
D. Strongly recommend MVA because she will not be exposed to the risks of general anaesthesia.
E. Strongly recommend EVA because it is more effective.

12.

A 23-year-old woman in her second pregnancy presents to you requesting surgical termination of the pregnancy. She is 11 weeks pregnant, verified by ultrasound scan.

What is the risk of uterine perforation in this case?

A. 1–4/1000.
B. 5–9/1000.
C. 10–14/1000.
D. 15–19/1000.
E. 20–24/1000.

13.

A 31-year-old woman is booked for surgical termination of pregnancy at nine weeks' gestation.

Which of the following options is correct regarding prevention of infective complications?

A. Augmentin 625 mg within two hours before the procedure.
B. Ceftriaxone 500 mg within two hours before the procedure.
C. Doxycycline 200 mg within two hours before the procedure.
D. Metronidazole 500 mg within two hours before the procedure.
E. No antibiotics are needed.

14.

The general practitioner calls you out of hours to ask what to do because she has an eight-week pregnant woman who is complaining of moderate right abdominal pain and slight vaginal bleeding.

What is your advice?

A. Book the woman to the earliest antenatal clinic appointment.
B. Book the woman for the earliest possible ultrasound scan.
C. Immediate referral to the emergency gynaecology unit.

D. Offer the woman an analgesic.
E. Refer the patient to the next day early pregnancy assessment unit.

15.

The midwife in the early pregnancy assessment unit asks you to review a woman who has seven weeks of amenorrhea but the previous and current ultrasound could not locate the pregnancy. The human chorionic gonadotropin (BhCG) increased from 800 IU/L to 1600 IU/L after 48 hours. The woman is fit and well with no signs or symptoms.

What is your next plan?

A. Ultrasound scan within four to seven days.
B. Ultrasound scan after 14 days.
C. Ultrasound scan after nine days.
D. Request an inhibin blood test.
E. Request a serum progesterone blood test.

16.

The serum BhCG of a symptomless woman with a pregnancy of unknown location (PUL) has dropped by more than 50% after 48 hours.

What is the next step you advise?

A. Ask her to submit a urine pregnancy test after 14 days if she stays asymptomatic.
B. Discharge her home.
C. Repeat the BhCG after another 48 hours.
D. Request a cancer antigen (CA-125) blood test.
E. Request a Doppler ultrasound scan.

17.

A woman who is eight weeks pregnant is offered laparoscopic surgical management of an ectopic pregnancy. She had a previous normal pregnancy and vaginal delivery.

How will you justify laparoscopic salpingectomy as opposed to salpingostomy?

A. Removing the diseased tube is easier and quicker to perform.
B. Removal of the diseased tube will not affect her future fertility.
C. Removing the ectopic pregnancy and keeping the tube will have a significantly higher incidence of a recurrent ectopic pregnancy requiring repeat surgery.
D. Removing the ectopic pregnancy and keeping the tube will require more follow-up visits and tests, currently.
E. There are no differences in the management options for the current or future pregnancies.

18.

A 15-year-old single teenage girl comes to see you because she had an unplanned pregnancy. She is nine weeks pregnant after failure of an emergency post-coital contraception. She explains her great inability to handle either the pregnancy care or the child, if born, for personal and social reasons.

How will you handle the situation?

A. Ask her to bring her parents to discuss the situation.
B. Ask her to bring her boyfriend to discuss the situation.

C. Advise her to involve her parents but endorse her request if two doctors agree that she has sufficient maturity and understanding to appreciate what is involved.
D. Refer her to a psychiatrist to assess her ability to understand what is involved.
E. She cannot have an abortion without her parents' consent because she is under age (16 years).

19.

The general practitioner calls to ask about the immediate follow-up of a woman who had a suction evacuation of a complete molar pregnancy.

What is your advice?

A. Do a urine or blood test for human chorionic gonadotropins (hCG) every two weeks for eight weeks.
B. Do a urine pregnancy test every two weeks for 24 weeks.
C. Do a urine check test every week until it is negative for four successive tests.
D. Do a urine or blood test for hCG every week until it normalizes.
E. No need for any follow-up if the urine pregnancy test is negative after one month.

20.

A woman has an evacuation of a partial molar pregnancy. She was 11 weeks pregnant.

What is your follow-up plan?

A. Chorionic gonadotropin (hCG) assessment until she starts a hormonal contraception after the tests have normalized.
B. Serum and urine hCG every two weeks until the levels are normal followed by one confirmatory normal urine sample after four weeks.
C. Serum hCG after four weeks.
D. Urine pregnancy test every two weeks.
E. Urine pregnancy test every four weeks.

21.

Following appropriate treatment of complete and partial molar pregnancies, what percentage of women need additional chemotherapy in each case, respectively?

A. 10% and 0.3%.
B. 15% and 0.5%.
C. 20% and 1.0%.
D. 25% and 2.0%.
F. 33% and 3.0%.

22.

A 36-year-old woman has had a suction evacuation because of a complete molar pregnancy. Her chorionic gonadotropin (hCG) levels started to rise six months after treatment. Her FIGO 2000 score was assessed as 6.

What is your management?

A. Intravenous multi-agent chemotherapy.
B. Needs treatment only if her score goes up to 7.
C. Single-agent intramuscular methotrexate.
D. Subtotal hysterectomy.
E. Total hysterectomy and bilateral salpingo-oophorectomy.

23.

A 28-year-old woman who has received single-agent chemotherapy because of a persistent rise in her chorionic gonadotropin levels after evacuation of a complete molar pregnancy asks about her future fertility options.

What will you tell her?

A. She cannot conceive because of the chemotherapy.
B. She can conceive but after one year of completion of her treatment and follow-up.
C. She can conceive after two years of undetectable gonadotropin levels (hCG) levels.
D. She can conceive after two years of a contraceptive.
E. She can conceive but only with oocyte donation.

24.

To improve the results of treatment of gestational trophoblastic disease (GTD), what audit topic would you recommend?

A. The proportion of women with GTD registered with the relevant screening centre.
B. The proportion of women with a histological diagnosis of molar pregnancy who were diagnosed by ultrasound before evacuation of the molar pregnancy.
C. The proportion of women who receive medical management for the evacuation of a molar pregnancy.
D. The proportion of women who had histological examination of the products of conception after an induced abortion.
E. The proportion of women who did not use contraception during the follow-up period.

25.

You are counselling a couple who have had two consecutive miscarriages. She is 22 years old and wants to know if there are any age-related risks of miscarriage.

Which of the following age groups is associated with the smallest risk of miscarriage?

A. 12–19 years.
B. 20–24 years.
C. 25–29 years.
D. 30–34 years.
E. 35–40 years.

26.

There are cases of women who have recurrent miscarriages.

What percentage of these women have antiphospholipid antibodies?

A. 5%.
B. 10%.
C. 15%.
D. 25%.
E. 40%.

27.

Your foundation year 2 trainee enquires about the different types of thrombophilia.

Which of the following is an acquired thrombophilia?

A. Antiphospholipid syndrome.
B. Activated protein C resistance.
C. Factor V Leiden.
D. Prothrombin gene mutation.
E. Protein S deficiency.

28.

A couple who have had three consecutive miscarriages have come to see you for advice after having a thrombophilia screen. The result showed that she was positive to one of the antiphospholipid antibodies.

Which of the following is an antiphospholipid antibody?

A. Anti-B2-glycoprotein-1 antibody.
B. Anti-B1-glycoprotein-1 antibody.
C. Anti-B2-glycoprotein-2 antibody.
D. Anti-B2-glycoprotein-3 antibody.
E. Anti-B3-glycoprotein-1 antibody.

29.

A couple who have had three consecutive miscarriages have come to see you for counselling. Genetic screening showed a paternal balanced translocation.

What is their chance of having a healthy baby?

A. 0%.
B. 10%–20%.
C. 20%–30%.
D. 40%–50%.
E. More than 80%.

30.

A 20-year-old woman presents to the family planning clinic. She is requesting termination of a 10-week pregnancy. She had a surgical termination of a 14-week pregnancy six months previously. She had problems attending and complying with the different family planning options offered to her after completion of the termination of her previous pregnancy.

What is your advice for an effective contraception in her situation?

A. Change to surgical termination so she can have a copper intrauterine device inserted at the end of the procedure.
B. Change to surgical termination so she can have a Mirena coil inserted at the end of the procedure.
C. Carry on with the medical termination but have the etonogestrel implant inserted at the time of mifepristone administration.
D. Carry on with any method of termination and resort to tubal ligation at the end of the procedure.
E. She should be able to revisit the family planning clinic after she gets her first period.

31.

A 25-year-old woman is referred to the clinic. She has a pituitary macroprolactinoma and has been treated with bromocriptine for a year. Her prolactin levels have been normal for the past six months. She is now 11 weeks pregnant and was advised to continue this medication. She is worried about any risks if she continues this medication while pregnant.

What will you tell her?

A. Bromocriptine can be continued during pregnancy safely.
B. She should discontinue this medication.
C. She has an increased risk of miscarriage.
D. She should not breast feed.
E. She has a higher risk of developing pre-eclampsia.

ANSWERS

Q1: B. Drink ginger syrup [evidence level 1b].[1,2]

- The incidence of hyperemesis gravidarum is 3.5/1000 deliveries [evidence level 3].[1]
- Hyperemesis gravidarum is severe morning sickness and vomiting requiring hospital admission. Symptoms can include persistent vomiting, dehydration, tiredness and dizziness. If symptoms are severe, admission to hospital is recommended to observe and treat dehydration and offer antiemetics. Symptoms start by eight weeks and usually disappear around 16 weeks. It occurs more commonly in multiple and molar pregnancies.
- Randomized controlled trials and systematic reviews confirmed that 250 mg four times a day, or one tablespoon of ginger syrup in four to eight fluid ounces (113–227 mL) of water four times daily, was effective ($P = 0.035$) for reducing or resolving nausea and vomiting of pregnancy.[1,2]
- Pregnancy nausea and vomiting will resolve spontaneously within 16–20 weeks.
- Pregnant women should be assured that nausea and vomiting are not usually associated with a poor pregnancy outcome.

Q2: D. Negative thyroid receptor antibodies titre [evidence level 3].[3]

- Transient THHG is a self-limiting condition with hyperthyroidism occurring in some cases of hyperemesis gravidarum.
- It usually resolves by 18 weeks of pregnancy with return of normal thyroid function tests.
- THHG might be responsible for 40%–70% of thyroid function abnormalities in pregnancy.
- Elevated levels of gonadotropins have a thyrotrophic activity (lower TSH and raised T4) causing the transient THHG.
- Although a negative past history and absence of clinical sings of hyperthyroidism is also useful to exclude Graves' disease, thyroid antibody tests are still essential to confirm the absence of Graves' disease.
- THHG does not require any specific treatment except the usual treatment for hyperemesis.

Q3: D. There is no strong evidence to recommend the use of any progesterone therapy.[4]

- Few, different meta-analyses have shown conflicting evidence for the benefit of progesterone therapy for threatened miscarriage.
- Studies that have shown a beneficial effect included small numbers; some had a high degree of bias, some had a poor follow-up rate and were all considered as low or very low quality and lacked long-term safety data.

- Consequently, the 2012 NICE guidelines development group concluded that there are no sufficient grounds to recommend oral or vaginal progesterone for threatened miscarriage.[4]

Q4: D. Her anxiety will most likely disappear in around four months when she gets over it [evidence level 3].[5,6]

- Available studies suggest that 30%–50% of miscarriage cases experience anxiety symptoms and 10%–15% experience depressive symptoms, which commonly persist for up to four months.[6]
- A study in Iran involving 278 women has shown that worrying about not being able to conceive again was the dominant psychological consequences of abortion.[6]
- Other studies have also found an anxiety concern about completeness of a future pregnancy in women who had a previous miscarriage.[6]

Q5: C. Explain that she is at a higher risk of bleeding.[4]

- You must respect a patient's wishes and offer different options but do not recommend any specific treatment if there are no contraindications to various other treatment options.

Q6: E. It avoids the need for surgery in over 70% of women.[4]

Q7: D. Respect her wishes but explain the limitations of a transabdominal (TAS) versus the transvaginal scan (TVS).[7]

- In the study of 46 normal intrauterine pregnancies, TVS showed additional information in 36 patients (78.3%) compared to TAS, and provided more information in 64% of abnormal pregnancies.
- In ectopic pregnancies, TVS gave additional information in 71.4%, which included detection of ectopic fetal pole, yolk sac, decidual cast, adnexal mass and fluid in cul-de-sac.
- TVS will offer more information in detection of gestation sac, yolk sac, double bleb sign or better visualization of embryonic anatomy.
- TVS avoids the discomfort of a full bladder and saves time waiting for the bladder to fill.
- TVS is also superior in obese patients or patients with a retroverted uterus, and it also bypasses obstacles such as bone, gas-filled bowel and extensive pelvic adhesions.[7]

Q8: A. Assure her that waiting for a repeat scan will have no detrimental effect on the outcome of the pregnancy or her health. [evidence level 3].[4]

- Human chorionic gonadotropin measurements are indicated if there is a pregnancy of unknown location or if there is a suspicion of ectopic pregnancy.
- A single human chorionic gonadotropin measurement is not helpful in confirming fetal demise because of the large variations in the normal values.[4]

Q9: E. Repeat a pregnancy test after three weeks [evidence level 3].[8]

- A repeat pregnancy test is less expensive and less time consuming than an ultrasound scan or a repeat serial human chorionic gonadotropin (beta-hCG/BhCG).
- The BhCG level rises from 60% to doubling approximately every 48 hours for 85% of intrauterine pregnancies.

- In the remaining 15%, the BhCG graph may change to have a different slope or plateau.
- In two studies involving a total of 41 patients, the clearance of hCG to a level of 2 mIU/mL averaged between two and three weeks.[8]

Q10: D. Vaginal 600 mcg misoprostol [evidence level 1−].[9]

- NICE guidelines do not recommend the use of mifepristone. It does not offer any advantage on the efficacy of treatment. It is not cost effective.
- A Cochrane study (4208 women) showed a high success rate for misoprostol alone. In the same study, there was no clear evidence of any one route of administration (vaginal, oral or sublingual) being superior to another. The vaginal route has fewer side effects [evidence level 1−].[9]

Q11: C. Explain that the median waiting time, the number of women requiring a blood transfusion, and the mean blood loss were all lower in an outpatient setting [evidence level 3].[4]

- NICE guidelines development group did not feel that any strong evidence supports one technique over the other, but felt that the reduced waiting time is strong enough to justify a recommendation that units should be able to offer outpatient surgical management in order to provide women with a choice.[1]
- Women should always be empowered to make their own informed consent without recommending any specific choice.
- This situation is a simple medical issue and does not require an experienced counsellor.
- All the examination questions test your own ability; you should offer your own response.

Q12: A. 1–4/1000.[10]

- Cervical trauma – the risk of damage is no more than 1/100 and is lower for first-trimester abortions.[10]
- Trauma is less likely if cervical preparation is undertaken in line with best practice.[10]

Q13: C. Doxycycline 200 mg within two hours before the procedure.[4]

- The following regimens are recommended for presurgical abortion antibiotic prophylaxis:
  - 200 mg doxycycline within two hours before the procedure.
    OR
  - 500 mg azithromycin within two hours before the procedure.

Q14: C. Immediate referral to the emergency gynaecology unit [good practice point].[11]

- Lowering the index of suspicion for the diagnosis of ectopic pregnancy is likely to be associated with a cost-effective reduction of loss of quality-adjusted life years (QALYs).
- The QALY is a measure of the value of health outcomes. A year of life lived in perfect health is worth one QALY, a year of life lived in a state of less than this perfect health is worth less than one QALY, while death or loss of life is associated with zero QALYs.[11]

Q15: A. Ultrasound scan within four to seven days.[12]

- Pregnancy of unknown location (PUL) is the absence of signs of intra- or extrauterine pregnancy or retained products of conception in a transvaginal ultrasound in spite of a positive pregnancy test.[12]
- Serum progesterone and inhibin levels may be useful in a resolving PUL but will not help to diagnose an ectopic pregnancy or locate the pregnancy. There are no well-established levels to discriminate between a viable intrauterine and an ectopic pregnancy.
- NICE guidelines recommend scanning within seven days if the BhCG is 1500 IU/mL or higher.
- There is no 100% accurate method to predict the clinical outcome of PUL.
- PUL should be managed conservatively with serial BhCG and transvaginal ultrasound scans until either the pregnancy is accurately located or intervention is necessary.

Q16: A. Ask her to submit a urine pregnancy test after 14 days if she stays asymptomatic.[4]

Q17: C. Removing the ectopic pregnancy and keeping the tube will have a significantly higher incidence of a recurrent ectopic pregnancy requiring repeat surgery [evidence level 1−].[4,13]

- There were no randomized controlled trials to offer firm evidence for the effectiveness of salpingostomy versus salpingectomy in improving future pregnancy outcomes.
- For answer (C), NICE guidelines are that the significantly higher interventions after salpingostomy would be a more important consideration for women than those given in answers (A) and (D).
- For answer (B), the NICE guidelines development group considered that the evidence from observational studies on improved future fertility outcomes was of poor quality, with a high possibility of bias.[4]
- Answer (E) is wrong.
- Women who have salpingotomy have up to 20% risk of needing further treatment. This treatment may include methotrexate and/or a salpingectomy.[4]
- Women who have had a salpingostomy should be followed up by one serum BhCG measurement seven days after surgery, then one weekly serum BhCG measurement until a negative result is obtained.

Q18: C. Advise her to involve her parents but endorse her request if two doctors agree that she has sufficient maturity and understanding to appreciate what is involved.[14]

According to the Gillick competence and Fraser guidelines

- In 1982, Mrs Victoria Gillick took her local health authority (West Norfolk and Wisbech Area Health Authority) and the Department of Health and Social Security to court in an attempt to stop doctors from giving contraceptive advice or treatment to under-16-year-olds without parental consent.
- The Fraser guidelines refer to those set out by Lord Fraser in his judgement of the Gillick case in the House of Lords (1985), which apply specifically to contraceptive advice. Lord Fraser stated that a doctor could proceed to give advice and treatment, 'provided he is satisfied in the following criteria:
  - that the girl (although under the age of 16) will understand his advice;
  - that he cannot persuade her to inform her parents or to allow him to inform the parents that she is seeking contraceptive advice;[14]

- that she is very likely to continue having sexual intercourse with or without contraceptive use;
- that unless she receives contraceptive advice or treatment her physical or mental health or both are likely to suffer;
- that her best interests require him to give her contraceptive advice, treatment or both without parental consent;
- that it is still a good practice to advise her to involve her parents or another adult, at least to care for her during and after the termination procedures'.

The Fraser guidelines may be applied to other conditions where treatment is required.

Q19: A. Do a urine or blood test for human chorionic gonadotropin (hCG) every two weeks for eight weeks [evidence level 4].[15]

- The three UK referral centres for molar pregnancies (Charing Cross Hospital in London, Weston Park Hospital in Sheffield and Ninewells Hospital in Dundee) recommend hCG estimation in urine or blood tests or both, every two weeks for 56 days (eight weeks).
- If hCG has reverted to normal within 56 days of the pregnancy event then follow-up will be for six months from the date of uterine evacuation.
- Once levels are normal, a urine test is done every two to four weeks for six months from the day hCG has fallen to normal levels.[15]
- If hCG has not reverted to normal within 56 days of the pregnancy event, follow-up will be for six months from subsequent normalization of the hCG level.
- The treatment centre will send all the kits that the patient needs for the follow-up tests so patients do not need to worry about remembering the timings.
- When hCG has normalized, the possibility of developing gestational trophoblastic neoplasia is very low.[15] Overall, the risk of recurrence of a vesicular mole is very low. [evidence level 2+].
- In a large retrospective review of database of registrations for gestational trophoblastic disease (2578 complete moles and 2627 partial moles), >98% of women who become pregnant following a molar conception will not have a further hydatidiform mole and these pregnancies are at no increased risk of other obstetric complications.[2]

Q20: B. Serum and urine hCG every two weeks until the levels are normal, followed by one confirmatory normal urine sample after four weeks.[15]

Q21: B. 15% and 0.5% [evidence level 3].[15]

- The need for chemotherapy is 15% following a complete mole and 0.5% after a partial mole.
- Before chemotherapy, assessment is carried out using the FIGO 2000 scoring system.
- Women with scores ≤6 are at low risk and should receive single-agent intramuscular methotrexate alternating daily with folinic acid for one week followed by six rest days.
- Women with scores ≥7 are at high risk and should be treated with intravenous multi-agent chemotherapy, which includes combinations of methotrexate, dactinomycin, etoposide, cyclophosphamide and vincristine.
- Treatment should continue until the hCG level has returned to normal, for a further six consecutive weeks.[15]
- The cure rate for women with a score ≤6 is almost 100%; the rate for women with a score ≥7 is 95%.

Q22: C. Single-agent intramuscular methotrexate [evidence level 3].[15]

- Surgical treatment is indicated in a placental site trophoblastic tumour because it is less sensitive to chemotherapy.[15]

Q23: B. She can conceive but after one year of completion of her treatment and follow-up.[15]

- If a woman who received chemotherapy starts having regular periods, and after completion of her one-year follow-up, she can conceive and the low risk of congenital anomalies (1.8%) is not increased beyond the background risk of 2%–3%.

Q24: A. The proportion of women with GTD registered with the relevant screening centre.[16]

- In the UK, the effective registration and treatment programme has achieved excellent results, with high cure (98%–100%) and low chemotherapy (5%–8%) rates.
- Histological examination of products of conception is not required for cases of induced abortion of spontaneous miscarriage if a viable pregnancy was diagnosed on ultrasound or fetal parts have been identified.
- Evacuation of a molar pregnancy is best carried out surgically, preferably without the use of syntocinon or prostaglandins to avoid the risk of embolization [evidence level 3].

Q25: B. 20–24 years [evidence level 2+].[4]

- A large prospective study reported the age-related risk of miscarriage in recognized pregnancies to be: 12–19 years: 13%, 20–24 years: 11%, 25–29 years: 12%, 30–34 years: 15%, 35–39 years: 25%, 40–44 years: 51%, 45 years and above: 93%. Advanced paternal age is also a risk factor.
- The risk is highest in women 35 or more and the man 40 or more years.[4]

Q26: C. 15%.[17]

- Antiphospholipid antibodies are present in 15% of women with recurrent miscarriage.
- In women with recurrent miscarriages associated with antiphospholipid antibodies, the live birth rate in pregnancies with no pharmacological intervention has been reported to be as low as 10%.[17]
- Aspirin plus unfractionated heparin have a 54% success rate [evidence level 1+].[17]

Q27: A. Antiphospholipid syndrome.[17]

- A meta-analysis of retrospective studies has reported a strong association between second trimester miscarriage and inherited thrombophilias: factor V Leiden, factor II (prothrombin) gene mutation and protein S deficiency [evidence level 2+].
- Congenital or hereditary thrombophilia refers to inborn conditions, with the development of unprovoked thrombosis or an increased tendency to develop thrombosis.
- Congenital thrombophilias typically are caused by a deficiency of natural anticoagulants, prothrombin G20210A, antithrombin III, protein C and protein S, and factors V Leiden and XIII mutation.
- Acquired thrombophilia arises later in life.

- Antiphospholipid syndrome is caused by antibodies against constituents of the cell membrane, particularly lupus anticoagulant, anti-cardiolipin antibodies, and anti-B2-glycoprotein antibodies; it is an autoimmune disease.
- Heparin-induced thrombocytopenia (HIT) is due to an immune system reaction against the anticoagulant drug heparin or its derivatives. HIT is strongly associated with risk of venous and arterial thrombosis. Diagnosis is based on the combination of clinical findings, thrombocytopenia, and laboratory studies of HIT antibodies.[17]

Q28: A. Anti-B2-glycoprotein-1 antibody.[17]

- The antiphospholipid antibodies are lupus anticoagulant, anticardiolipin, and anti-B2-glycoprotein-1 antibody.[17]

Management
- A combination of low-dose aspirin and low-molecular weight heparin (LMWH) [evidence level 1+].
- There is accumulating evidence that LMWH is at least as effective and safe as unfractionated heparin with potential advantages during pregnancy as they cause less heparin-induced thrombocytopenia, can be administered once daily, and are associated with a lower risk of heparin-induced osteoporosis.

Q29: E. More than 80%.[17]

- Couples with balanced translocation have a low risk (0.8%) of pregnancies with unbalanced karyotyping surviving into the second trimester, and their chance of having a healthy child is 83%.
- In the UK, an audit of four UK centres examining more than 20 000 parents with recurrent miscarriages reported balanced translocation in 1.9%.

Q30: C. Carry on with the medical termination but have the etonogestrel implant inserted at the time of mifepristone administration [evidence level 1+].[18]

- Randomized controlled trials have shown that the application of the implanon implant at the time of medical abortion had a 90.7% continuation of the method against only 48% in the control groups.[18]

Q31: A. Bromocriptine can be continued during pregnancy safely [evidence level 3].[19]

- Approximately 80% of patients with hyperprolactinaemia achieve pregnancy on dopamine agonist treatment.
- There is no increase in the rates of spontaneous miscarriage or other complications of pregnancy.
- Breastfeeding may be undertaken normally.
- Enlargement of microprolactinomas in pregnancy is low (approximately 2.6%). This risk is much higher with macroprolactinomas (30%–35%).
- Bromocriptine is usually discontinued early in pregnancy in women with microprolactinaemia and most will have a very low risk of tumour expansion during the pregnancy.
- An MRI should be performed if the woman develops visual symptoms.
- Bromocriptine can be safely started/restarted in pregnancy without adversely affecting the pregnancy or fetal development.

References

1. National Institute for Health and Clinical Excellence. *Antenatal Care, Routine Care for the Healthy Pregnant Woman.* March, 2008. [https://www.nice.org.uk/guidance/cg62]

2. Jewell D, Young G. Interventions for nausea and vomiting in early pregnancy. *Cochrane Database Syst Rev* 2000;(2):CD000145.

3. Tan JY, Loh KC, Yeo GS, Chee YC. Transient hyperthyroidism of hyperemesis gravidarum. *Brit J Obstet Gynycol* 2002;109(6):683–8.

4. National Institute of Health and Clinical Excellence. *Diagnosis and Initial Management in Early Pregnancy of Ectopic Pregnancy and Miscarriage.* December, 2012. [https://www.nice.org.uk/guidance/cg154]

5. Pourreza A, Batebi A. Psychological consequences of abortion among the post abortion care seeking women in Tehran. *Iran J Psychiatry* 2011;6(1):31–6.

6. Woods-Giscombé CL, Lobel M, Crandell JL. The impact of miscarriage and parity on patterns of maternal distress in pregnancy. *Res Nurs Health* 2010;33(4):316–28.

7. Kaur A, Kaur, A. Transvaginal ultrasonography in first trimester of pregnancy and its comparison with transabdominal ultrasonography. *J Pharm Bioallied Sci* 2011; 3(3):329–38.

8. van der Lugt B, Drogendijk AC. Disappearance of HCG after induced abortion. *Acta Obstet Gynecol Scand* 1985;64(7):547–52.

9. Neilson JP, Gyte GM, Hickey M, Vazquez JC, Dou L. Medical treatments for incomplete miscarriage. *Cochrane Database Syst Rev* 2013;(3):CD007223.

10. Royal College of Obstetricians and Gynaecologists. *Best Practice in Comprehensive Abortion Care.* June, 2015. [https://www.rcog.org.uk/globalassets/documents/guidelines/best-practice-papers/best-practice-paper-2.pdf]

11. National Institute of Health and Clinical Excellence. *Measuring Effectiveness and Cost Effectiveness: the QALY,* 2010. [https://www.nice.org.uk/proxy]

12. Haritha S, Kamel M. Pregnancy of unknown location: an evidence-based approach to management. *Obstet Gynaecol* 2008;10(4): 224–30.

13. Mol F, van Mello NM, Strandell A, et al. Salpingotomy versus salpingectomy in women with tubal pregnancy (ESEP study): an open-label, multicentre, randomised controlled trial. *Lancet* 2014;383(9927):1483–9.

14. Gillick Competency and Fraser Guidelines. *A Child's Legal Rights.* [https://www.nspcc.org.uk/preventing-abuse/child-protection-system/legal-definition]

15. Charing Cross Hospital. *Follow-up After a Molar Pregnancy.* [www.hmolehorio.org.uk]

16. Royal College of Obstetricians and Gynaecologists. *The Management of Gestational Trophoblastic Disease.* February, 2010. [https://www.rcog.org.uk/en/guidelines-research-services/guidelines/gtg38]

17. Royal College of Obstetricians and Gynaecologists. *Recurrent Miscarriage, Investigation and treatment of couples.* May, 2011. [https://www.rcog.org.uk/en/guidelines-research-services/guidelines/gtg17]

18. Raymond EG, Weaver MA, Tan YL, et al. Effect of immediate compared with delayed insertion of etonogestrel implants on medical abortion efficacy and repeat pregnancy: a randomized controlled trial. *Obstet Gynecol* 2016;127(2):306–12.

19. Hamoda H, Khalaf Y, Carroll P. Hyperprolactinaemia and female reproductive function: what does the evidence say? *Obstet Gynaecol* 2012;14:81–6.

Chapter 2

Second and Third Trimester Pregnancy

QUESTIONS

1.

A 32-year-old nulliparous woman sees you in the antenatal clinic at 22 weeks' gestation. She has just had a transvaginal scan that showed the cervix to be 22 mm in length. She has a past history of a cone biopsy of the cervix six years previously with normal follow-up smears.

Which of the following options would you recommend for her?

A. Cervical cerclage surgery.
B. Follow-up scan in one week.
C. Follow-up scan in two weeks.
D. Rectal progesterone tablets.
E. Vaginal progesterone tablets.

2.

A 29-year-old woman in her first pregnancy presents to the labour ward with some vaginal discharge at 27 weeks and two days. The pregnancy has been uneventful. Speculum examination reveals the cervix to be partially effaced and dilated 3 cm with bulging amniotic membranes. She is not in pain, and her observations are normal. The cardiotocograph (CTG) is reassuring.

Which of the following options is the most appropriate in her management?

A. Admit for bed rest and await events.
B. Admit and give steroids.
C. Admit, give steroids and book for emergency cerclage.
D. Admit and give steroids and erythromycin tablets.
E. Admit and perform fetal fibronectin test.

3.

A 35-year-old healthy woman in her second pregnancy at 27 weeks presents to the labour ward with abdominal pain. She had a normal vaginal delivery at term in her first pregnancy three years previously. All observations are within normal limits. A CTG shows one to two irregular contractions every 10 minutes. The fetal heart trace is normal. Vaginal examination reveals the cervix to be 50% effaced but closed.

Which of the following is the most appropriate management option?

A. Perform transvaginal scan to check the cervical length.
B. Perform a fetal fibronectin test.
C. Start treatment with intravenous beta-mimetics.
D. Start treatment with oxytocin receptor antagonists.
E. Start treatment with oral nifedipine.

4.

A 35-year-old healthy woman in her second pregnancy at 30^{+6} weeks presents to the labour ward with abdominal pain. She had a normal vaginal delivery at term in her first pregnancy three years previously. All observations are within normal limits. A CTG shows one to two irregular contractions every 10 minutes. The fetal heart trace is normal. Vaginal examination reveals the cervix to be 50% effaced but closed.

What should you do next?

A. Perform transvaginal scan to check the cervical length.
B. Perform fetal fibronectin test.
C. Start treatment with intravenous beta-mimetics.
D. Start treatment with oxytocin receptor antagonists.
E. Start treatment with oral nifedipine.

5.

A 26-year-old woman in her first pregnancy presents to the labour ward at 28 weeks and four days gestation with abdominal pain. Maternal observations are all within normal limits. A CTG reveals she is contracting at a rate of three times in 10 minutes, with a normal fetal heart rate. Speculum examination shows the cervix is effaced and dilated 3 cm. The ST3 obstetric trainee wants to know the correct dose of magnesium sulfate for neuroprotection for the baby.

Which of the following statements is the most appropriate answer?

A. 4 g intravenous bolus of magnesium sulfate over five minutes, followed by an intravenous infusion of 1 g per hour until the birth or for 24 hours.
B. 4 g intravenous bolus of magnesium sulfate over 10 minutes, followed by an intravenous infusion of 1 g per hour until the birth or for 24 hours.
C. 4 g intravenous bolus of magnesium sulfate over 15 minutes, followed by an intravenous infusion of 1 g per hour until the birth or for 24 hours.
D. 4 g intravenous bolus of magnesium sulfate over 20 minutes, followed by an intravenous infusion of 1 g per hour until the birth or for 24 hours.
E. No need for magnesium sulfate.

6.

A 28-year-old primigravida with monochorionic diamniotic (MCDA) twins undergoes an ultrasound scan at 24 weeks. Twin 1 has an estimated weight at the 20th centile with the deepest pool of liquor of 1.6 cm. Twin 2 is growing at the 80th centile with the deepest pool of liquor measuring 9.5 cm. Doppler studies on both twins are normal. The bladders of both twins are visible.

Which of the following options is the most likely diagnosis?

A. Discordant fetal growth restriction.
B. Twin-to-twin transfusion syndrome (TTTS) Quintero Stage 1.
C. Twin-to-twin transfusion syndrome Quintero Stage 2.
D. Twin-to-twin transfusion syndrome Quintero Stage 3.
E. Twin-to-twin transfusion syndrome Quintero Stage 4.

7.

A 28-year-old primigravida presents to the antenatal clinic with headache.

Which of the following headaches in pregnancy is classified as primary headache?

A. Anaemia.
B. Caffeine withdrawal.
C. Hypertension.
D. Stroke.
E. Tension headache.

8.

A 29-year-old woman in her first pregnancy presents at the antenatal clinic complaining of recurrent attacks of migraine. She is now 20 weeks pregnant and is concerned as she has these attacks once every 10 days. She is enquiring if there is any medication that she can safely use during the pregnancy to stop these attacks.

Which of the following medications would you consider most appropriate?

A. Amitriptyline.
B. 5-hydroxytryptamine.
C. 5-hydroxytryptophan.
D. Ibuprofen.
E. Propranolol.

9.

A 28-year-old woman is admitted with slight lower abdominal pains and a watery vaginal discharge. A beta-methasone course is prescribed.

By how much will this management reduce the risk of neonatal death?

A. 10%–20%.
B. 21%–30%.
C. 31%–40%.
D. 41%–50%.
E. 51%–60%.

10.

A 36-year-old woman with uncontrolled diabetes and who is 29 weeks pregnant is admitted because of threatened preterm labour.

What is your advice regarding steroids for lung maturity?

A. Steroids are contraindicated because of her uncontrolled diabetes.
B. Steroids can be administered but only after her glycosylated haemoglobin has been controlled to 6.1.

C. Steroids can be administered if her pre- and postprandial blood glucose level is stable at 5 mmol/L and 7 mmol/L.
D. Steroids are administered with additional insulin and close monitoring.
E. Uncontrolled diabetes is not a contraindication.

11.

A 32-year-old woman who is 36 weeks pregnant comes to the labour ward because of upper abdominal pain and slight vaginal bleeding. Her two previous pregnancies ended in Caesarean section because of placental abruption. She has a normal blood pressure (BP) and a reactive non-stress test.

What are her chances of having another placental abruption?

A. 4%–5%.
B. 10%–16%.
C. 19%–25%.
D. 30%–42%.
E. Over 45%.

12.

A 29-year-old pregnant woman has just booked for her antenatal care. Her first pregnancy ended in a Caesarean section birth because of placenta praevia.

What are her risks (odds ratio, OR) for a recurrence?

A. 2.2.
B. 3.2.
C. 4.1.
D. 9.7.
E. 22.4.

13.

A non-sensitized Rh-negative pregnant woman is admitted at 34 weeks with a moderate amount of vaginal bleeding. She is stable and the bleeding has stopped.

What specific test should you request?

A. Anti-D titre.
B. Full blood count.
C. Full blood count, a coagulation profile, liver and renal function tests.
D. Kleihauer count.
E. Platelet count.

14.

A 33-year-old woman who is 34 weeks pregnant and under community care is referred to the antenatal clinic because of recurrent mild vaginal spotting over the last week. Her antenatal care has been uneventful. She has a normal fundal placenta. Her history and your clinical examination of her did not reveal any abnormality. Your speculum examination revealed a small ectropion. Her last cervical smear 18 months previously showed mild dyskaryosis. She has screened negative for human papilloma virus (HPV).

How will you conduct the rest of her antenatal care and delivery?

A. Admit her for observation.
B. Offer her a course of steroids and refer her back to her community care.
C. Refer her back to her community antenatal care and delivery.

D. Refer her to a consultant-led care delivery.
E. Repeat the cervical smear.

15.

A 33-year-old woman who is 33 weeks pregnant is admitted with severe abruption and an estimated blood loss of 1500 mL. An emergency ultrasound scan showed a large retro-placental haematoma. Fetal heart pulsations were not seen on the ultrasound scan. She is stabilized with intravenous saline infusions and prepared for an emergency Caesarean section.

What is your first line empirical treatment while waiting for the coagulation profile results?

A. Intramuscular injection of 250 μg carboprost.
B. One litre of fresh frozen plasma and 10 units of cryoprecipitate.
C. Rapid infusion of 3 L saline.
D. Rapid infusion of 500 μg carboprost.
E. Transfusion of 4 L of cross-matched whole blood.

16.

A 23-year-old para 2 woman presented with vague abdominal pains when she was 29 weeks pregnant. General and abdominal examination did not reveal any abnormality. She had a normal BP. Fetal Doppler and CTG could not demonstrate the fetal heart. A real-time ultrasound scan augmented with colour Doppler of the fetal heart and umbilical artery confirmed intrauterine fetal demise. It also showed collapse of the fetal skull with overlapping bones. These findings were confirmed by a second scan. She insisted she still feels fetal movements.

How will you handle the situation?

A. Arrange for a 3D or 4D ultrasound.
B. Explain that some pregnant women may sometimes have false positive perceptions of fetal movements, but the baby is definitely dead.
C. Explain that some pregnant women may sometimes have false positive perceptions of fetal movements, and offer a third opinion and a repeat scan.
D. Refer her to the fetal medicine unit.
E. Repeat the CTG after asking her to drink a fruit juice.

17.

A 36-year-old woman comes to the labour ward with absent fetal movements for the last six hours. She is 36 weeks pregnant. All investigations confirmed intrauterine death. She has had two previous vaginal births. After counselling, she was still undecided about the period of waiting before active intervention.

What is the incidence of the most serious complication if she waits for four or more weeks?

A. Five in every 100 women.
B. 10 in every 100 women.
C. 12 in every 100 women.
D. 19 in every 100 women.
E. 22 in every 100 women.

18.

A 31-year-old woman presents to the antenatal clinic when she is 22 weeks pregnant. She has had normal antenatal care until her last visit two weeks previously with no medical history or medications. At this visit, her BP is 145/98 mmHg with significant proteinuria.

What is your management?

A. Admit and treat.
B. Admit and measure BP every four hours.
C. Arrange for home blood measurements daily.
D. Arrange for home BP measurements every other day.
E. Arrange for antenatal clinic visit reviews every week.

19.

You are admitting a 33-year-old woman with a BP of 170/115 mmHg. Her urine dipstick showed 1+ proteinuria.

What is the quickest and most convenient method to quantify her proteinuria?

A. Automated reagent-strip urine testing daily.
B. Automated reagent-strip urine testing twice weekly.
C. A spot urinary protein: creatinine ratio.
D. Urine dipstick twice daily.
E. Urine dipstick once daily.

20.

A 29-year-old primiparous woman complains of pruritus in the palm of the hands and soles of the feet when 32 weeks pregnant.

What is the risk of perinatal mortality because of this obstetric cholestasis?

A. 5.7/1000.
B. 6.7/1000.
C. 8.5/1000.
D. 13.4/1000.
E. >14/1000.

21.

A 38-year-old primigravida undergoes first trimester screening and the result shows a low placental-associated plasma protein (PAPP-A) of <0.4 MoM (multiples of the median).

What is the implication of this result?

A. She is at no risk of any pregnancy complications.
B. She is at a higher risk of multiple pregnancy complications.
C. She is at a low risk of multiple pregnancy complications.
D. She is at a high risk of developing a small-for-gestational-age (SGA) pregnancy.
E. She is not at any risk of developing any fetal complications.

22.

A 32-year-old pregnant woman had a history of a previous small-for-gestational-age baby. Her uterine artery Doppler shows notching at 22 weeks' gestation, which normalizes when repeated two weeks later.

How will you continue her antenatal care?

A. Routine usual antenatal care.
B. Repeat uterine artery Doppler twice weekly.
C. Start serial ultrasound measurements of the biparietal diameter.

D. Start serial ultrasound biometry and umbilical artery Doppler at 26–28 weeks of pregnancy.
E. Start fetal biometry every week from the 34th week.

23.

You are caring for a 33-year-old pregnant woman who is diagnosed with a small-for-gestational-age fetus. At 31 weeks she showed an umbilical flow plasticity index of >+2 standard deviations (SDs) above the mean for gestational age.

What indices should you use to time delivery?

A. Daily umbilical artery Doppler.
B. Ductus venosus Doppler.
C. Middle cerebral artery Doppler.
D. Ultrasound assessment of the deepest vertical pool.
E. Weekly uterine artery Doppler.

24.

A young couple comes to see you at the antenatal clinic. She is 29 years old and 23 weeks pregnant. They have to travel to a ZIKA virus endemic area. She shows you a National Health Service (NHS) advice about how to avoid mosquito bites, but asks you if you have any further advice.

What else will you tell her?

A. Ask her to sign a form to indicate she is travelling on her own responsibility.
B. Advise condom use during vaginal, anal and oral sex during travel and for the duration of the pregnancy.
C. Advise local assistance during the travel period.
D. No need for any extra precautions if she is not bitten by a mosquito.
E. She is fine if neither of the couple is bitten by a mosquito.

ANSWERS

Q1: A. Cervical cerclage surgery.[1]

• Consider prophylactic cervical cerclage for women in whom a transvaginal ultrasound scan between 16^{+0} and 24^{+0} weeks of pregnancy shows a cervical length of less than 25 mm and who have had either preterm pre-labour rupture of membranes in a previous pregnancy or a history of cervical trauma.

• Offer prophylactic vaginal progesterone to women with no history of spontaneous preterm birth or mid-trimester loss in whom a transvaginal ultrasound scan between 16^{+0} and 24^{+0} weeks of pregnancy reveals a cervical length <25 mm.

• Offer either prophylactic vaginal progesterone or prophylactic cervical cerclage to women with a history of spontaneous preterm birth or mid-trimester loss between 16^{+0} and 34^{+0} weeks, in whom a transvaginal ultrasound scan between 16^{+0} and 24^{+0} weeks of pregnancy reveals a cervical length <25 mm.

Q2: C. Admit, give steroids and book for emergency cerclage.[1]

• Consider 'rescue' cervical cerclage for women between 16^{+0} and 27^{+6} weeks of pregnancy with a dilated cervix and exposed, none-ruptured fetal membranes.

Q3: E. Start treatment with oral nifedipine.[1]

- Offer nifedipine for tocolysis to women between 24^{+0} and 33^{+6} weeks of pregnancy who have intact membranes and are in suspected or diagnosed preterm labour.
- The suggested dose of nifedipine is an initial oral dose of 20 mg followed by 10–20 mg three to four times daily, adjusted according to uterine activity for up to 48 hours. A total dose above 60 mg appears to be associated with a three- to four-fold increase in adverse events.
- Nifedipine and atosiban have comparable effectiveness in delaying birth for up to seven days.
- If nifedipine is contraindicated, offer oxytocin receptor antagonists for tocolysis.[1]

Q4: A. Perform transvaginal scan to check the cervical length.[1]

- If the clinical assessment suggests that the woman is in suspected preterm labour and she is 30^{+0} weeks pregnant or more, consider transvaginal ultrasound measurement of cervical length as a diagnostic test to determine the likelihood of birth within 48 hours.

Act on the results as follows
- If the cervical length is >15 mm, it is unlikely that she is in preterm. Discuss the benefits and risks of going home versus staying in hospital.
- If the cervical length is 15 mm or less, view the woman as being in diagnosed preterm labour and offer treatment of nifedipine or atosiban.
- If there is no expertise in transvaginal scanning or the woman declines the scan, use fetal fibronectin if the patient is >30 weeks.
- If fetal fibronectin testing is positive (concentration >50 ng/mL), start preterm labour treatment. If the woman declines both tests, treat as in preterm labour.

Q5: C. 4 g intravenous bolus of magnesium sulfate over 15 minutes, followed by an intravenous infusion of 1 g per hour until the birth or for 24 hours.[1]

- Offer intravenous magnesium sulfate for neuroprotection of the baby to women between 24^{+0} and 29^{+6} weeks of pregnancy who are in established preterm labour or having a planned preterm birth within 24 hours.
- For women who are between 30^{+0} and 33^{+6} weeks of pregnancy and are either in preterm labour or are for a planned preterm birth in the next 24 hours, consider magnesium sulphate for neuroprotection.[1]

Q6: B. Twin-to-twin transfusion syndrome (TTTS) Quintero Stage 1.[2]

- TTTS is the most important cause of death and disability in a MCDA twin pregnancy.
- In TTTS, the diagnosis is based on the presence of polyhydramnios with a distended bladder in the recipient and oligohydramnios (deepest vertical pocket (DVP) <2 cm) with a small or empty bladder in the donor.
- Discordant fetal growth restriction may be differentiated from TTTS by the absence of polyhydramnios in the amniotic sacs, although the small twin may have oligohydramnios owing to placental insufficiency.
- The normal range for the DVP is 2–8 cm in singleton gestations.
- The normal range for the single DVP in twin gestation appears to be 2.2–7.5 cm.
- Fetoscopic laser coagulation of the anastomoses leads to a 50%–60% survival for both twins and an 80% survival for at least one twin.

Q7: E. Tension headache.[3]

Primary headache
- Migraine and tension headache.

Secondary headache
- Hypertension, subarachnoid haemorrhage, drug-related (e.g. nifedipine), medication overuse, epidural tap, meningitis, cerebral venous thrombosis, anaemia, caffeine withdrawal, idiopathic intracranial hypertension, stroke, enlargement of a pituitary tumour, enlargement of a hormone-sensitive tumour (e.g. meningioma), bleeding into a pre-existing tumour, cerebral metastasis of choriocarcinoma.

Q8: E. Propranolol.[3]

- Women experiencing three to four headaches a month may be considered for prophylactic treatment, especially when the headache is unresponsive to simple analgesia.
- Propranolol (10–40 mg three times a day) has the best evidence of safety in pregnancy and lactation.

Q9: C. 31%–40% [evidence level 1++].[4]

- Steroids will reduce the respiratory distress syndrome by 44% [evidence level 1++].[5]
- It will reduce intraventricular haemorrhage by 46% [evidence level 1++].[4]

Q10: D. Steroids are administered with additional insulin and close monitoring [evidence level 3].[5]

- There are no randomized trials to assess the safety or efficacy for steroids in diabetic pregnant women.
- Option (E) is correct, but not the best answer.

Q11: C. 19%–25%.[6]

- Other risk factors for placental abruption include pre-eclampsia, fetal growth restriction, polyhydramnios, advanced maternal age, multiparity, low body mass index (BMI), pregnancy following assisted reproductive techniques, intrauterine infection, premature rupture of membranes, abdominal trauma (both accidental and resulting from domestic violence), smoking and drug misuse (e.g. cocaine and amphetamines) during pregnancy and maternal thrombophilia.[1]

Q12: D. 9.7 [evidence level 2–].[6]

- The OR for recurrence of placenta praevia after a previous episode is 9.7.[6]
- Other risk factors include previous termination of pregnancy, multiparity, advanced maternal age (>40 years old), multiple pregnancies, smoking, deficient endometrium due to assisted conception.
- OR represents the odds of an outcome (recurrence of placenta praevia) because of an exposure (previous placenta praevia) compared to no exposure.

Q13: D. Kleihauer count [evidence level 3].[6]

- All the suggested investigations are required in all antepartum haemorrhage cases.

- In Rhesus D (RhD)-negative women, the Kleihauer test is the specific test to access the amount of fetomaternal haemorrhage and adjust the anti-D immunoglobulin (anti-D Ig) dose.

Q14: C. Refer her back to her community antenatal care and delivery.[7]

- It is clear that the ectropion is the cause of bleeding. She is at a low risk because she does not have an unexplained antepartum haemorrhage, placenta praevia, or placental abruption. RCOG guidelines recommend no alteration of antenatal care if the bleeding is due to a cervical ectropion.[6]
- There is no need to repeat the cervical smear. In the UK screening programme, if she has a mild or borderline dyskaryosis and is HPV negative, she is back to her routine call–recall system with no need for any interventions.

Q15: B. One litre of fresh frozen plasma and 10 units of cryoprecipitate.[8]

Q16: B. Explain that some pregnant women may sometimes have false positive perceptions of fetal movements, but the baby is definitely dead.[9]

- Be sympathetic in your approach.
- Do not use auscultation and cardiotocography (CTG) to investigate suspected intrauterine fetal death (IUFD).
- Real-time ultrasonography, which should be available at all times, is essential for the accurate diagnosis of IUFD.
- A repeat scan should be carried out to confirm the diagnosis.
- In counselling couples with an IUFD, you should recognize their emotions.[9]

Q17: B. 10 in every 100 women.[9]

- The most serious complication is coagulopathy, which rises to 30% after four weeks.
- She should be monitored with blood platelet count and fibrinogen measurement [evidence level 3].
  - A combination of mifepristone (single 200 mg dose) and a prostaglandin preparation is the first-line intervention.
  - Vaginal misoprostol for induction of labour is equally effective as gemeprost or prostaglandin E2 but is less expensive [evidence level 1+].
- Vaginal birth can be achieved within 24 hours of induction of labour for IUFD in about 90% of women.
  - The dose is 100 µg six hourly before 26^{+6} weeks, 25–50 µg four hourly at 27^{+0} weeks or more.
- Vaginal administration of misoprostol is as effective as oral administration but is associated with fewer side effects (diarrhoea, vomiting, shivering and pyrexia).[9]

Q18: B. Admit and measure BP every four hours.[10]

Gestational hypertension: new hypertension presenting after 20 weeks without significant proteinuria.
Mild hypertension: 140–149/90–99 mmHg; **moderate hypertension:** 150–159/100–109 mmHg; **severe hypertension:** 160/110 mmHg or greater.
Severe pre-eclampsia: pre-eclampsia with severe hypertension and/or with symptoms, and/or with biochemical or haematological impairment.
Significant proteinuria: if the urinary protein:creatinine ratio is greater than 30 mg/mmol or a 24-hour urine collection result shows >300 mg protein.

Q19: C. A spot urinary protein: creatinine ratio.[10]

      If an automated reagent-strip reading device is used to detect proteinuria and a result of 1+ or more is obtained, use a spot urinary protein:creatinine ratio or 24-hour urine collection to quantify proteinuria.

- Once proteinuria is quantified, there is no need for further quantification. Women should be continually monitored for BP every four hours with kidney function, electrolytes, full blood count, transaminases and bilirubin three times weekly.
- Repeat ultrasound fetal growth scan, amniotic fluid volume assessment, and umbilical artery Doppler velocimetry every two weeks.

Q20: A. 5.7/1000 [evidence level 2+].[11]

- In recent studies between 2001 and 2011, the perinatal mortality rate for obstetric cholestasis was not any higher than the UK national average.

Q21: D. She is at a high risk of developing a small-for-gestational-age (SGA) pregnancy [evidence level 1+].[12]

- A low PAPP-A is associated with a higher risk of an SGA baby.
- The odds ratio for a birthweight <10th centile is 2.7 while her odds ratio of developing a severe SGA (birthweight <3rd centile) is 3.66.[12]

Q22: D. Start serial ultrasound biometry and umbilical artery Doppler at 26–28 weeks of pregnancy [evidence level 1++].[12]

- Women who have an abnormal uterine artery Doppler at 20–24 weeks (pulsatility index (PI) >95th centile and/or notching) should be scheduled for serial ultrasound measurements of fetal size and assessment of well-being with umbilical artery Doppler commencing at 26–28 weeks of pregnancy.
- Pregnant women with a normal uterine artery Doppler do not require serial follow-up measurements of fetal size and or serial umbilical artery Doppler to assess fetal well-being unless they develop specific pregnancy complications (e.g. antepartum haemorrhage or hypertension).
- However, they should be offered a scan for fetal size and umbilical artery Doppler during the third trimester.

Q23: B. Ductus venosus Doppler [evidence level 2−].[12]

- On the basis of the Growth Restriction Intervention Trial (GRIT) study, it is reasonable to recommend delivery when the ductus venosis Doppler becomes abnormal after completion of a steroid course.[12]
- In the preterm SGA fetus, middle cerebral artery Doppler has limited value for the prediction of acidaemia and adverse outcomes. It should not be used to time delivery.
- In fetuses with absent end-diastolic velocity in the umbilical artery, the presence of umbilical vein pulsations identifies a subgroup of fetuses with a more severe compromise of acid-base status.
- In the term SGA fetus with normal umbilical artery Doppler, an abnormal middle cerebral artery Doppler (PI <5th centile) has moderate predictive accuracy to detect acidosis at birth and should be used to time delivery.
  - Delivery should not be delayed beyond 37 weeks.

Q24: B. Advise condom use during vaginal, anal and oral sex during travel and for the duration of the pregnancy.[13]

- Zika virus can be transmitted during sexual intercourse. Approximately 80% of infections are asymptomatic.
- They should be advised to use condom contraception for any form of sexual relations during the period of travel and until the end of pregnancy even if they do not develop any symptoms of infection.

References

1. National Institute for Health and Clinical Excellence. *Preterm Labour and Birth*. November, 2015. [https://www.nice.org.uk/guidance/ng25]
2. Quintero RA, Morales WJ, Allen MH, et al. Staging of twin–twin transfusion syndrome. *J Perinatol* 1999;19(8 Pt 1):550–5.
3. Revelle K, Morrish P. Headaches in pregnancy. *Obstet Gynaecol* 2014;16(3):179–84.
4. Roberts D, Dalziel SR. Antenatal corticosteroids for accelerating fetal lung maturation for women at risk of preterm birth. *Cochrane Database Syst Rev* 2006;(3): CD004454.
5. National Institute for Health and Clinical Excellence. *Diabetes in Pregnancy. Management of Diabetes and its Complications from Pre-conception to the Postnatal Period*. March, 2008. [https://www.nice.org.uk/guidance/ng63]
6. Royal College of Obstetricians and Gynaecologists. *Antepartum Haemorrhage*. November, 2011. [https://www.rcog.org.uk/en/guidelines-research-services/guidelines/gtg63]
7. National Health Service. *Choices, Cervical Screening*. [www.nhs.uk/Conditions/Cervical-screening-test]
8. Royal College of Obstetricians and Gynaecologists. *Postpartum Haemorrhage, Prevention and Management*. December, 2016. [https://www.rcog.org.uk/en/guidelines-research-services/guidelines/gtg52]
9. Royal College of Obstetricians and Gynaecologists. *Late Intrauterine Fetal Death and Stillbirth*. October, 2010. [https://www.rcog.org.uk/en/guidelines-research-services/guidelines/gtg55]
10. National Institute for Health and Clinical Excellence. *Hypertension in Pregnancy: Diagnosis and Management*. August, 2010. [https://www.nice.org.uk/guidance/cg107]
11. Royal College of Obstetricians and Gynaecologists. *Obstetric Cholestasis*. April, 2011. [https://www.rcog.org.uk/en/guidelines-research-services/guidelines/gtg43]
12. Royal College of Obstetricians and Gynaecologists. *The Investigation and Management of the Small-for-Gestational-Age Fetus*. February, 2013. [https://www.rcog.org.uk/en/guidelines-research-services/guidelines/gtg31]
13. Travel Health Programme. *Zika Virus – Update and Advice for Travellers Including Pregnant Women and Those Planning Pregnancy*. [http://travelhealthpro.org.uk/zika-virus-update-and-advice-for-travellers]

Chapter 3

Aneuploidy and Anomaly Screening

QUESTIONS

1.

A 25-year-old, G1 P0 woman attends the antenatal clinic for her 12-week scan. She accepted the offer of undergoing a combined test. However, she has queried the accuracy of the test.

Which of the followings best describes the detection rate (DR) and the screen positive rate (SPR) of a combined test?

A. DR >75% and SPR <3%.
B. DR >75% and SPR <1%.
C. DR >90% and SPR <2%.
D. DR >95% and SPR <1%.
E. DR >99% and SPR <5%.

2.

A 37-year-old pregnant woman has been diagnosed with monochorionic diamniotic (MCDA) twins. She agreed to screening for Down syndrome at 13^{+4} weeks.

Which of the following screenings best describes her available option?

A. Either combined or quadruple test.
B. Triple test.
C. Nuchal translucency.
D. Nuchal translucency and maternal age.
E. Quadruple test.

3.

A 25-year-old has just had her 20-week scan. The fetus is found to have holoprosencephaly and bilateral cleft palate. The cardiac ultrasound scan shows a ventricular septal defect.

Which of the following is most likely to be associated with these ultrasound scan findings?

A. Down syndrome.
B. DiGeorge syndrome.
C. Edward syndrome.
D. Patau syndrome.
E. Turner syndrome.

4.

The screening midwife has shown you a result of a combined test for a 19-year-old woman. It reads as follows:
bHCG: 0.2 MoM
PAPP-A: 0.3 MoM
NT: 2.5 mm
Risk of Down syndrome: 1:170.

What will be your next step?

A. Book a growth scan.
B. Offer chorionic villus sampling to exclude Down syndrome.
C. Repeat the blood test for confirmation.
D. The woman to be sent a letter confirming a low risk.
E. The woman should be counselled about Edward and Patau syndromes.

5.

A woman has just had her dating ultrasound scan. The sonographer has clearly documented two gestational sacs (T-sign) and confirmed 10-week MCDA viable twins. The woman asks you for further information about MCDA twins.

Which of the following statements can you quote in your counselling?

A. A special fetal echocardiographic assessment should be done routinely in MCDA twins' pregnancies.
B. MCDA twins are 1% of twins' pregnancies.
C. MCDA twins' pregnancy has around a 15% chance of developing twin-to-twin transfusion syndrome (TTTS).
D. She may require an extra scan at 15 weeks as chorionicity is assessed better after 14 weeks.
E. The risk of twin-to-twin transfusion is less than in cases of monochorionic monoamniotic (MCMA) twins.

6.

A 28-year-old low-risk pregnant woman attends the antenatal clinic for the 18–20-week ultrasound anomaly scan. She asks about the chance of finding a structural abnormality.

Which of the following describes best the risk of structural abnormalities in all pregnancies?

A. 1%–2%.
B. 2%–3%.
C. 4%–5%.
D. 5%–8%.
E. 5%–10%.

7.

A 17-year-old woman attends the antenatal clinic for her 20-week scan. The sonographer has confirmed the presence of an isolated large gastroschisis. The woman is committed to her pregnancy.

What is your next step?

A. Offer amniocentesis.
B. Offer chorionic villus sampling.
C. Offer termination of the pregnancy.
D. Offer serial growth scans.
E. Offer Caesarean section at term.

8.

A woman attends the antenatal clinic for her 18–20-week scan. The sonographer has demonstrated 'lemon and banana' sign and the baby is diagnosed with Arnold–Chiari syndrome.

What is the 'banana' sign?

A. Congenitally malformed thalamus.
B. Deformed cerebellum.
C. Deformed skull.
D. Malformed cerebellum.
E. Open spina bifida.

9.

A pregnant woman has just had her 20-week anomaly scan. Her baby is diagnosed with ventricular septal defect and its femur length is at the 5th centile.

What is the most appropriate next step?

A. Offer serial growth scans.
B. Offer delivery arrangements at a tertiary hospital.
C. Offer amniocentesis.
D. Offer termination of the pregnancy for ground E.
E. Offer a repeat of the cardiac scan at 32 weeks.

10.

A pregnant woman complaining of reduced fetal movements at 26 weeks is referred for an ultrasound scan. The scan shows fetal hydrothorax, ascites and massive skin oedema. She is rhesus positive and all her antibody tests are negative.

What is the proportion of this condition as a cause of perinatal mortality?

A. 1%.
B. 3%.
C. 5%.
D. 8%.
E. 10%.

11.

A pregnant woman has just had her 12-week ultrasound scan. The scan shows a live severely hydropic baby.

What is the most appropriate investigation you would like to offer next?

A. Karyotyping.
B. Maternal blood group and Rhesus status.
C. Middle cerebral artery Doppler study.
D. Parvovirus B19 antibodies.
E. Sabin–Feldman dye test.

12.

A woman has booked her pregnancy at 27 weeks' gestation. She has an ultrasound scan that shows multiple congenital abnormalities. She is offered amniocentesis and the baby is diagnosed with Edward syndrome (Trisomy 18). She asks for termination of the pregnancy.

Based on the 1967 United Kingdom Abortion (amended in 1990), which ground will support her request?

A. Ground A.
B. Ground B.
C. Ground C.
D. Ground D.
E. Ground E.

13.

A pregnant woman has just had her 12-week scan. She is diagnosed with a dichorionic diamniotic (DCDA) twin pregnancy. She queries the chance of having them prematurely.

What proportion of all twins deliver before 37 weeks?

A. 25%.
B. 30%.
C. 40%.
D. 50%.
E. 60%.

14.

A pregnant woman with MCDA twins has just had a scan at 21 weeks in the fetal medicine unit. Twin 1's estimated weight is 40% less than the estimated weight for twin 2, and is diagnosed with sacral agenesis and right diaphragmatic hernia. No obvious anomaly is seen in twin 2 and it's growth and amniotic fluid are normal.

What is the management option you would like to offer her?

A. Expectant management.
B. Selective fetocide with intracardiac potassium choloride for twin 1.
C. Selective fetocide with cord occlusion for twin 1.
D. Termination of the pregnancy.
E. Weekly growth and Doppler scans.

15.

A woman has had her scan at 24 weeks as the symphysiofundal height (SFH) height measures more than for the estimated date. The scan demonstrates severe polyhydramnios. The sonographer could not see one of the fetal organs.

What is the most likely missing organ/s in the scan?

A. Fetal bladder.
B. Fetal kidneys.

C. Fetal ureters.
D. Fetal stomach.
E. Fetal oesophagus.

16.

A woman has had her first trimester combined risk calculated as 1:50. Chorionic villus sampling is offered and accepted. An uncomplicated procedure is performed and she is informed that the first result will be within 72 hours.

What type of test is usually used to give the first cytogenetic result?

A. Array comparative genomic hybridization (CGH).
B. Fluorescence *in situ* hybridization (FISH).
C. Karyotyping.
D. Microarray comparative genomic hybridization (aCGH).
E. Quantitative fluorescent polymerase chain reaction (QF-PCR).

17.

A 36-year-old woman with a BMI of 19 kg/m^2 has become pregnant following a successful second attempt at in vitro fertilization. She is healthy but smokes 5–10 cigarettes a day. The 19-week anomaly scan did not show any obvious abnormality.

What further management would you like to recommend?

A. Growth and Doppler scans at 36 weeks.
B. Middle cerebral artery Doppler scan at 24 weeks.
C. Serial growth and Doppler scans from 28 weeks.
D. Serial symphysiofundal measurements.
E. Uterine artery Doppler scan at 20–24 weeks.

18.

A 26-week pregnant woman is referred for an ultrasound scan after she presented with an episode of reduced fetal movements. The fetal Doppler assessment shows middle cerebral artery peak velocity multiple of the mean (MoM) at 2 and mild fetal ascites. You noted that her booked blood results show anti-K antibodies level of 2 IU/mL.

What is the most appropriate management?

A. Arrange for daily ultrasound assessments.
B. Arrange for daily cardiotocography (CTG).
C. Arrange for delivery by Caesarean section.
D. Arrange for fetal blood sampling and/or transfusion.
E. Arrange for weekly ultrasound assessments.

19.

A pregnant woman has just had her 20-week anomaly scan. There is no obvious fetal anomaly seen on the scan but the umbilical cord contains only two blood vessels.

What further management would you like to recommend?

A. Amniocentesis for karyotyping.
B. Reassure.
C. Referral to tertiary fetal medicine unit.
D. Third trimester growth scan and neonatal cranial scan.
E. Third trimester growth scan and neonatal renal and cardiac scan.

20.

The airport authorities are on the phone. A woman has refused to go through the airport body scanner as she is seven weeks pregnant and worried about fetal radiation exposure.

What would be your advice?

A. Advise body scanning with shield protection.
B. Advise allowing the woman to pass without body scanning at this gestation.
C. Advise the woman to rearrange her journey if possible to later in her pregnancy.
D. Advise hand-held scanner to avoid fetal exposure.
E. Reassure the woman.

ANSWERS

Q1: C. DR >90% and SPR <2%.[1,2]

- For first trimester combined screening, the current UK National Screening Committee (UKNSC) Model of Best Practice standard is a DR >90% of affected pregnancies with a SPR <2% of unaffected pregnancies.
- For the second trimester quadruple test, the standard is a DR greater than>75% for a SPR <3%.
- First trimester combined screening is offered between 10^{+0} and 14^{+1} weeks' gestation. The maternal serum sample can be taken between 10^{+0} and 14^{+1} weeks' gestation and the nuchal translucency measured between 11^{+2} and 14^{+1} weeks' gestation.
- For women presenting late, or with a crown–rump length (CRL) >84 mm, or between 14^{+2} and 20^{+0} weeks, the quadruple test is offered.
- Cell free fetal DNA testing is a screening test and is not diagnostic for Down syndrome.[2]

For definitive diagnoses, invasive tests, chorionic villus sampling (CVS) or amniocentests are required.

- Amniocentesis should be performed after 15 weeks of gestation [evidence level 1+].
- Amniocentesis before 14 weeks of gestation has a higher fetal loss rate and increased incidence of fetal talipes and respiratory morbidity.
- CVS should not be performed before 10 (10^{+0}) completed weeks of gestation.
- If the risk of having a term pregnancy affected with Down syndrome is 1 in 150 or higher, calculated by either a combined or quadruple test, the pregnancy is regarded as higher risk and the woman will be offered a diagnostic test.
- The risk of miscarriage following amniocentesis is around 1%.
- The risk of miscarriage following CVS is slightly higher than that of amniocentesis.

Q2: A. Either combined or quadruple test.[3]

- For twin pregnancies (monochorionic diamniotic, MCDA; dichorionic diamniotic, DCDA), the 'combined test' is to be used.
- However, second trimester serum screening can be considered if a woman books too late for first trimester screening.
- We should explain the potential problems of screening and diagnostic testing, because of the increased likelihood of pregnancy loss associated with double invasive testing as the risk cannot be calculated separately for each baby.

- For triplet pregnancies, only nuchal translucency and maternal age can be used. We do not use second trimester serum screening.

Q3: D. Patau syndrome.[4]

Q4: E. The woman should be counselled about Edward and Patau syndromes.[4]

- The woman should be seen by a fetal medicine consultant because her pregnancy is at high risk of trisomy 13 and 18.
- The cut-off risk for Down syndrome is 1 in 150, above which a diagnostic test should be offered.[5]
- In the screening programmes, markers' levels are described in multiples of the median (MoM) to allow for the fact that levels vary with gestational age.[1]
- The calculation of risk using a combined test includes maternal age, nuchal translucency measurement, beta-human chorionic gonadotropin (BhCG) and placental-associated plasma protein (PAPP-A) levels.[1]
- The calculation of risk using a quadruple test includes BhCG, uE3 (unconjugated estriol), alpha-fetoprotein (AFP) and inhibin-A.[1]
- The biochemical markers of the common aneuploidies.[5]

Aneuploidy	BhCG	PAPP-A	uE3	AFP	Inhibin-A
Trisomy 21	High	Low	Low	Low	High
Trisomy 13	Low/normal	Low	Normal	Increased	Normal
Trisomy 18	Low	Very low	Low	Normal	Normal
Turner (XO)	Normal/mildly high	Low	Normal	Normal	High
Diandric triploidy	Very high	Mildly low	–	–	–
Digynic triploidy	Very low	Very low	–	–	–

Q5: C. MCDA twin pregnancy has around a 15% chance of developing twin-to-twin transfusion syndrome (TTTS).[6]

- TTTS complicates 10%–15% of monochorionic diamniotic twins.
- TTTS is more common in MCDA pregnancies than MCMA pregnancies, most probably because of the protective artery–artery anastomoses in the latter.
- Chorionicity is better assessed by ultrasound before 14 weeks.
- All monochorionic twins should have a detailed ultrasound scan which includes extended views of the fetal heart. A special fetal echocardiographic assessment should be considered in the assessment of severe TTTS.

Q6: B. 2%–3%.[7]

- Structural fetal abnormalities occur in approximately 2%–3% of all pregnancies.
- Structural fetal abnormalities account for almost 10% of stillbirths and 25% of all neonatal deaths.

Q7: D. Offer serial growth scans.[6]

Gastroschisis
- In gastroschisis, free loops of bowel are seen floating in the amniotic cavity on ultrasound examination, as there is no covering membrane.

- Gastroschisis, unlike exomphalos, is rarely associated with chromosomal abnormality.
- Caesarean section is usually reserved for obstetric indication.
- Babies with gastroschisis are at high risk of growth restriction (30%); growth scans should be arranged.[6]
- If it is an isolated defect, the prognosis following early neonatal surgery is generally very good (80%–90% survival).
- Gastroschisis: approximately one in 2500–3000 live births.
- The risk of aneuploidy is not increased (<1%).

Exomphalos
- It is a midline defect in which the herniated contents are covered by a membrane and the umbilical cord inserts into the apex of the lesion.
- The incidence is approximately one in 5000 live births.
- It is associated with chromosomal (up to 60%) and additional structural abnormalities (30%–70%).

Q8: B. Deformed cerebellum.[7]

- The 'lemon' and 'banana' signs describe the cranial features seen on ultrasound that are associated with spina bifida.
- The **Arnold–Chiari** malformation (type II) is a descent of the cerebellum, pons and medulla through the foramen magnum, leading to obliteration of the cisterna magna.
- **Prune belly syndrome**: lower urinary tract obstruction with an enlarged bladder, bilateral hydronephrosis and reduced amniotic fluid.
- It is associated with high mortality from pulmonary hypoplasia.

Q9: C. Offer amniocentesis.[7]

- Up to 44% of congenital heart lesions are associated with anomalies in one or more body systems.
- There is a strong association between congenital heart disease and aneuploidy (35%–48%).
- Amniocentesis should be offered to exclude an associated chromosomal abnormality.

Q10: B. 3%.[7]

- Non-immune hydrops fetalis (NIHF) is an uncommon condition accounting for around 3% of overall perinatal mortality.
- With the decline in rhesus isoimmunisation, non-immunological causes have become responsible for the majority of fetal hydrops.
- The major causes of NIHF are chromosomal abnormality, structural cardiovascular disease, cardiac dysrhythmias, abnormalities of the fetal thorax, haematological disorders and infections.

Q11: A. Karyotyping.[7]

- Hydrops fetalis in the first trimester is most likely to be associated with chromosomal abnormality; karyotyping is needed to exclude the possibility before allowing the pregnancy to continue.

Q12: D. Clause D.[8]

- A pregnancy may be terminated at any stage for fetal abnormality if there is a substantial risk that if the child were born, it would suffer from such physical and mental abnormalities as to be severely handicapped.

- Each of the grounds for termination of pregnancy has to be recognized by two medical practitioners in good faith, except for ground F, which can be approved by only one registered medical practitioner.
- There is no legal definition of what comprises a 'substantial' risk or 'serious handicap'.
- A pregnancy may be terminated at any stage for fetal abnormality if there is a substantial risk that if the child were born, it would suffer from such physical and mental abnormalities as to be severely handicapped.
- The 24-week limit is for ground C and D. For ground A, B, E, F and G, there is no limit as the termination can be performed at any time during pregnancy if the conditions are met.

Grounds for Abortion under Section 1 of the Abortion Act subject to the provisions of this section, a person shall not be guilty of an offence under the law relating to abortion when a pregnancy is terminated by a registered medical practitioner if two registered medical practitioners are of the opinion, formed in good faith, that:

A   The continuance of the pregnancy would involve risk to the life of the pregnant woman greater than if the pregnancy were terminated (Abortion Act, 1967, as amended, section 1(1)(c))

B   The termination is necessary to prevent grave permanent injury to the physical or mental health of the pregnant woman

C   The pregnancy has not exceeded its twenty-fourth week and that the continuance of the pregnancy would involve risk, greater than if the pregnancy were terminated, of injury to the physical or mental health of the pregnant woman (section 1(1)(a))

D   The pregnancy has not exceeded its twenty-fourth week and that the continuance of the pregnancy would involve risk, greater than if the pregnancy were terminated, of injury to the physical or mental health of any existing children of the family of the pregnant woman (section 1(1)(a))

E   There is a substantial risk that if the child were born it would suffer from such physical or mental abnormalities as to be seriously handicapped (section 1(1) (d)); or, in an emergency, certified by the operating practitioner as immediately necessary

F   To save the life of the pregnant woman (section 1(4))

G   To prevent grave permanent injury to the physical or mental health of the pregnant woman (section 1(4))

Q13: E. 60%.[3]

- About 60% of twin pregnancies result in spontaneous birth before 37 weeks and 0 days.
- NICE recommends elective birth from 36 weeks and 0 days for monochorionic twins and 37 weeks and 0 days for dichorionic twins, after a single course of steroids.
- Continuing twin pregnancies beyond 38 weeks and 0 days increases the risk of fetal death.
- About 75% of triplet pregnancies result in spontaneous birth before 35 weeks and 0 days.
- For triplet pregnancies, NICE recommends elective birth from 35 weeks and 0 days, after a course of corticosteroids.

Q14: C. Selective fetocide with cord occlusion for twin 1.[6]

- In MCDA twins, the structural abnormality affects only one twin in 80% of cases.
- Anomalies such as anencephaly or diaphragmatic hernia are typically complicated by polyhydramnios and place the normal co-twin at risk of severe preterm delivery owing to uterine distension.
- In monochorionic twins, selective feticide by intracardiac potassium chloride cannot be used owing to the vascular anastomoses between the two fetoplacental circulations.
- Cord occlusive techniques by interstitial laser, bipolar diathermy or ligation are the only 'selective' option for feticide in monochorionic twin pregnancies.
- These procedures carry a significant risk of membrane rupture (10%–30%) and loss of the structurally normal twin.[6]

Q15: D. Fetal stomach.[7]

- In polyhydramnios, prenatal diagnosis of oesophageal atresia is suspected when repeated ultrasonographic examinations fail to demonstrate the fetal stomach.[7]
- Routine symphysiofundal height (SFH) measurement is a sound method for detecting small-for-gestational-age babies in developing countries and may be recommended as standard practice.[9]
- A 'double bubble' sign is a sonographic feature of duodenal atresia.

Q16: E. Quantitative fluorescent polymerase chain reaction (QF-PCR).[10]

- QF-PCR marker analysis does not require cell culture whereas karyotyping does.
- PCR results can be available within 48–72 hours. The results are nearly 100% accurate.
- PCR testing usually only looks for three specific defined chromosomal conditions in the fetus: trisomy 21 (Down syndrome), trisomy 18 (Edward syndrome) and trisomy 13 (Patau syndrome).

Q17: E. Uterine artery Doppler scan at 20–24 weeks [good practice point].[14]

- Women who have three or more minor risk factors for a small-for-gestational-age (SGA) baby should be referred for a uterine artery Doppler scan at 20–24 weeks of gestation.
- Women with an abnormal uterine artery Doppler scan at 20–24 weeks (defined as a pulsatility index [PI] >95th centile) and/or notching should be referred for serial ultrasound measurements of fetal size and assessment of well-being with umbilical artery Doppler scans commencing at 26–28 weeks of pregnancy.
- Women with three minor risk factors and a normal uterine artery Doppler scan require third trimester growth and umbilical artery Doppler scans during the third trimester.
- Risk factors for SGA:[11]

Type of risk	Risks	Management
Minor Risks	Age >35 IVF BMI <20 or 25–34.9 Smoking 1–10/day Pregnancy interval <6 months Pregnancy interval >60 months Previous pre-eclampsia	≥3 risk factors: offer uterine artery Doppler at 20–24 weeks If abnormal: offer serial growth and umbilical artery Doppler scans from 26–28 weeks If normal: offer third trimester growth and Doppler scan
Major Risk Factors	Age >40, smokes >11/day Cocaine diabetic vasculopathy Maternal/paternal SGA Previous SGA/stillbirth Renal impairment Antiphospholipid syndrome. PAPPA<0.4 MoM Chronic hypertension Echogenic (bright) bowels	One risk factor: offer serial growth and umbilical artery Doppler scans from 26–28 weeks
Unsuitable for Serial SFH	BMI >35 Fibroids	Offer serial growth and umbilical artery Doppler scans from 26–28 weeks

Q18: D. Arrange for fetal blood sampling and/or transfusion.[12]

- For anti-K antibodies, referral should take place once detected, as severe fetal anaemia can occur even with low titres.
- Refer to a fetal medicine specialist for invasive treatment if the middle cerebral artery peak velocity rises above 1.5 MoM or if there are other signs of fetal anaemia.
- Red cell preparations for intrauterine transfusion should be group O (low titre haemolysin) or ABO identical with the fetus (if known) and negative for the antigen(s) corresponding to maternal red cell antibodies.

Q19: E. Third trimester growth scan and neonatal renal and cardiac scan.[13]

- An isolated single umbilical artery does not warrant invasive testing for fetal aneuploidy, but consider third trimester ultrasonography for fetal growth.

Q20: E. Reassure the woman.[14]

- The Health Protection Agency (HPA) concludes that the potential doses received from the use of a correctly installed and used X-ray backscatter body scanner are likely to be very low and are unlikely to exceed 20 micro-Sv/year.[14]
  - For the pregnant women, the advice is 'the backscatter technology ensures that negligible doses are absorbed into the body, the fetal dose is thus much lower than the dose to a pregnant woman.
- The radiation levels of such machines is equivalent to two minutes of air travel.
- Emission levels are 10 000 times lower than that of a mobile phone.[14]

References

1. National Screening Committee. *NHS Down's Syndrome Screening (Trisomy 21) Programme*. November, 2012. [www.doh.gov.uk/nsc/index/htm]
2. Royal College of Obstetricians and Gynaecologists. *Non-invasive Prenatal Testing for Chromosomal Abnormality using Maternal Plasma DNA*. March, 2014. [https://www.rcog.org.uk/en/guidelines-research-services/guidelines/sip15]
3. National Institute for Health and Clinical Excellence. *Multiple Pregnancy: The Management of Twin and Triplet Pregnancies in the Antenatal Period*. September, 2011. [https://www.nice.org.uk/guidance/cg129]
4. Cameron A, Brennand J, Crichton L, Gibson J. Routine Anomaly Scan. In: Higham J, ed. *Fetal Medicine for MRCOG and Beyond*, 2nd edn. London, UK: RCOG Press, 2011; p. 35.
5. Nicolaides KH. Screening for fetal aneuploidies at 11 to 13 weeks. *Prenat Diagn* 2011;31:7–15. [www.fetalmedicine.com/synced/fmf/aneuploidies.pdf]
6. Royal College of Obstetricians and Gynaecologists. *Monochorionic Twin Pregnancy, Management*. November, 2016. [https://www.rcog.org.uk/en/guidelines-research-services/guidelines/gtg51]
7. National Health Service. *Fetal Anomaly Screening. Programme Handbook*. July, 2015. [https://www.gov.uk/government/publications/fetal-anomaly-screening-programme-handbook]
8. Department of Health. *Guidance in Relation to Requirements of the Abortion ACT 1967*. [https://www.gov.uk/government/uploads/system/uploads/attachment_data/file/313459/20140509_-_Abortion_Guidance_Document.pdf]
9. World Health Organization Reproductive Health Library. *Routine Symphysis–Fundal Height Measurement During Pregnancy*. December, 2016. [https://extranet.who.int/rhl]
10. National Screening Committee. *Chorionic Villus Sampling (CVS) and Amniocentesis Information for Health Professionals*. July, 2009. [www.doh.gov.uk/nsc/index/htm]
11. Royal College of Obstetricians and Gynaecologists. *Small-for-Gestational-Age Fetus, Investigation and Management*. March, 2013. [https://www.rcog.org.uk/en/guidelines-research-services//guidelines/gtg_31]
12. Royal College of Obstetricians and Gynaecologists. *The Management of Women with Red Cell Antibodies during Pregnancy*. May, 2014. [https://www.rcog.org.uk/en/guidelines-research-services/guidelines/gtg65]
13. Royal College of Obstetricians and Gynaecologists. *Single Umbilical Artery* (Query Bank), April, 2013. [https://www.rcog.org.uk/en/guidelines-research-services/guidelines/single-umbilical-artery]
14. MacDonald A, Tattersall P, O'Hagan J, et al. *Assessment of Comparative Ionising Radiation Doses from the Use of Rapiscan Secure 1000 X-ray Backscatter Body Scanner*. Health Protection Agency, Centre for Radiation, Chemical and Environmental Hazards. February, 2010. [https://www.rcog.org.uk/en/guidelines-research-services/guidelines/airport-full-body-scanners-and-pregnancy—query-bank]

Chapter 4

Labour Ward Management

QUESTIONS

1.

Your year ST 1 junior colleague wants to know why electronic fetal monitoring (EFM) is the recommended method of intrapartum fetal surveillance for high-risk pregnancies.

What will you tell him?

A. It has low sensitivity and specificity in detecting abnormalities.
B. It is sensitive in detecting abnormalities in fetal heart rate pattern.
C. It is specific in detecting abnormalities in fetal heart pattern.
D. It is sensitive in detecting fetal hypoxia.
E. It is specific in detecting fetal hypoxia.

2.

A 33-year-old woman is induced at 38 weeks because of mild pre-eclampsia. She wants to know how she would benefit from continuous electronic fetal monitoring as she felt it may limit her freedom of movement during labour.

What will you tell her?

A. It will help reduce the incidence of neonatal seizures.
B. It will help reduce the incidence of cerebral palsy.
C. It will help reduce the incidence of ischemic hypoxic encephalopathy.
D. It will improve the overall perinatal mortality.
E. It will reduce the incidence of cerebral palsy, encephalopathy and seizures of the newborn.

3.

A 28-year-old woman in her first pregnancy is 36 weeks with an uncomplicated pregnancy. She would like to have a home delivery and wants to know more information about choosing the place to have her baby.

What will you tell her according to the Birthplace Study of 2011?

A. Planning birth in an obstetric unit is associated with a lower rate of interventions.
B. Planning birth in a stand-alone midwifery-led unit is associated with a small increase of poor outcome for the baby.
C. Planning birth at home is associated with an overall small increase in the risk of a baby having a poor outcome.
D. Planning birth in an alongside midwifery-led unit is associated with an overall small risk of a baby having serious medical complications.
E. Planning homebirth is associated with the highest rate of Caesarean section compared to having birth in an obstetrics unit.

4.

A 37-year-old primigravida attends the labour ward complaining of irregular contractions. She is 38 weeks pregnant. The ultrasound scan performed at 36 weeks showed the placenta to be posterior and high, with a normally grown baby. She conceived by in vitro fertilization (IVF). Her admission cardiotocography (CTG) shows a baseline rate of 145 beats per minute (bpm), variability of 10–15 bpm, accelerations, no decelerations, and she is contracting once every 10 minutes. Vaginal examination showed the cervix to be partially effaced and dilated 2 cm with intact membranes. The head is 5/5 palpable. All her observations are normal.

Which of the following options would you do next?

A. Admit her to the antenatal ward.
B. Admit her to the labour ward and keep her on continuous monitoring.
C. Admit her to the labour ward and perform artificial rupture of membranes.
D. Admit her to the labour ward and book her for a category 2 Caesarean section.
E. Reassure her that all is well and discharge her home.

5.

A 28-year-old in her first pregnancy is induced at term plus 10 days. The CTG was normal before induction of labour; she was dilated 6 cm four hours previously and now is dilated 8 cm on vaginal examination. She has uterine contractions at a rate of two every 10 minutes. The CTG shows a baseline rate of 150 bpm, good variability and infrequent shallow variable deceleration.

What is the next most appropriate action?

A. Assess in 30 minutes without augmentation.
B. Assess in two hours without augmentation.
C. Assess in four hours without augmentation.
D. Start syntocinon and assess in two hours.
E. Start syntocinon and assess in four hours.

6.

A 32-year-old woman at 37 weeks in her first pregnancy is admitted for induction of labour as her baby has ultrasound-confirmed intrauterine growth restriction. In early labour, the CTG shows a baseline rate of 150 bpm, variability of 5 bpm, and infrequent variable decelerations, dropping from baseline by 60 bpm or less and taking 60 seconds to recover, recorded over the previous 45 minutes. She is contracting once every 10 minutes and the cervix is dilated 1 cm and 2 cm long.

What is the most appropriate next step?

A. Artificial rupture of membranes (ARM).
B. Artificial rupture of membranes and syntocinon augmentation.

C. Induction by prostaglandins in a vaginal pessary.
D. No action, but continue monitoring.
E. Perform an immediate Caesarean section.

7.

A woman in her first pregnancy, presents with decreased fetal movements for 24 hours. She is 34 weeks pregnant. A non-stress CTG shows the fetal heart rate is 180 bpm, variability is 3 bpm, and there have been unprovoked persistent decelerations for the last 20 minutes.

What is the most appropriate management option?

A. Admit her to the labour ward and repeat the CTG in an hour.
B. Category 1 Caesarean section.
C. Category 2 Caesarean section.
D. Induction of labour with prostaglandin.
E. Reassure and discharge her.

8.

A low-risk woman in her first pregnancy is in advanced labour. She is progressing well. One hour previously the cervix was dilated 7 cm and the head was at the spines. She has epidural analgesia for pain relief. The midwife is concerned about the CTG, and asks for your input.

The CTG shows a baseline rate of 155 bpm and has recorded a sinusoidal pattern for the last 30 minutes.

What is the most appropriate management option?

A. Category 1 Caesarean section.
B. Category 2 Caesarean section.
C. No action required.
D. Obtain a fetal blood sample.
E. Put the woman in a left lateral position.

9.

A 28-year-old nulliparous woman on the midwifery-led unit is in advanced labour. She has had an uncomplicated pregnancy. She has made acceptable progress in the first stage of labour. She is now contracting three times every 10 minutes, the cervix is fully dilated and the head is 1 cm above the ischial spines in occipitotransverse position. She has been in the second stage of labour for 30 minutes.

Which of the following management options would you recommend?

A. Category 1 Caesarean section.
B. Category 2 Caesarean section.
C. Instrumental delivery.
D. Conservative follow-up for the next 60 minutes.
E. Start syntocinon.

10.

A 34-year-old nulliparous woman in the second stage of labour has been pushing for the last two hours and is exhausted. The CTG is normal; the head is 1 cm above the ischial spines, in occipitoanterior position.

Which of the following would be the most appropriate action?

A. Emergency Caesarean section.
B. Increase syntocinon.
C. Perform fetal blood sampling.
D. Trial of forceps in theatre.
E. Trial of forceps in the delivery room.

11.

A 36-year-old nulliparous woman in the second stage of labour has been pushing for 30 minutes. The CTG shows a fetal heart rate of 170 bpm, reduced variability and late decelerations having occurred for the last 25 minutes. Vaginal examination shows the head to be at the ischial spines in occipitoposterior position.

Which of the following management options would be most appropriate?

A. Continue pushing for another 30 minutes.
B. Fetal blood sampling.
C. Category 1 emergency Caesarean section.
D. Start syntocinon infusion.
E. Trial of instrumental delivery in theatre.

12.

A 32-year-old primigravida is in labour at term. She was started on an oxytocin infusion four hours previously because of slow progress. There is clear liquor draining. The CTG shows five contractions every 10 minutes, a baseline rate of 155 bpm, variability of 5-10 bpm, early decelerations in more than 50% of the contractions, and occasional accelerations for the last 90 minutes. Vaginal examination shows the head to be 1 cm above the ischial spines, in a right occipitoposterior position, and the cervix is dilated 7 cm. She has progressed 3 cm over the last four hours.

Which of the following options would be most appropriate for her management?

A. Book for category 2 Caesarean section.
B. Fetal blood sampling.
C. Reassure and examine in four hours.
D. Reduce syntocinon.
E. Stop syntocinon.

13.

A 36-year-old woman with three previous Caesarean sections was booked for repeat elective Caesarean section at 39 weeks. She declined tubal ligation as she wishes to have more children.

What is her risk of placenta praevia in her next pregnancy?

A. 1.1%.
B. 2.8%.
C. 7.5%.
D. 11%.
E. 60%.

14.

A 27-year-old woman in her second pregnancy presents to the labour ward at 39 weeks' gestation with painful uterine contractions. Her first baby was delivered by emergency Caesarean section due to slow progress in labour three years previously. She is very keen to have a vaginal delivery. Your junior registrar asks you about the signs of uterine rupture.

Which of the following findings is the most common in women with uterine rupture during labour?

A. Abnormal CTG.
B. Acute onset of scar tenderness.
C. Cessation of previously efficient uterine contractions.
D. Haematuria.
E. Severe abdominal pain persisting between the contractions.

15.

A 23-year-old nulliparous woman has been pushing for two hours. The head is not palpable abdominally, the cervix is fully dilated, and on vaginal examination, the head is in right occipitoposterior position with minimal caput. The station is 1 cm below the ischial spine. The CTG is reassuring.

Which of the following management options would be the most appropriate?

A. Continue pushing for another 30 minutes.
B. Emergency Caesarean section.
C. Instrumental delivery in the delivery room.
D. Instrumental delivery in theatre.
E. Start syntocinon.

16.

You are teaching the ST 2 trainee the basic principles of forceps delivery.

Which type of episiotomy would be most appropriate to reduce the risk of severe perineal tear?

A. A mediolateral episiotomy with an angle of 60 degrees away from the midline.
B. A mediolateral episiotomy with an angle of 45 degrees away from the midline.
C. A mediolateral episiotomy with an angle of 30 degrees away from the midline.
D. A midline episiotomy.
E. A mediolateral episiotomy with an angle of 90 degrees away from the midline.

17.

A 32-year-old woman had a forceps delivery due to maternal exhaustion. All her observations are normal, and the placenta was delivered complete. Perineal examination revealed a torn external anal sphincter to about 80%. She was counselled, consented and taken to theatre for repair.

Which techniques do you recommend to accomplish the repair of the external anal sphincter?

A. End-to-end method using 3/0 PDS.
B. End-to-end method using 2/0 PDS.
C. End-to-end method using 3/0 vicryl.
D. Overlapping method using 2/0 vicryl.
E. Overlapping method using 3/0 PDS.

18.

A 32-year-old woman has a forceps delivery due to maternal exhaustion. All her observations are normal, and the placenta is delivered complete. Perineal examination revealed partial thickness torn external and internal anal sphincters. She was counselled, consented and taken to theatre for repair. The internal anal sphincter was identified separately when the patient was examined under anaesthesia.

Which techniques do you recommend to accomplish the repair of the anal sphincters?

A. Each sphincter should be repaired separately using the overlap method.
B. Each sphincter should be repaired separately using the end-to-end method.
C. Only the external anal sphincter should be repaired as the internal anal sphincter would heal concomitantly.
D. The two sphincters should be repaired jointly using the overlap method.
E. The internal sphincter should be repaired separately using the overlap method while the external sphincter should be repaired using the end-to-end method.

19.

A 30-year-old woman in her second pregnancy presents in the antenatal clinic at 28 weeks' gestation for counselling. Her first pregnancy ended in a spontaneous vaginal delivery at 41 weeks. This was complicated by a third degree tear, which was repaired in theatre.

She had mild incontinence of flatus during the first three months after delivery but recovered completely by the end of five months. She would like to know about the risk of faecal incontinence.

What is her risk of faecal incontinence if she has a normal vaginal delivery in this pregnancy without complications?

A. 10%.
B. 17%.
C. 30%.
D. 40%.
E. 50%.

20.

A 33-year-old woman in her second pregnancy presents to the labour ward at 39 weeks with painful uterine contractions every three minutes. Vaginal examination shows the cervix to be dilated 6 cm and effaced. The head is 3 cm above the ischial spines. The membranes are ruptured. You could easily feel the anterior fontanel and the supraorbital ridges. Fetal heart rate is normal. Her first pregnancy ended in a normal uncomplicated vaginal delivery.

Which of the following is the best management option?

A. Augmentation with oxytocin.
B. Category 1 Caesarean section.
C. Category 2 Caesarean section.
D. Reassess in two hours.
E. Reassess in four hours.

21.

A 24-year-old woman had a normal vaginal delivery 20 minutes previously; this was complicated by brisk postpartum haemorrhage. She lost 1500 mL blood and is responding to medical management but is still bleeding slightly. A decision is made to transfuse.

Which of the following should she receive?

A. Cytomegalovirus (CMV)-seronegative red cells and platelets.
B. CMV-seronegative whole blood and platelets.
C. Leucocyte-depleted red cells.
D. Platelet-depleted red cells.
E. Plasma-depleted red cells.

22.

You are called to assist in a case of massive obstetric haemorrhage. The patient is 60 kg and has already had six units of red cells.

Which of the following is the appropriate dose of fresh frozen plasma?

A. 700 mL.
B. 800 mL.
C. 950 mL.
D. 1100 mL.
E. 1500 mL.

23.

A patient in early labour enquires about the risk of accidental dural puncture if she has epidural analgesia.

What is the risk of dural puncture?

A. 0.5%–2.5%.
B. 6%–10%.
C. 11%–15%.
D. 16%–20%.
E. 21%–25%.

24.

As an ST 5 preparing for your completion of a certified training, you are asked to look into the department Caesarean section rate, compare it with other low-Caesarean section rate countries and propose some changes in the practices at your department. You find that the rate of vaginal birth after Caesarean section in your unit is 30%.

To how much should this practice be increased in order to reduce the overall Caesarean section rate substantially?

A. 40%–50%.
B. 50%–60%.
C. 70%–75%.
D. 80%.
E. 90%.

25.

As an ST 5 preparing for your completion of a certified training, you are asked to look into the department Caesarean section rate, compare it with other low-Caesarean section rate countries and propose some changes in the practices at your department. You find that the rate of vaginal delivery for breech presentation was very low at only 7%.

To how much should vaginal delivery for breech presentations be increased in order to reduce the overall Caesarean section rate substantially?

A. 9%.
B. 15%.
C. 17%.
D. 19%.
E. 21%.

ANSWERS

Q1: B. It is sensitive in detecting abnormalities in fetal heart pattern [evidence level 3].[1]

- Although cardiotocography (CTG) is sensitive in detecting abnormalities of fetal heart rate, its specificity for detection of fetal hypoxia remains low and therefore confirmatory tests such as fetal scalp blood sampling become necessary.
- Combination of abnormalities on the CTG (e.g. reduced variability, with fetal tachycardia, and late decelerations) may increase the specificity.

Q2: A. It will help reduce the incidence of neonatal seizures [evidence level 2+][2]

- In a review of studies including over 37 000 women, comparing intermittent auscultation with continuous CTG, there was no significant difference in cerebral palsy or perinatal death rate but there was halving of neonatal seizures in the continuous CTG arm of the study.
- In the CTG group, there was a significant increase in Caesarean sections and instrumental vaginal delivery.

Q3: C. Planning birth at home is associated with an overall small increase (0.4%) in the risk of a baby having a poor outcome.[1,3]

- In low-risk nulliparous women, planning to give birth in a midwifery-led unit (freestanding or alongside) has the lowest rate of intervention with no difference in the perinatal outcome for the baby if it is delivered in an obstetric unit.
- For multiparous women, the incidence of episiotomy, Caesarean section and instrumental birth is considerably reduced in home, freestanding or alongside midwifery-led units than in obstetric units.[1,3]

Q4: A. Admit to the antenatal ward [evidence level 3].[4]

- She is still in the latent phase of labour but the high head indicates high risk of cord prolapse.
- There is more than a 10-fold increase of perinatal mortality and morbidity if cord prolapse occurs outside the hospital [evidence level 3].[4]

Q5: B. Assess in two hours without augmentation.[1]

- She is dilated 8 cm and progressing well; there is no need for augmentation, but review in two hours.
- In normally progressing labour, do not perform amniotomy or combined early amniotomy with use of oxytocin routinely.[1]

Q6: A. Artificial rupture of membranes (ARM).

- The recorded variable deceleration indicates a non-reassuring trace with need for conservative measures.
- ARM allows checking liquor for blood or meconium and fetal blood sampling if required.
- Non-reassuring CTG is not enough to decide to book a Caesarean section.[1]

New NICE guidelines classifies CTG into four categories[1]
- Normal/reassuring.
- Non-reassuring and suggests the need for conservative measures.

- Abnormal and indicates the need for observation AND further testing.
- Abnormal and indicates the need for urgent intervention.

Q7: B. Category 1 Caesarean section.[5]

- We do not know for how long the CTG was abnormal, and she is complaining of diminished fetal movements with multiple CTG abnormalities.[5]
- Category 1 is urgent delivery when there is immediate threat to life of woman or fetus. The decision-to-delivery interval should not exceed 30 minutes.
- Category 2 is the need for early delivery when there is maternal or fetal compromise but no immediate threat to life of woman or fetus, e.g. failure to progress in labour.
- Category 3 is when there is no maternal or fetal compromise but early delivery is required, e.g. breech presentation in early labour.
- Category 4 is no compromise and Caesarean section is carried out at a time to suit the woman and maternity services.[5]

Q8: A. Category 1 Caesarean section.

- A sinusoidal trace is suspicious of fetal anaemia. Fetal blood sampling will not detect fetal anaemia, therefore category 1 Caesarean section is required.

Q9: E. Start syntocinon.[1]

- She has made slow progress as the head is still above the spines.
- The management of slow progress in the first or second stage of labour in low-risk women is augmentation.[1]

Q10: A. Emergency Caesarean section.[6]

- It is too dangerous to perform trial of instrumental delivery if the head is above the ischial spines.
- She is exhausted and has pushed for two hours, thus it is unlikely that there would be any further progress.[1,6]

Q11: B. Fetal blood sampling.[6]

- Trial of instrumental delivery should not be performed if there is an abnormal CTG, unless the fetal blood sampling result is normal.
- Normal fetal blood sampling result is reassuring. She can keep pushing or have a trial of instrumental delivery if the result is normal.
- However, even if the fetal blood sampling result is normal, an anticipated difficult instrumental delivery is best avoided.
- In an abnormal fetal blood sampling result, there is no place for a trial of instrumental delivery.

Q12: C. Reassure and examine in four hours.

- Early decelerations are normal during labour.
- A progress of 3 cm in four hours is acceptable.[1]

Q13: B. 2.8% [evidence level 2++].[7]

- A systematic review reported that women with one, two, three or more previous Caesarean deliveries experience a 1%, 1.7% or 2.8% risk, respectively.
- In women with placenta praevia and five or more prior Caesarean deliveries, the incidence of placenta accreta is up to 67%.[7]

Q14: A. Abnormal CTG.[8]

- Abnormal CTG is the most consistent finding in uterine rupture and is present in 66%–76% of cases.
- Over half of cases present with a combination of findings (most often abnormal CTG and abdominal pain).
- Scar rupture risk is 0.5%.[8]

Q15: D. Instrumental delivery in theatre.[6]

- She is station plus 1 cm (mid-cavity) and with occipitoposterior position. Instrumental delivery in theatre allows for immediate Caesarean section if it fails.
- **Low instrumental**: leading point of the skull (not caput) is at station plus 2 cm or more and not on the pelvic floor.
- **Mid-cavity instrumental**: fetal head is no more than one-fifth palpable per abdomen and the leading point of the skull is station zero or plus 1 cm.

Q16: A. A mediolateral episiotomy with an angle of 60 degrees away from the midline [evidence level 2−].[9]

Q17: A. End-to-end method using 3/0 PDS [evidence level 1++].[10]

- For repair of a full thickness external anal sphincter tear, either an overlapping or an end-to-end approximation method can be used with equivalent outcomes.
- For partial thickness (all 3a and some 3b) tears, use end-to-end technique.
- For anal sphincter injuries, either monofilament sutures such as 3-0 PDS or modern braided sutures such as 2-0 polyglactin can be used with equivalent results.

Q18: B. Each sphincter should be repaired separately using the end-to-end method [evidence level 1++].[9]

Q19: B. 17% [evidence level 4].[9]

- There are no systematic reviews or randomized controlled trials to suggest the best method of delivery following obstetrical anal sphincter injuries.
- The risk of sustaining a further third- or fourth-degree tear after a subsequent delivery is 5%–7%.
- There is a 17% risk of developing worsening faecal symptoms after a second vaginal delivery.[8]

Q20: D. Reassess in two hours.

- This is a brow presentation and in most cases the head either flexes back to vertex presentation or extends more to become a face presentation.
- Depending on what happens over the next two hours, you can decide your further management then.

Q21: C. Leucocyte-depleted red cells [evidence level 4].[11]

- Universal leucocyte depletion substantially reduces the risk of cytomegalovirus (CMV) transmission.
- In an emergency, standard leucocyte-depleted components should be given to avoid delay searching of CMV-negative blood.[11]
- If intraoperative cell saver is used in non-sensitised RhD-negative blood, and where the cord blood group is confirmed as RhD positive (or

unknown), a minimum dose of 1500 IU anti-D immunoglobulin should be administered.

- In the event of life-threatening haemorrhage, even if a woman has red blood cell antibodies, the transfusion of group O Rh-negative red cells or group-specific red cells must not be delayed.[11]

Q22: B. 800 mL.[11]

- Fresh frozen plasma at a dose of 12–15 mL/kg should be administered for every six units of red cells during major obstetric haemorrhage.[11]
- Cryoprecipitate at a standard dose of two five-unit pools should be administered early in major obstetric haemorrhage and subsequent cryoprecipitate transfusion should be guided by fibrinogen results, aiming to keep a fibrinogen level of more than 1.5 g/L.
- The subsequent fresh frozen plasma transfusion should be guided by the results of clotting tests if they are available in a timely manner, aiming to maintain prothrombin time and activated partial thromboplastin time ratios at less than one and a half times normal.
- The fibrinogen level should be maintained above 1.5 g/L.[11]

Q23: A. 0.5%–2.5%.[12]

- Epidural headache is usually in the fronto-occipital regions and radiates to the neck. It is characteristically worse on standing and typically develops 24–48 hours post-puncture.
- Conservative management includes hydration and simple analgesics.
- Untreated epidural puncture headache typically lasts for 7–10 days but can last up to 6 weeks.

Q24: C. 70%–75% [evidence level 2+].[13]

- In a cross-sectional study in a total of 685 452 births in The Netherlands from 2007 to 2010, the Caesarean section rate was one of the lowest worldwide at 15.6%.
- One of the main factors that contributed to this low rate was a high rate of 71% of vaginal births after a previous Caesarean section, of which 75% was a successful vaginal birth. This has eventually accounted for a low rate of repeat Caesarean sections.

Q25: E. 21% [evidence level 2+].[13]

- In this study in The Netherlands, the vaginal breech delivery rate was 21%, which has also contributed substantially towards the overall low Caesarean section rate.

References

1. National Institute for Health and Clinical Excellence. *Intrapartum Care for Healthy Women and Babies*. December, 2014. [https://www.nice.org.uk/guidance/cg190/resources/intrapartum-care]
2. Alfirevic Z, Devane D, Gyte GML. Continuous cardiotocography (CTG) as a form of electronic fetal monitoring (EFM) for fetal assessment during labour. *Cochrane Database Syst Rev* 2006;(3):CD006066.
3. National Perinatal Epidemiology Unit. *Birthplace in England Research Programme*. June, 2015. [https://www.npeu.ox.ac.uk/birthplace]

4. Royal College of Obstetricians and Gynaecologists. *Umbilical Cord Prolapse.* November, 2014. [https://www.rcog.org.uk/en/guidelines-research-services/guidelines/gtg50]

5. Lucas DN, Yentis SM, Kinsella SM, et al. Urgency of caesarean section: a new classification. *J R Soc Med* 2000;93:346–50.

6. Royal College of Obstetricians and Gynaecologists. *Operative Vaginal Delivery.* February, 2011. [https://www.rcog.org.uk/en/guidelines-research-services/guidelines/gtg26]

7. Royal College of Obstetricians and Gynaecologists. *Placenta Praevia, Placenta Praevia Accreta and Vasa Praevia, Diagnosis and Management.* January, 2011. [https://www.rcog.org.uk/en/guidelines-research-services/guidelines/gtg27]

8. Royal College of Obstetricians and Gynaecologists. *Birth After Previous Caesarean Birth.* October, 2015. [https://www.rcog.org.uk/en/guidelines-research-services/guidelines/gtg45]

9. Royal College of Obstetricians and Gynecologists. *Third- and Fourth-Degree Perineal Tears, Management.* June, 2015. [https://www.rcog.org.uk/en/guidelines-research-services/guidelines/gtg29]

10. Fernando RJ, Sultan AH, Kettle C, Thakar R. Methods of repair for obstetric anal sphincter injury. *Cochrane Database Syst Rev* 2013;(12):CD002866.

11. Royal College of Obstetricians and Gynaecologists. *Blood Transfusion in Obstetrics.* May, 2015. [https://www.rcog.org.uk/en/guidelines-research-services/guidelines/gtg47]

12. Revelle K, Morrish P. Headaches in pregnancy. *Obstet Gynaecol* 2014;16(3):179–84.

13. Zhang J, Geerts AC, Hukkel Hoven BC,et al. Caesarean section rates in subgroups of women and perinatal outcomes. *Brit J Obstet Gynaecol* 2016;123:754–61.

Chapter 5

Obstetric Emergencies

Ahmed Elbohoty

QUESTIONS

1.

A 31-year-old woman who was infertile for three years is now pregnant on in vitro fertilization (IVF).

What is the risk of occurrence of vasa praevia during the current pregnancy?

A. 1/100.
B. 1/300.
C. 1/600.
D. 1/1000.
E. 1/3000.

2.

A 35-year-old woman achieved her second pregnancy after IVF.

What is her increased risk of developing placenta praevia compared to her first naturally conceived pregnancy?

A. Two-fold.
B. Three-fold.
C. Five-fold.
D. Six-fold.
E. There is no increased risk.

3.

A 27-year-old Asian woman in her first pregnancy is known to have thalassemia major. She is 28 weeks pregnant. She comes to the emergency department with shortness of breath that has rapidly deteriorated. Despite resuscitation, she died within 20 minutes.

What is the most likely cause of death?

A. Amniotic fluid embolism.
B. Cardiac failure.
C. Eclampsia.
D. Placental abruption.
E. Pulmonary embolism.

4.

A 19-year-old woman in her first pregnancy presents to the emergency department with sudden breathlessness. On examination, her lips are swollen. Her pulse is 110 beats/minute (bpm) and her blood pressure (BP) is 100/60 mmHg. Chest examination shows generalized diminished air entry. She denies any medical history of any illnesses.

What would be the best immediate action?

A. 0.5 ml of 1:1000 adrenaline intramuscularly.
B. 0.5 ml of 1:1000 adrenaline intravenously.
C. 10 mg chlopheniramine intramuscularly.
D. 10 ml 10% calcium gluconate by slow intravenous injection.
E. 200 mg hydrocortisone intramuscularly.

5.

A 35-year-old primigravida pregnant at 32 weeks presents to the emergency department with severe vaginal bleeding. She collapses and is unresponsive. Cardiopulmonary resuscitation (CPR) has been started but there is no response for four minutes.

Which of the following is the most appropriate course of action?

A. Aggressive intravenous fluid and packed red blood cell transfusion.
B. Caesarean section immediately with no interruption to administer CPR.
C. Continue CPR and move rapidly to the operating theatre for category 1 Caesarean section.
D. Stop CPR and check for fetal life and, if it is found to be +ve, deliver immediately by category 1 Caesarean section.
E. Ultrasound scan to establish fetal well-being.

6.

A 24-year-old woman in her fifth pregnancy has delivered normally 20 minutes previously. She had active management of the third stage. The midwife noticed severe vaginal bleeding just after the placental birth and the uterus was lax. The blood loss was estimated as 1500 ml. After the emergency call, the anaesthetist arrived and is controlling her airway, has inserted two wide-bore cannulas, is running in crystalloid rapidly, and has requested cross-matched blood.

What is your next step?

A. Administer prostaglandin F2-alpha-intramyometrial.
B. Bimanual uterine massage.
C. Laparotomy and stepwise devascularization.
D. Laparotomy and hysterectomy.
E. Transfuse O-negative blood.

7.

A 33-year-old woman in her fifth pregnancy has just delivered a living baby of 4 kg by the midwife. Upon delivery of the placenta, there was excessive blood loss and the midwife feels a lump in the vagina. You arrived and diagnosed an acute uterine inversion. She is vitally stable and you are attempting to reverse the position of the uterus, but the cervix is tightly contracted, preventing the fundus of the uterus from being repositioned.

What is your next step?

A. Examination under anaesthesia and manual placental separation.
B. Examination under anaesthesia and hydrostatic replacement in theatre.
C. Laparotomy and supravaginal hysterectomy.
D. Laparotomy and Huntington's operation.
E. Laparotomy and Haultain's operation.

8.

A 33-year-old woman presents to the emergency department on day 5 after a Caesarean birth with a disturbed level of consciousness, pulse of 120 bpm, respiratory rate of 26/min and BP of 90/50 mmHg. There was no vaginal bleeding. On assessment, the multidisciplinary team decided to draw blood for cultures and lactate and start intra-venous antibiotic, intravenous fluids, and assisted ventilation.

What is the suitable level of care?

A. Level 1 care.
B. Level 2 care.
C. Level 3 care.
D. Level 4 care.
E. Level 5 care.

9.

A 25-year-old healthy woman has a normal labour and a spontaneous delivery of the fetal head. On expulsion of the head, the head remains tightly applied to the vulva. The midwife activated the emergency buzzer and declared that there is shoulder dystocia. You attended immediately.

How will you confirm your diagnosis?

A. Ask the woman to push.
B. Change the position of the woman to the all-four position.
C. Do a mild traction in an axial direction to confirm the diagnosis.
D. Do a mild traction in different directions.
E. Inform the consultant.

10.

A 24-year-old woman with three previous Caesarean deliveries comes to the antenatal clinic at 32 weeks' gestation with confirmed diagnosis of placenta praevia with no evidence of morbid adherence. However, the Doppler scan showed there is vasa praevia.

What is your plan of care?

A. Elective delivery by Caesarean section at 34 weeks with immediate umbilical cord clamping.
B. Elective delivery by Caesarean section at 35 weeks and defer umbilical cord clamping for one minute.
C. Elective delivery by Caesarean section at 37 weeks with immediate umbilical cord clamping.

D. Elective delivery by Caesarean section at 38 weeks and defer umbilical cord clamping for one minute.

E. Elective delivery by Caesarean section at 38 weeks with immediate umbilical cord clamping.

11.

A 24-year-old woman in her third pregnancy with two previous uneventful full-term vaginal deliveries presents to the emergency department at 37 weeks of gestation with nausea, occasional vomiting and a severe pain in the right iliac region. She is generally unwell. On examination she was normotensive at 100/50 mmHg, with a pulse of 100 bpm and a temperature of 37.8°C. Her abdomen showed localized rigidity and tenderness in the right iliac region. Ultrasound scan showed enlarged non-compressible appendix. The general surgeon decided to do an appendectomy and asks your advice regarding the need to deliver.

What will be your advice to him?

A. Caesarean section would be considered only if the appendix appeared inflamed.
B. Do appendectomy and wait for spontaneous onset of labour.
C. She should have a Caesarean section prior to the appendectomy.
D. She should have a Caesarean section after the appendectomy.
E. She should have a Caesarean section at the time of the appendectomy.

12.

You are an ST5 on call for the labour ward. You are asked to review a primigravid woman in induced labour at 41 weeks plus five days of gestation. She received epidural anaesthesia and she is free of pain. She is on an oxytocin drip at 10 mU/min. The woman has been in the active 2nd stage for two and a half hours. On abdominal examination, the head is 0/5 palpable per abdomen. Estimated fetal weight is 4 kg. Cardiotocography (CTG) is reassuring with five uterine contractions in the last 10 minutes, each lasted for 30–40 seconds. Vaginal examination shows left occipitotransverse position ++ station with diffuse caput ++ and molding ++. You decide to deliver by a Caesarean section.

What can you do to deliver the baby safely?

A. Deliver the fetal head with forceps.
B. Deliver the fetal head with ventouse.
C. Patwardhan technique.
D. Reverse breech extraction.
E. The fetal disimpaction system.

13.

A 32-year-old woman is on her third pregnancy with two previous uncomplicated vaginal deliveries. She presented in labour. She has a twin pregnancy and both babies are in a cephalic presentation. The pregnancy has been uncomplicated to date and both twins are above the 50th centile for growth with no discordant growth. The CTG has been normal throughout labour. The first twin is delivered uneventfully. The second twin is found to be transverse.

What would be the best immediate action?

A. Breech extraction.
B. Caesarean section.
C. External cephalic version.
D. Rupture of membranes and commence syntocinon.
E. Wait for another 30 minutes.

14.

A 38-year-old woman, on her third pregnancy, presents to the emergency department at 37 weeks of gestation with a stabbing pain in the epigastrium that radiates to the back and left arm.

What is the most relevant laboratory marker to be requested?

A. Alanine aminotransferase.
B. Creatinine kinase isoenzyme.
C. Creatine phosphokinase.
D. Myoglobin.
E. Tropinin I.

ANSWERS

Q1: B. 1/300 [evidence level 2−].[1]

- The reported incidence of vasa praevia is one in 2000 to one in 6000 pregnancies, but in in vitro fertilization (IVF) pregnancies it has been reported to be as high as one in 300.
- Other risk factors for vasa praevia include placental anomalies, such as a bilobed placenta or succenturiate lobe where the fetal vessels run through the membranes joining the separate lobes together, a history of low-lying placenta in the second trimester and multiple pregnancy.[1]

Q2: B. Three-fold [evidence level 2−].[1]

- Among mothers who had conceived after IVF, the risk of placenta praevia was nearly three-fold higher in this pregnancy compared to the previous naturally occurring pregnancies (adjusted odds ratio (OR) 2.9, 95% confidence interval (CI) 1.4–6.1).
- Among mothers who conceived by IVF who did not have a previous natural pregnancy, there was a six-fold higher risk compared to naturally conceived pregnancies (adjusted OR 5.6, 95% CI 4.4–7.0).

Q3: B. Cardiac failure [evidence level 3].[2]

Cardiac failure is the primary cause of death in over 50% of thalassemia cases.

- All women should be assessed by a cardiologist with expertise in thalassaemia and/or iron overload prior to embarking on a pregnancy.
- An echocardiogram and an electrocardiogram (ECG) should be performed as well as a T2* cardiac MRI.

Q4: A. 0.5 ml of 1:1000 adrenaline intramuscularly.[3]

- Anaphylaxis is a severe, life-threatening, generalized or systemic hypersensitivity reaction resulting in respiratory, cutaneous, and circulatory changes and, possibly, gastrointestinal disturbance and collapse. Its incidence varies between 3/1000 and 10/1000, with a mortality rate of around 1%.
- Anaphylaxis is likely when there is sudden onset and rapid progression of symptoms, life-threatening airway and/or breathing and/or circulation problems and skin and/or mucosal changes (flushing, urticaria, angio-oedema). Exposure to a known allergen supports the diagnosis but many cases occur with no previous history.
- The definitive treatment for anaphylaxis is 500 µg (0.5 ml) of 1:1000 adrenaline intramuscularly, which can be repeated after five minutes if there is no effect.

In experienced hands, it can be given intravenously as a 50 µg bolus (0.5 ml of 1:10 000 solution).

- Adjuvant therapy consists of chlopheniramine (10 mg) and hydrocortisone (200 mg) given intramuscularly or by slow intravenous injection.

Q5: B. Caesarean section immediately with no interruption to administer CPR [evidence level 4].[3,4]

- If there is no response to correctly performed CPR within four minutes of maternal collapse in women beyond 20 weeks of gestation, immediate delivery should be undertaken to assist maternal resuscitation.
- Delivery improves cardiac output beyond that achieved with closed chest compressions.
- Perimortem Caesarean section should be considered a resuscitative procedure to be performed primarily in the interests of maternal, not fetal, survival.

Q6: B. Bimanual uterine massage.[5]

- Uterine atony is the most common cause of primary postpartum haemorrhage (PPH). Simple mechanical and physiological measures of 'rubbing up the fundus', bimanual uterine compression and emptying the bladder to stimulate uterine contraction, represent time-honoured first-line management of PPH.[5]

Q7: B. Examination under anaesthesia and hydrostatic replacement in theatre.[6]

- Acute uterine inversion is a rare and unpredictable obstetric emergency. Once the diagnosis is made, manual uterine replacement should be attempted promptly.
- If it fails, she should be transferred to the operating room to exclude rupture of the uterus after which the hydrostatic method should be considered. Warm sterile water or isotonic sodium chloride solution is rapidly instilled into the vagina via a rubber tube or intravenous giving set, while the accoucheur's hand blocks the introitus.
- The fluid distends the vagina and pushes the fundus upwards into its natural position by hydrostatic pressure. The bag of fluid should be elevated approximately 100–150 cm above the level of the vagina to ensure sufficient pressure for insufflation. The problem with this method is the difficulty in maintaining a tight seal at the introitus. This can be overcome by the use of a silastic ventouse cup, although a hand may still be necessary to ensure a tight seal.

Q8: C. Level 3 care.[7]

- The level of care in the hospital can vary from 0 to 3.
- Level 0: hospital admission only.
- Level 1: a higher degree of observation or monitoring, special expertise or facility, downgrade from a higher level of care.
- Level 2: having an uncorrected major physiological abnormality or downgrade from level 3.
- Level 3: needing ventilation.

Q9: C. Do a mild traction in an axial direction to confirm the diagnosis [evidence level 3].[8]

- Shoulder dystocia is a challenging obstetric emergency; it needs a prompt recognition and timely management.

- Clinical signs include difficulty with delivery of the face and chin, the head remaining tightly applied to the vulva or even retracting (turtle-neck sign), failure of restitution of the fetal head, failure of the shoulders to descend.
- The confirmation of diagnosis needs traction in an axial direction; any other traction should be avoided.
- Routine traction is that traction required for delivery of the shoulders in a normal vaginal delivery where there is no difficulty with the shoulders.
- Axial traction is traction in line with the fetal spine, i.e. without lateral deviation.

Q10: C. Elective delivery by Caesarean section at 37 weeks with immediate umbilical cord clamping.[9]

- In the presence of confirmed vasa praevia, elective Caesarean section should be carried out between 35 and 37 weeks.
- The umbilical cord is clamped as soon as possible after delivery.

Q11: B. Do appendectomy and wait for spontaneous onset of labour [evidence level 3].[10]

- Caesarean section is not usually indicated at the time of appendectomy. Opening the uterus within an abdominal cavity affected by potential infection increases the risk of infection and adhesions, which may cause secondary problems with fertility.
- Caesarean section may be considered in some cases, e.g. critically ill woman or over 37 weeks if there is a concomitant obstetric indication for Caesarean section.

Q12: D. Reverse breech extraction [evidence level 2+].[11]

- The 'push' method or the fetal disimpaction system describes the woman being placed in the semi-lithotomy position and the fetal head being pushed up from the vagina by an assistant after incision of the uterus while the operating surgeon applies upward displacement of the fetal head.
- A recent systematic review showed that the reverse breech extraction (grasping one or both fetal feet at the fundus of the uterus and applying steady traction in the downward direction) carries a significantly lower risk of extension of the uterine incision compared to the push fetal disimpaction method. It is also associated with a lower risk of infection, a lower operative time, and less operative blood loss. In practice, it is best to use whatever the obstetrician has been accustomed to do.
- However, there is no difference in blood transfusion rate and neonatal outcome from the push disimpaction method. The operator is entitled to use either method according to his experience.
- In the second stage of labour after full dilatation, the deeply engaged head, along with a raised bladder and an elevated thinned out lower segment, are the main reasons for the increased difficulty and increased morbidity if Caesarean section is carried out after full dilatation.

Q13: C. External cephalic version.[12]

- After the delivery of the first twin, the lie and presentation of the second twin should be confirmed preferably with an ultrasound scan.
- When the second twin is transverse, the obstetrician may choose one of the three following options: external cephalic or internal podalic version of the second twin into a cephalic presentation or, rarely, resort to Caesarean section.

- The obstetrician should take the opportunity of the period of uterine quiescence after the birth of the first twin to accomplish the version.
- The reported success rate of external cephalic version varies from 60% to 80%. Once the version is successful, an oxytocin infusion may be started to promote engagement of the fetal head in the pelvis.
- There is a risk of cord prolapse and fetal well-being should be established throughout the procedure.
- Internal podalic version and breech extraction can be performed for the second twin, after a failed cephalic version attempt, if the obstetrician is experienced in vaginal breech delivery.

Indications for Caesarean section for the second twin
- If the second twin is significantly larger than the first.
- The attending obstetrician lacks the expertise to deal with the birth of a non-cephalic presentation of the second twin.
- Complications in the form of fetal distress, cord prolapse or abruption.
- If there is no progress after delivery of the first twin in spite of adequate uterine contractions.
- If external or internal podalic version fails.

Q14: E. Tropinin I.[13]

- Cardiac disease remains the largest single cause of indirect maternal deaths in 2011–2013.
- Diagnosis of acute myocardial infarction (AMI) in pregnancy may be difficult because of its low prevalence and consequent low index of suspicion. Two consecutive Maternal and Child Enquiries (CMACE) reports have shown a consistent failure to consider AMI as a cause of chest pain in women with risk factors.
- ECGs are classically the first-line test in making a diagnosis of AMI in any patient presenting with chest pain. The most sensitive and specific ECG marker is ST elevation, which normally appears within a few minutes of onset of symptoms.
- Cardiac-specific troponin I and troponin T are the specific biomarkers of choice for diagnosing myocardial infarction.
- In contrast, other cardiac markers – myoglobin, creatinine kinase, creatinine kinase isoenzyme – can be increased significantly in labour or Caesarean section.

References

1. Romundstad LB, Romundstad PR, Sunde A, et al. Increased risk of placenta previa in pregnancies following IVF/ICSI; a comparison of ART and non-ART pregnancies in the same mother. *Hum Reprod* 2006;21(9):2353–8.
2. Royal College of Obstetricians and Gynaecologists. *Thalassaemia in Pregnancy, Management of Beta.* March, 2014. [https://www.rcog.org.uk/en/guidelines-research-services/guidelines/gtg66]
3. Royal College of Obstetricians and Gynaecologists. *Maternal Collapse in Pregnancy and the Puerperium.* February, 2011. [https://www.rcog.org.uk/en/guidelines-research-services/guidelines/gtg56]
4. Elkady AA, Keith L, Sinha P. Peri-mortem caesarean section delivery: a literature review and comprehensive overview. *Enliven Gynecol Obstet* 2015;2(2):005.
5. Royal College of Obstetricians and Gynaecologists. *Postpartum Haemorrhage, Prevention and Management.* May, 2009. [https://www.rcog.org.uk/en/guidelines-research-services/guidelines/gtg52]

6. Bhalla R, Wuntakal R, Odijinmi F, Khan RU. Acute inversion of the uterus. *Obstet Gynaecol* 2009;11:13–18.]

7. National Institute for Health and Care Excellence. *Acutely Ill Patients in Hospital, Overview.* August, 2016. [https://pathways.nice.org.uk/pathways/acutely-ill-patients-in-hospital]

8. Royal College of Obstetricians and Gynaecologists. *Shoulder Dystocia.* March, 2012. [https://www.rcog.org.uk/en/guidelines-research-services/guidelines/gtg42]

9. Royal College of Obstetricians and Gynaecologists. *Antepartum Haemorrhage.* December, 2011. [https://www.rcog.org.uk/en/guidelines-research-services/guidelines/gtg63]

10. Weston P, Moroz P. Appendicitis in pregnancy; how to manage and whether to deliver. *Obstet Gynaecol* 2015;17:105–10.

11. Jeve YB, Navti OB, Konje JC. Comparison of techniques used to deliver a deeply impacted fetal head at full dilation: a systematic review and meta-analysis. *Brit J Obstet Gynaecol* 2016;123(3):337–45.

12. Webster SNE, Loughney AD. Internal podalic version with breech extraction. *Obstet Gynaecol* 2011;13:7–14.

13. Wuntakal R, Shetty N, Ioannou E, et al. Myocardial infarction and pregnancy. *Obstet Gynaecol* 2013;15:247–55.

Chapter 6

Obstetric Medicine

Alexandra Rees and Amy Shacaluga

QUESTIONS

1.

A 29-year-old primigravida in her first pregnancy attends the antenatal clinic at 32 weeks' gestation. She is fit and well with no comorbidities. She had a vasovagal fainting episode and underwent an electrocardiogram (ECG), which was normal.

Which of the following features would have prompted suspicion of an underlying abnormality?

A. Atrial ectopic beats.
B. Right shift in the QRS axis.
C. ST segment depression and T wave inversion in the inferior and lateral leads.
D. Small Q wave and inverted T wave in lead III.
E. Ventricular ectopics.

2.

A 34-year-old Pakistani woman in her third pregnancy attends the antenatal clinic at 36 weeks for a labour plan. She tells you she is on a beta-blocker as she suffered from rheumatic heart disease as a child.

Which of the following therapies should she avoid in the second stage of labour?

A. Intravenous benzylpenicillin.
B. Intravenous ergometrine.
C. Intravenous oxytocin.
D. Intramuscular oxytocin.
E. Intravenous sodium chloride with potassium chloride.

3.

37-year-old primigravida of African origin with a BMI of 38 kg/m^2 attends the emergency department with shortness of breath, oedema and tachycardia. She has no proteinuria but admits to a family history of hypertrophic cardiomyopathy. It becomes apparent she is hypertensive at 153/100 mmHg and needs treatment prior to investigations.

Which of the following antihypertensive would be most appropriate?

A. Amlodipine.
B. Hydralazine.
C. Labetalol.
D. Methyldopa.
E. Nifedipine.

4.

While on the delivery suite, you are called to the emergency department to assess a 30-week pregnant woman known to be a brittle asthmatic. She complains of shortness of breath, widespread wheeze and is tachycardic at 98 bpm. She takes salbutamol 100 mcg two puffs as required, a salmeterol/fluticasone 50/500 inhaler twice daily and theophylline 500 mg twice daily. On this admission, there is no evidence of pneumonia and her oxygen saturations are 98%.

How would you change her medication?

A. Continue the current treatment plan but tell her to rest.
B. Increase salmeterol/fluticasone to two puffs twice a day.
C. Salbutamol 2.5 mg nebulizer and prednisolone 20 mg orally for five days.
D. Salbutamol 2.5 mg nebulizer and prednisolone 40 mg orally for five days.
E. Salbutamol 5 mg nebulizer and prednisolone 40 mg orally for five days.

5.

A 24-year-old woman in her second pregnancy presents at 12 weeks' gestation with confirmed venous thromboembolism (VTE).

How would you advise her with regard to her treatment?

A. Commence warfarin for the initial three weeks then convert to low-molecular weight heparin (LMWH) until delivery.
B. Commence therapeutic LMWH for six weeks.
C. Commence therapeutic LMWH for one month in total then convert to a prophylactic dose.
D. Commence therapeutic LMWH for three to six months and then convert to a prophylactic dose.
E. Commence therapeutic LMWH for the entire pregnancy.

6.

A 29-year-old woman in her third pregnancy attends the obstetric day unit with persistent vomiting. She is known to have type 2 diabetes and does not recall how much insulin she is taking. On examination, she has a respiratory rate of 22/min, she is tachycardic (110 bpm) and appears dehydrated. She is apyrexial. You perform an arterial blood gas test.

Which of the following are you likely to find?

Answer	pH	pO$_2$ (mmHg)	pCO$_2$ (mmHg)	HCO$_3$ (mEq/L)
A	7.25	129	16	9
B	7.37	80	20	18
C	7.42	90	15	19
D	7.46	99	13	10
E	7.49	129	10	9

7.

A 20-year-old woman, a known epileptic, attends the medical antenatal clinic for preconceptual counselling. She has been seizure free for two years.

Which of the following medications would you advise her against because of the risk of congenital malformation?

A. Carbamazepine.
B. Levetiracetam.
C. Lamotrigine.
D. Phenytoin.
E. Sodium valproate.

8.

A 34-year-old woman presents to the obstetric unit via ambulance after collapsing in the supermarket. She has previously suffered two miscarriages and is 28 weeks pregnant. On examination, she appears confused and complains she is dizzy. You elicit a right-sided hemiparesis. She is apyrexial and all observations are stable.

What would be your first investigation of choice?

A. Computed tomography (CT).
B. Computed tomography venogram.
C. Full blood count and thrombophilia screen.
D. Lumbar puncture.
E. Magnetic resonance imaging (MRI).

9.

A 39-year-old woman presents with right upper quadrant pain and polydipsia in her third trimester. She appears jaundiced and tells you that she has been vomiting for two days. On examination, she has a BMI of 35 kg/m^2 and blood tests show a raised alanine transaminase with hyperuricemia. Her creatinine is normal and she shows a mild leucocytosis. Her BP is 149/100 mmHg and she has 3+ proteinuria.

Which of the following is most likely the cause of her clinical picture?

A. Acute fatty liver of pregnancy.
B. Diabetic ketoacidosis.
C. Hepatitis.
D. Obstetric cholestasis.
E. Pre-eclampsia.

10.

A 32-year-old diabetic woman had an instrumental delivery two hours previously. Antenatally she complained of severe lethargy but is found to have normal haemoglobin. You are called to see her as she has become confused and bradycardic. Her observations record a temperature of 35°C, heart rate of 45 bpm and oxygen saturations of 80% on air. Blood glucose level is 4 mmol/L, she is hyponatraemic and has decreased reflexes.

What will the patient need following initial supportive treatment?

A. Intravenous (IV) dextrose.
B. IV insulin.
C. IV labetalol.
D. IV levothyroxine.
E. IV phenylephrine.

11.

A primigravida in her second trimester attends your antenatal clinic complaining of palpitations and tremors. Her heart rate is 110 bpm. She is fit and well otherwise but explains she has lost a lot of weight and has been vomiting excessively in the mornings. Her mother suffers with arthritis but there is no other family history of note.

What is the most likely blood picture you will see?

Answer	TSH level (mIU/L)	Free tri-iodothyronine (pmol/L)	Free thyroxine (pmol/L)
A	0.5	8	<1
B	0.6	20	4
C	5	3	8
D	12	15	15
E	<1	32	20

12.

A 17-year-old primigravida attends the early pregnancy assessment unit at six weeks' gestation. She complains of a headache and blood-stained vomiting, stating she has been feeling awful for several days and 'unable to keep anything down'. Her boy-friend tells you she has not stopped vomiting.

Which of the following is likely to be the results of her arterial blood gas?

Answers	pH	pO$_2$ (mmHg)	pCO$_2$ (mmHg)	HCO$_3$ (mEq/L)
A	7.59	90	37	35
B	7.50	45	38	22
C	7.25	100	49	26
D	7.20	80	30	29
E	7.30	70	32	4

13.

Sickle cell disease (SCD) is the most common inherited condition worldwide.

The recommended daily dose of folic acid for pregnant women with SCD is:

A. 400 μg daily up to 12 weeks.
B. 400 μg daily throughout pregnancy.
C. 1 mg daily to 12 weeks.
D. 5 mg daily to 12 weeks.
E. 5 mg daily throughout pregnancy.

14.

A 26-year-old woman with SCD is admitted at 18 weeks with symptoms of chest pain, tachypnoea, cough and shortness of breath. Chest X-ray shows a new infiltrate throughout the lung fields.

What is the most likely diagnosis?

A. Acute chest syndrome.
B. Acute pulmonary embolus.
C. Dissecting aortic aneurysm.
D. Myocardial infarction.
E. Pneumonia.

15.

A 28-year-old woman with a BMI of 25 kg/m^2 books into the antenatal clinic at 12 weeks. Two years previously she had a confirmed unprovoked iliofemoral thrombosis in her left leg.

Your advice regarding thromboprophylaxis during this pregnancy is:

A. To use low-dose aspirin (LDA) throughout the pregnancy and for six weeks postpartum.
B. To use LMWH throughout the pregnancy and for six weeks postpartum.
C. To use LMWH from 28 weeks and for 10 weeks postpartum.
D. To use LDA and LMWH throughout the pregnancy and for six weeks postpartum.
E. To use LMWH only if other risk factors arise in pregnancy.

16.

A 28-year-old woman with a BMI of 25 kg/m^2 books into the antenatal clinic at 12 weeks. Two years previously she had a confirmed iliofemoral thrombosis in her left leg after major knee surgery.

Your advice regarding thromboprophylaxis should be:

A. To use LDA throughout the pregnancy and for six weeks postpartum.
B. To use LMWH throughout the pregnancy and for six weeks postpartum.
C. To use LMWH from 28 weeks and for 10 days postpartum.
D. To use LDA and LMWH throughout the pregnancy and for six weeks postpartum.
E. To use LMWH only if other risk factors arise in pregnancy.

17.

A 28-year-old woman with a BMI of 35 kg/m^2 presents to the antenatal clinic for a booking. She has confirmed anti-phospholipid syndrome (APLS). She has no previous history of venous thrombosis, but was tested after a stillbirth at term and was found to have a positive lupus anticoagulant test on two occasions, 12 weeks apart. She is a non-smoker.

She asks about the risk of venous thrombosis and the role of LMWH in her pregnancy.

You advise her that she should

A. Commence with LMWH as soon as possible and continue for six weeks postpartum.
B. Commence with LMWH at 28 weeks and for six weeks postpartum.
C. Have no increased risk of venous thrombosis and does not require routine treatment with LMWH.
D. Commence with LMWH at 28 weeks and continue until 10 days postpartum.
E. Only use LMWH if she has other risk factors.

18.

A pregnant woman attends antenatal clinic at 12 weeks. She has systemic lupus erythematosus (SLE). Her disease is well controlled and she has not had a flare for six months. She asks about her risk of a flare of SLE in pregnancy.

You tell her that

A. Pregnancy reduces the risk of a flare of her SLE.
B. She has a 5%–10% increased risk of a flare in pregnancy.
C. She has a 25%–60% increased risk of a flare in pregnancy.
D. She has a 60%–80% increased risk of a flare in pregnancy.
E. There is no increased risk above her background risk.

19.

A pregnant woman attends the antenatal clinic at 12 weeks. She has SLE. She is currently in remission. She asks about live birth rates in women with SLE.

You tell her that the chances of a live birth are

A. The same as in the general population.
B. 60%–70%.
C. 70%–80%.
D. 80%–90%.
E. 90%–100%.

20.

A primigravida who has anti-Ro antibodies attends antenatal clinic. She asks you about the risk of her baby having congenital heart block (CHB).

You tell her the risk is:

A. 2%.
B. 5%.
C. 10%.
D. 20%.
E. 50%.

21.

A 24-year-old primigravida with SLE asks about drug therapy in pregnancy as she is planning to become pregnant soon.

With regard to hydroxychloroquine therapy, you tell her that she should:

A. Continue therapy because of the beneficial effects of the drug on her SLE.
B. Stop the drug because of potential harmful effects to her pregnancy.
C. Stop the drug during pregnancy but can recommence it while breastfeeding.
D. Stop the drug during pregnancy and while breastfeeding.
E. That it is impossible to give her accurate advice as there is no clear evidence either way.

22.

A 24-year-old primigravida with SLE asks about drug therapy in pregnancy as she is planning to become pregnant soon.

With regard to non-steroidal anti-inflammatory drug (NSAID) therapy, you tell her that

A. They are safe throughout pregnancy.
B. They are safe only in the third trimester.
C. They are safe in the first and second trimester only.
D. They are not safe and should be avoided throughout pregnancy.
E. She should stop treatment pre-pregnancy and avoid them throughout pregnancy.

23.

A 26-year-old woman with rheumatoid arthritis (RA) attends antenatal clinic at 10 weeks. She is concerned about a flare up of her RA during pregnancy.

You tell her that during her pregnancy the risk of a disease flare up is:

A. Increased by 5%–10%.
B. Increased by 20%–60%.
C. Increased by 60%–80%.
D. Reduced.
E. The same as if she were not pregnant.

24.

A 26-year-old woman consults you because she is contemplating a pregnancy. She has RA and is taking methotrexate.

Your advice regarding methotrexate and pregnancy is:

A. To continue treatment as there is no known adverse effect.
B. To take the treatment up to 12 weeks and then discontinue.
C. To avoid treatment in the first trimester but to restart it after 12 weeks.
D. To stop treatment for at least three months prior to pregnancy and during pregnancy.
E. To stop treatment for at least six months prior to pregnancy and during pregnancy.

25.

A woman with RA has delivered normally one week previously and is now experiencing a flare of her disease. Her rheumatologist advises a course of prednisolone, starting at 20 mg twice daily. She is breastfeeding and is concerned about the risks to her baby.

With regard to steroid therapy and breastfeeding:

A. Any dose can be safely used and breastfeeding continued.
B. She should express and discard until she has reduced to a lower dose.
C. She should express and discard for four hours after taking the medication.
D. She should express and discard for eight hours after taking the medication.
E. She should avoid breastfeeding until she has stopped the prednisolone treatment.

ANSWERS

Q1: B. Right shift in the QRS axis.[1]

- It is normal to see a left shift in QRS axis but a right shift may indicate right ventricular hypertrophy as the right ventricle is enlarged and generates more electrical activity.[1]

Q2: B. Intravenous ergometrine.[2]

- Rheumatic endocarditis causes mitral stenosis in 75% of cases.
- Ergometrine causes rapid autotransfusion and can precipitate pulmonary oedema.

Q3: C. Labetalol.[2]

- Nifedipine should be avoided owing to vasodilation.
- Methyldopa will take a while to work.
- Amlodipine is not used as a first-line antihypertensive.
- Hydralazine promotes hyperdynamic circulation with adverse cardiac function.

Q4: D. Salbutamol 2.5 mg nebulizer and prednisolone 40 mg orally for five days [evidence level 1−].[3,4]

- No clinically significant difference is seen at the higher dose of 5 mg salbutamol.
- Doses lower than 40 mg prednisolone are not as effective.
- Owing to the small risk associated with oral corticosteroid and cleft lip and palate ($<0.3\%$ in the first trimester), 40 mg prednisolone should be for the shortest time (five days).[4]

Q5: D. Commence therapeutic LMWH for three to six months and then convert to a prophylactic dose.[5]

- Low-molecular weight heparin (LMWH) is the drug of choice; warfarin poses a teratogenic risk.
- She is at increased risk of further thromboembolism during the rest of her pregnancy and still requires a prophylactic dose following her treatment for current venous thromboembolism (VTE).[5]

Q6: A.[6]

Correct answer	pH	pO$_2$ (mmHg)	pCO$_2$ (mmHg)	HCO$_3$ (mEq/L)
A	7.25	129	16	9

- Diabetic ketoacidosis is characterized by hyperglycaemia (glucose >11 mmol/L), acidosis (venous pH <7.3 +/− venous bicarbonate <15 mmol/L) and ketonuria ($>3+$).[6]
- In this case the only acidotic picture is A; this coupled with a very low bicarbonate level gives the answer.

Q7: E. Sodium valproate.[7]

- Sodium valproate has been associated with an increased cognitive impairment in children aged three years when compared to those cases of women who took carbamazepine, lamotrigine or phenytoin. [7]
- Spina bifida is reported in 1%–2% of patients taking sodium valproate. Up to 10% of women taking sodium valproate had babies with congenital malformations. [7]

Q8: B. Computed tomography venogram.[8]

- A history of recurrent miscarriages should prompt you to think about thrombophilias, most likely causing a venous sinus thrombosis.
- CT venography does not suffer from the in-plane flow artefact that causes signal loss on 2D MRI with venography.
- Not all units will have access to an MRI and so MRI venogram was omitted from the answer options. This would be an equally valid option.
- Moving forwards, one should think about investigating for thrombophilias but this would not help the acute management picture in this instance.

Q9: A. Acute fatty liver of pregnancy.[9]

- Pre-eclampsia usually has an element of renal compromise if liver function tests are abnormal.
- Hypertension with no history of diabetes mellitus makes it unlikely to be diabetic ketoacidosis.
- Hepatitis does not cause hypertension.

Q10: D. IV levothyroxine.[6]

- This patient is likely to have myxoedema coma from undiagnosed hypothyroidism.[6]
- She is known to have diabetes and this could mean autoimmune hypothyroidism.

Q11: E.[6]

Correct answer	TSH level (mIU/L)	Free tri-iodothyronine (pmol/L)	Free thyroxine pmol/L
E	<1	32	20

- She is hyperthyroid.
- A family history of rheumatoid arthritis suggests an autoimmune propensity.

Q12: A.[6]

Answer	pH	pO_2 (mmHg)	pCO_2 (mmHg)	HCO_3 (mEq/L)
A	7.59	90	37	35

- This patient has hyperemesis and is losing stomach acid from vomiting.
- The pH is >7.45 making it alkalotic, as also reflected by the alkalotic HCO_3 >26.
- This is suggestive of a metabolic alkalosis. It is metabolic as the bicarbonate matches the pH.

Q13: E. 5 mg daily throughout pregnancy.[10]

- Pregnant women with sickle cell disease (SCD) should take folic acid through pregnancy (5 mg) and pre-conception (1 mg) to reduce the risk of neural tube defects.[10]

Q14: A. Acute chest syndrome.[10]

- Acute chest syndrome is the most common complication in women with SCD in pregnancy after acute pain.
- In 7%–20% of pregnant women, the signs and symptoms are the same as pneumonia and the two diagnoses should be considered simultaneously.[10]

Q15: B. To use LMWH throughout the pregnancy and for six weeks postpartum.[5]

- Any woman who has a previous unprovoked (or oestrogen-related) VTE should have LMWH throughout the pregnancy and for six weeks postpartum.[5]
- There is no role for low-dose aspirin (LDA) in this scenario in pregnancy.[5]

Q16: C. To use LMWH from 28 weeks and for 10 days postpartum.[5]

- In women where the previous VTE was related to major surgery and there are no other risk factors, thromboprophylaxis can be withheld until 28 weeks.[5]

Q17: B. Commence with LMWH at 28 weeks and for six weeks postpartum.[5]

- APLS is considered a risk factor for VTE in otherwise asymptomatic women. Women with three other risk factors for VTE should receive thromboprophylaxis throughout the antenatal period and for six weeks postpartum.
- Those with two risk factors (as in this question, i.e. previous stillbirth and raised BMI), should be offered VTE prevention from 28 weeks and for six weeks postpartum.[5]
- Those with one risk factor should be offered LMWH for 10 days postpartum.

Q18: C. She has a 25%–60% increased risk of a flare in pregnancy.[11]

- The risks of a flare are multifactorial depending on her disease state prior to pregnancy and medication.[11]
- Musculoskeletal flares are less common but renal and haematological flares more common.
- Active disease in the six months prior to pregnancy, discontinuation of anti-malarial medication and a history of lupus nephritis increase the risk.

Q19: D. 80%–90%.[11]

- Main issues with systemic lupus erythematosus (SLE) are the higher rate of fetal loss, pre-eclampsia, fetal growth restriction and neonatal lupus.[11]

Q20: A. 2% [evidence level 2+l].[12]

- Anti-Ro antibodies are anti-nuclear autoantibodies, and are associated with many autoimmune diseases, such as SLE and rheumatoid arthritis (RA).
- In pregnant women with SLE, having anti-Ro antibodies is a major aetiological factor of neonatal lupus. It is able to interrupt the atrioventricular conduction.
- Complete congenital heart block is the most severe manifestation of neonatal lupus syndrome and is associated with mortality of up to 30%.
- It causes irreversible damage to the fetal cardiac conducting system secondary to transplacental passage of maternal antibodies.

Q21: A. Continue therapy because of the beneficial effects of the drug on her SLE [evidence level 1−].[13]

- The benefits of hydroxychloroquine during pregnancy in women with SLE are reduction in flare and in neonatal CHB and neonatal lupus.

Q22: C. They are safe in the first and second trimester only.[13]

- NSAIDs are widely used by women with SLE and are considered safe in the first and second trimesters.
- They may result in premature closure of the ductus when used after 32 weeks.
- There is an increased risk to the fetal renal function if used after 20 weeks.

Q23: D. Reduced.[14]

- The reason for the reduced risk of flare ups in RA is unclear, but may be due to the effect of pregnancy on cell-mediated immunity, the elevated levels of anti-inflammatory cytokines and the effect of hormonal changes in pregnancy such as increases in oestrogen and cortisol.[14]

Q24: D. To stop treatment for at least three months prior to pregnancy and during pregnancy.[15]

- Methotrexate is a folate antagonist and should be stopped in pregnancy.
- It is an abortifacient and is associated with congenital anomalies.
- Because its active metabolites have a long half-life, it must be stopped at least three months before conception.

Q25: C. She should express and discard for four hours after taking the medication.[16]

- Prednisolone can be safely used while breastfeeding but only in smaller doses as about 5% crosses into breast milk.
- At a dose above 20 mg twice daily, the milk should be discarded for four hours following the dose as it minimizes any effects on the fetus.
- Hydroxychloroquine can be used to treat RA in pregnancy. Its use appears to be safe during pregnancy and while breastfeeding.

References

1. Tomlinson MW. Rheumatic heart disease. In: James, DK, Steer, PJ, Weiner, CP, et al., eds. *High Risk Pregnancy*, 4th edn. St Louis, MO: Elsevier, 2011; p. 624.
2. National institute of Clinical Excellence Guidelines. *Hypertension in Pregnancy, Diagnosis and Management.* August, 2010. [https://www.nice.org.uk/guidance/cg107]
3. British Thoracic Society. *British Guideline on the Management of Asthma.* October, 2014. [https://www.brit-thoracic.org.uk/document-library/clinical-information/asthma/btssign-asthma-guideline-2014]
4. Park-Whyllie L, Mazotti P, Pastuszak A, et al. Birth defects after maternal exposure to corticosteroids. Prospective cohort study and meta analysis of epidemiological studies. *Teratology* 2000;62:385–92.
5. Royal College of Obstetricians and Gynaecologists. *Thrombosis and Embolism During Pregnancy and the Puerperium, Reducing the Risk.* April, 2015. [https://www.rcog.org.uk/en/guidelines-research-services/guidelines/gtg37a]
6. Turner H, Wass J, eds. Endocrine disorders of pregnancy. *Oxford Handbook of Endocrinology and Diabetes.* Oxford, UK: Oxford University Press, 2009; Pt. 5.
7. Royal College of Obstetricians and Gynaecologists. *Epilepsy in Pregnancy.* June, 2016. [https://www.rcog.org.uk/en/guidelines-research-services/guidelines/gtg68]
8. Fujii Y, Tasaki O, Yoshiya K, et al. Evaluation of posttraumatic venous sinus occlusion with CT venography. *J Trauma* 2009;66(4):1002–6; discussion 1006–7.

9. Cammu H. Idiopathic acute fatty liver of pregnancy associated with diabetes insipidus. *Brit J Obstet Gynaecol* 1987;94:173–8.
10. Royal College of Obstetricians and Gynaecologists. *Sickle Cell Disease in Pregnancy, Management.* August, 2011. [https://www.rcog.org.uk/en/guidelines-research-services/guidelines/gtg61]
11. Lateef A, Petri M. Managing lupus patients in pregnancy. *Best Pract Res Clin Rheumatol* 2013;27(3):435–47.
12. Brucato A, Doria A, Frassi M, et al. Pregnancy outcome in 100 women with Ro/SSA antibodies: a prospective case controlled study. *Lupus* 2002;11(11):716–21.
13. Sperber K, Hom C, Chao CP, Shapiro D, Ash J. Systemic review of hydroxychloroquine use in pregnancy patients with autoimmune disease. *Pediatr Rheumatol Online J* 2009;7:9.
14. Barrett JH, Brennan P, Fiddler M, Silman AJ. Does rheumatoid arthritis remit during pregnancy and relapse postpartum? Results from a nationwide study in the United Kingdom performed prospectively from late pregnancy. *Arthritis Rheum* 1999;42(6):1219–27.
15. Temprano KK, Bandlamudi R, Moore TL. Anti-rheumatic drugs in pregnancy and lactation. *Semin Arthritis Rheum* 2005;35(2):112–21.
16. Ost L, Wettrell G, Björkhem I, Rane A. Prednisolone excretion in human milk. *J Pediatr* 1985;106(6):1008–11.

Chapter 7

Saving Mothers' Lives

Roshni R Patel

QUESTIONS

1.

You are teaching students regarding maternal death.

The World Health Organization (WHO) defines indirect maternal death as that resulting from:

A. New disease developed during the pregnancy and not the result of direct obstetric causes but aggravated by the physiological effects of pregnancy.
B. Previous existing disease only and not the result of direct obstetric causes but aggravated by the physiological effects of pregnancy.
C. Previous existing disease or developed during the pregnancy and further complicated by direct obstetric labour complications.
D. Previous existing disease or developed during the pregnancy and not the result of direct obstetric causes but aggravated by the physiological effects of pregnancy.
E. Previous existing disease or developed during the pregnancy and which occur in the puerperium.

2.

You have read the recent MBRRACE UK 2012–2014 report, *Mothers and Babies: Reducing Risk.*

What is the leading cause of late maternal death in that report?

A. Cardiac disease.
B. Haemorrhage.
C. Malignancy.
D. Psychiatric causes.
E. Thrombosis and thromboembolism.

3.

In the 2016 MBRRACE-UK report into maternal deaths, in the years 2009–2014, 191 women died before completion of 24 weeks.

What was the percentage of deaths due to ectopic pregnancy?

A. 2%.
B. 3.2%.
C. 4.8%.
D. 6.4%.
E. 7.4%.

4.

With regard to the MBRRACE-UK report:

Which statement is true regarding the trends in incidence of direct maternal deaths?

A. Direct maternal deaths have not fallen as expected.
B. Direct maternal deaths have fallen every year since 2004.
C. Direct maternal deaths have fallen every year since 1985.
D. Direct maternal deaths have fallen every three years since 1980.
E. Direct maternal deaths were more common than indirect deaths in 2012–2013.

5.

You have been fast bleeped to the accident and emergency department to attend to a woman who is 28 weeks pregnant and has just had a cardiac arrest. She requires a perimortem Caesarean section.

What is the most essential piece of equipment to start this surgery?

A. Cord clamps.
B. Cutting diathermy.
C. Doyen retractor.
D. Scalpel.
E. Suction.

6.

A 33-year-old woman who is 33 weeks pregnant was involved in a road traffic accident. She is cardiovascularly stable, her blood clotting profile is normal and there is no fetal distress but she has a pelvic fracture and needs a Caesarean section in the operating theatre.

Why is regional anaesthesia preferable over general anaesthesia?

A. Altered maternal physiology in relation to pregnancy.
B. Greater maternal satisfaction with faster skin-to-skin contact to promote breastfeeding.
C. Lower transfer of anaesthetic drugs to the fetus.
D. Lower risk of maternal hypoxaemic events.
E. Superior analgesic effect.

7.

You are teaching student midwives on the topic of maternal mortality.

What is your explanation for the most likely cause of maternal deaths secondary to anaesthesia?

A. Anaphylaxis to anaesthetic drugs.
B. Failure to secure adequate airway with general anaesthesia.
C. Local anaesthetic toxicity.
D. Sepsis secondary to epidural abscess.
E. Underestimation of maternal blood loss.

8.

You have just reviewed the MBRRACE-UK 2012–2014 report.

What is the rate of amniotic fluid embolism?

A. 0.68/100 000.
B. 0.87/100 000.
C. 0.97/100 000.
D. 1/100 000.
E. 1.02/100 000.

9.

Which obstetric intervention is most strongly associated with amniotic fluid embolism?

A. External cephalic version.
B. Fetal blood sampling.
C. Induction of labour.
D. Manual removal of placenta.
E. Vacuum-assisted vaginal delivery.

10.

A pregnant woman sees her general practitioner with a sore throat and palpable lymph nodes in her neck. One day later she attends the emergency department with severe diarrhoea and vomiting and feeling very unwell. While there she becomes hypotensive, tachycardic and then collapses.

What is the most likely diagnosis?

A. Amniotic fluid embolism.
B. Acute myocardial infarction.
C. Group A streptococcal sepsis.
D. Influenza B infection.
E. Pulmonary embolism.

11.

You are asked to review a severely ill woman who is 35 weeks pregnant. Her pulse is 102 bpm. You suspect systemic inflammatory response (SIRS).

What other finding is the most strongly associated diagnostic feature?

A. Blood glucose over 9.7 mmol/L in the absence of known diabetes.
B. New onset confusion or altered mental state.
C. Respiratory rate >30/min.
D. Temperature <35.0°C.
E. Temperature >39.8°C.

12.

A woman with a BMI of 37 kg/m^2 and asthma had an elective Caesarean section for breech at term with blood loss of 1300 ml. She was discharged home three days later. One week later, she became acutely short of breath and collapsed.

What is the most likely diagnosis?

A. Acute asthma.
B. Congestive cardiac failure.
C. Fulminating sepsis.
D. Pulmonary embolism.
E. Supra-ventricular tachycardia.

13.

You are called urgently to see a collapsed woman in room 4 on the labour ward. She has just had a prolonged labour and instrumental delivery. The midwife says the woman complained of slight headache, became short of breath and then said she had chest pain before she collapsed.

Which of these symptoms is not suggestive of a pulmonary embolism?

A. Chest pain.
B. Dizziness.
C. Headache.
D. Sudden onset breathlessness.
E. Tachycardia.

14.

A fit, 39-year-old, 18-week pregnant woman presented with non-specific abdominal pain, left-sided leg pain and oedema to the emergency department following a recent safari holiday in Africa. Doppler ultrasound scan of the leg is normal.

What is the most likely diagnosis?

A. Acute arterial embolus.
B. Deep vein thrombosis.
C. Musculoskeletal injury.
D. Ovarian mass.
E. Symphysiopelvic dysfunction.

15.

You have just briefed your juniors of the WHO maternal mortality reports.

What is the leading cause of maternal mortality worldwide?

A. Amniotic fluid embolism.
B. Haemorrhage.
C. Sepsis.
D. Thromboembolism.
E. Uterine rupture.

16.

Haemoglobin levels are tested in the UK at booking. If the level is below the normal range, the woman should be investigated further.

The abnormal range is less than:

A. 90 g/L.
B. 95 g/L.
C. 100 g/L.
D. 110 g/L.
E. 115 g/L.

17.

A woman has a postpartum haemorrhage following a forceps delivery. Uterotonics (syntocinon, intramuscular syntometrine and oral misoprostol) have been used but uterine atony remains. An intrauterine balloon tamponade is inserted but the post-partum haemorrhage continues. The estimated blood loss is 2100 ml.

What is the next management step?

A. IV ergometrine.
B. Laparotomy.
C. Misoprostol rectally.
D. Recombinant factor VIII.
E. Transfusion of packed cells.

18.

A 31-year-old woman who is 33 weeks pregnant presented with acute weight loss and fatigue in pregnancy. A malignancy is suspected but the primary is not identified. A category 3 Caesarean section for maternal deterioration is performed. The placenta is sent for histology as it looks and feels abnormal.

Which malignancy is most likely to show metastatic involvement of the placenta?

A. Acute myeloid leukaemia.
B. Breast carcinoma.
C. Gastric carcinoma.
D. Hodgkin's lymphoma.
E. Malignant melanoma.

19.

In the 2016 report, case notes were available for in-depth review of the care offered in 183 deaths.

What is the percentage of women in whom improvements to care may have made a difference to the outcome?

A. 40%.
B. 42%.
C. 46%.
D. 51%.
E. 53%.

20.

You are following up a 22-week pregnant woman in the antenatal clinic. Her epileptic fits are well controlled on medications.

What is the most common cause of maternal death secondary to epilepsy?

A. Accident.
B. Antiepileptic drug toxicity.
C. Aspiration secondary to seizure.
D. Head injury secondary to trauma.
E. Sudden unexpected death in pregnancy (SUDEP).

21.

Women who are victims of domestic abuse are more likely to suffer obstetric complications.

Which one of the following is not associated with domestic violence?

A. Antepartum haemorrhage.
B. Low-birthweight infant.
C. Preterm labour.
D. Pregnancy-induced hypertension.
E. Stillbirth.

22.

A general practitioner calls you about a postnatal woman who delivered two weeks previously. He thinks she should be admitted to a mother-and-baby psychiatric unit and gives you a full history.

Which of these reasons is not an indication for admission?

A. Beliefs of inadequacy as a mother.
B. Evidence of psychosis.
C. Persistent insomnia over three nights.
D. Pervasive guilt or hopelessness.
E. Suicidal ideation.

23.

What is the most common respiratory cause of maternal death in the UK in the three MBRRACE-UK reports?

A. Asthma.
B. Bronchiectasis.
C. Cystic fibrosis.
D. Pulmonary hypotension.
E. Tuberculosis.

24.

You are reviewing a woman who is 16 weeks pregnant and has asthma. Her antenatal care has been uneventful to date but she had an exacerbation of her asthma with the recent cold weather, which has now improved.

What is your immediate advice?

A. Ensure she has the seasonal influenza vaccine.
B. Offer the measles, mumps and rubella (MMR) vaccination.
C. Not to use Entonox in labour.
D. Replace her asthma inhalers with oral bronchodilators.
E. Should be closely managed by her general practitioner and midwife.

25.

You are reviewing a 23-year-old pregnant woman with long-standing type 1 diabetes in the combined pregnancy diabetic clinic. She has good control of her blood sugar levels.

Which of these complications most increases her risk of dying during this pregnancy?

A. Hypoglycaemia.
B. Infection.
C. Ketoacidosis.
D. Nephropathy.
E. Ulceration.

26.

What is the most common cardiac cause of late maternal death in the UK in the latest MBRRACE-UK report?

A. Acute myocardial infarction.
B. Aortic dissection.
C. Cardiomyopathy.
D. Mitral valve thrombosis.
E. Sudden arrhythmic cardiac deaths with a morphologically normal heart.

27.

A previously well 37-year-old patient with a metal mitral valve who is anti-coagulated, presents at 15 weeks' gestation on a cold day with an acute onset cough and frothy pink sputum. She becomes more short of breath and deteriorates very rapidly and has a cardiac arrest.

At postmortem, what is the most likely cause of death?

A. Acute asthma attack.
B. Acute myocardial infarction.
C. Cardiac tamponade.
D. Pulmonary embolism.
E. Heart failure.

28.

A previously well 26-year-old UK-born woman presents to her antenatal clinic at 18 weeks' gestation with a history of palpitations in recent weeks.

What is the most likely diagnosis?

A. Anxiety disorder.
B. Ectopic cardiac beats.
C. Previous rheumatic fever.
D. Supra-ventricular tachycardia.
E. Thyrotoxicosis.

29.

A 31-year-old smoker with no medical history comes for booking in the antenatal clinic and a systolic murmur is heard.

What is the most likely diagnosis?

A. Aortic stenosis.
B. Flow murmur of pregnancy.
C. Mitral valve prolapse.
D. Rheumatic fever.
E. Undiagnosed congenital cardiac disease.

30.

A 34-year-old woman who books in her pregnancy gives a history of her mother dying of a heart attack at 39 years old and her maternal grandfather dying of a heart attack at 38 years old. Her 27-year-old brother recently had a cardiac arrest while playing football, but survived after resuscitation.

What is the most likely condition, which increases her high risk of dying?

A. Congenital cardiac disease.
B. Clotting disorder.
C. Hypercholesterolemia.
D. Inherited cardiomyopathy.
E. Wolf–Parkinson–White syndrome.

31.

What is the difference in death rates reported in the UK confidential enquiry into maternal deaths for the years 2011–2013 compared to the previous 2010–2012 report?

A. There was a decrease from 11.3 deaths per 100 000 maternities to 9.02 deaths per 100 000 maternities.
B. There was no difference in the death rate.
C. The death rate remained stable at 10/100 000 maternities.
D. The death rate increased from 10.2/100 000 maternities in the 2010–1012 report to 10.6/100 000 maternities in the 2011–2013 report.
E. There was a reduction from 10.12 to 9.02 deaths per 100 000 maternities.

32.

In the 2012–2014 confidential enquiry report, what was the rate of the most common cause of death?

A. Amniotic fluid embolism at a rate of 4.9/100 000 maternities.
B. Cardiac disease at a rate of 2.18/100 000 maternities.
C. Haemorrhage at a rate of 3.10/100 000 maternities.
D. Neurological causes at a rate of 2.01/100 000 maternities.
E. Psychological causes at a rate of 2.08/100 000 maternities.

33.

A 33-year-old woman comes to the antenatal booking clinic. She is 14 weeks pregnant. On checking on her mental health, you find she had a previous mental health problem. She has improved and is not currently under any treatment.

What is the highest risk time for a recurrent episode?

A. At 20 weeks pregnancy when she feels the fetal movement.
B. If she has a threatened miscarriage.
C. In the immediate postpartum period.
D. If she is told that she has a condition which will require Caesarean section delivery.
E. If she develops a viral infection.

34.

The midwife in the postnatal ward calls you to review a woman who is doubtful about her competence as a mother and is not sure she will be able to look after her baby. She has no history of any past illnesses or any special medications.

How will you deal with the situation?

A. Assure her that all is well and she should not consider these thoughts any more.
B. Arrange for urgent senior psychiatric assessment.
C. Do not discharge and keep in the ward for a week under close observation.
D. Discharge her with a letter to the general practitioner.
E. Discharge with a recommendation she should be seen by the community mid-wife after 24 hours.

ANSWERS

Q1: D. Previous existing disease or developed during the pregnancy and not the result of direct obstetric causes but aggravated by the physiological effects of pregnancy [evidence level 4].[1]

- Coincidental deaths can be due to any unrelated cause.
- Direct deaths include those that result from interventions, omissions or incorrect treatment.
- Late deaths are those occurring between 42 days and 1 year postpartum.

Q2: C. Malignancy [evidence level 2+].[2]

- In the 2016 report, there were 23% coincidental malignancies. However, these are separate from 'indirect malignancies', which also contributed a further 8% of deaths.
- In the 2012–2014 report, 15% of women who died between six weeks and one year after the end of pregnancy, died from psychiatric disorders.[2]
- Cardiac disease is a leading cause of indirect maternal death.

Q3: C. 4.8% [evidence level 2+].[2]

- The prevalence of ectopic pregnancy among women who attend the emergency department is 6–16.
- In 98% of these women, the pregnancy is located in the Fallopian tube, with the remainder distributed variously in the ovary, cervix or structures within the abdomen.

Q4: B. Direct maternal deaths have fallen every year since 2004 [evidence level 2+].[2]

- Since 1985, maternal deaths increased slightly in 1988, then fell and increased again in the 1994–1996 and 2003–2005 reports.
- There is a higher rate of indirect deaths compared to direct deaths since 1994.

Q5: D. Scalpel.[3,4]

- The only essential equipment to start a perimortem section is a mounted scalpel.[2-4] This should ideally be pre-mounted and be on the resuscitation trolley.
- Cord clamps should be available, but can be replaced with suture material if cord clamps are not available.[3]
- There may not be time for anaesthesia.
- There will be minimal bleeding, as the patient does not have a circulation.

Q6: D. Lower risk of maternal hypoxaemic events [evidence level 1−].[5]

- All of the other options are correct but the main reason for regional anaesthesia is to minimize the risk of maternal hypoxaemic events, which occur more frequently with general anaesthesia and are more commonly associated with maternal death.[5]

Q7: B. Failure to secure adequate airway with general anaesthesia [evidence level 2++].[1]

- The main risk associated is of failed intubation with general anaesthesia, although the other causes listed can also cause maternal death.[5]

Q8: A. 0.68/100 000. [evidence level 2+].[6]

Q9: C. Induction of labour [evidence level 2−].[6,7]

Q10: C. Group A streptococcal sepsis [evidence level 3].[3]

- This combination of symptoms and signs is associated with sepsis.
- The most likely diagnosis is Group A streptococcus, which often presents with a sore throat/urinary tract infection.

Q11: B. New onset confusion or altered mental state [evidence level 4].[8]

- Systemic inflammatory response syndrome (SIRS) is an inflammatory state affecting the whole body, frequently a response of the immune system to infection, trauma, pancreatitis and surgery.[8]
- SIRS can compromise the function of various organs and systems resulting in multiple organ dysfunction.
- Sepsis can be defined as the presence of infection together with SIRS.
- Other criteria for SIRS: temperature $<36°C$ or $>38.3°C$, respiratory rate >20/min, blood glucose over 7.7 mmol/L in the absence of known diabetes, white cell count $>12x10^9$/L or $<4x10^9$/L.

Q12: D. Pulmonary embolism [evidence level 2+].[2,3]

- Risk factors for pulmonary embolism include elevated BMI, operative delivery, postpartum haemorrhage, postsurgical immobility.[2]
- The majority of pulmonary emboli occur in the first six weeks postnatally.

Q13: C. Headache [evidence level 4].[2,3]

- Chest pain, collapse, syncope, dizziness, hypoxia, tachycardia and sudden onset breathlessness are typically associated with pulmonary embolism.[2]
- Headache is not typically associated with pulmonary embolism but is related to cerebral vein thrombosis.

Q14: B. Deep vein thrombosis [evidence level 2−].[9]

- She has several risk factors for venous thromboembolism (age, pregnancy, air travel).[1]
- Deep vein thrombosis cannot be excluded by the presence of a negative Doppler scan if strong clinical suspicion remains.[2]
- Typical symptoms include redness, oedema, leg pain, non-specific abdominal/groin/buttock pain.[2]
- Dimer testing is sensitive but not specific for diagnosing deep venous thrombosis. It is not always reliable. It is of more value if it is negative.
- If the D-dimer test is negative, it rules out the possibility of deep venous thrombosis in up to 97% of cases.[9,10]

Q15: B. Haemorrhage [evidence level 2++].

- Obstetric haemorrhage is the leading cause of maternal death worldwide, accounting for up to 50% of deaths in some countries.[2]
- It accounts for 10% of all maternal direct deaths in the UK.

Q16: D. 110 g/L [evidence level 2+].[11]

- Haemoglobin <110 g/L at booking in the UK should be investigated.[11,]
- Anaemia is defined as haemoglobin <110 g/L during the first trimester, <105 g/L during the second trimester and <105 g/L in the third trimester/postpartum.

Q17: B. Laparotomy [evidence level 2++].[12]

- If pharmacological interventions fail to control the haemorrhage and there is a negative test to balloon tamponade, the next step must be to proceed to laparotomy.[12]

Q18: E. Malignant melanoma [evidence level 2++].[13]

- Malignant melanoma is most likely to metastasize to the placenta although other malignancies can also do this.[13]
- Transplacental spread is very rare but most cases are due to malignant melanoma.

Q19: B. 42% [evidence level 3].[2]

- The standard of care is determined following thorough review of the case notes by independent MBRRACE assessors across a range of specialties. The cases are then further reviewed by another team before individual chapters are written for the report and includes an assessment on the standard of care.
- The percentage of women in whom improvement of care would not have had an effect was 12%.
- However, the percentage of women who died in spite of good care was 46%.

Q20: E. Sudden unexpected death in pregnancy (SUDEP) [evidence level 2+].[14]

- SUDEP remains the major cause of maternal death among women with epilepsy.[14]
- At booking, women with epilepsy should be seen in a pregnancy multidisciplinary specialist clinic [evidence level 4].
- Women with epilepsy should continue their medication until advised otherwise by a specialist.[15]
- There is no indication for early induction due to the epilepsy.
- Women should not be managed in single rooms because of the risk of fitting.[14]

Q21: D. Pregnancy-induced hypertension [evidence level 2−].[2,5]

- The other four complications are associated with domestic violence.[2]

Q22: C. Persistent insomnia over three nights [evidence level 2−].

- The other symptoms (and also rapidly changing mental health) should lead to considering a mother-and-baby unit admission.[5]

Q23: A. Asthma [evidence level 2+].[5]

- Asthma has remained the most common respiratory cause of maternal death in the last three MBRRACE UK reports.[5]

Q24: A. Ensure she has the seasonal influenza vaccine [evidence level 3].[5]

Q25: A. Hypoglycaemia [evidence level 4].

- The patient and family needs education regarding hypoglycaemia because of the increased risk and how to manage it.
- In the MBRRACE-UK 2014 report, women with long-standing diabetes mellitus were noted to be more at risk of severe hypoglycaemia.[5]

Q26: E. Sudden arrhythmic cardiac deaths with a morphologically normal heart [SADS/MNH].[2]

- Cardiovascular disease was the leading cause of maternal death in the UK (over a quarter of women who died during pregnancy or up to 6 weeks after pregnancy).
- SADS/MNH was the cause of death in 38% of cardiac deaths.
- All women dying from sudden cardiac arrest with a morphologically normal heart should have molecular studies done at postmortem, with the potential for family screening.

Q27: E. Heart failure [evidence level 3].

- Heart failure is likely to be secondary to mitral valve stenosis.[5]

Q28: B. Ectopic cardiac beats [evidence level 4].[15]

- Ectopic beats are very common in everyone and increase in pregnancy.
- Coupled with the increased heart rate of pregnancy, these can become symptomatic.
- In pregnancy, the heart rate increases by 25%; thus sinus tachycardia, particularly in the third trimester, is not uncommon.
- Ectopic beats and non-sustained arrhythmia are encountered in more than 50% of pregnant women investigated for palpitations.[16]
- Most of these are benign sinus tachycardias or bradycardias or atrial and ventricular ectopic beats.
- Sustained tachycardias are less common at around 2–3/1000.[16]
- In general, arrhythmias during pregnancy can be managed safely conservatively or medically with little risk to mother or fetus.
- During pregnancy, treatment should be initiated only for severe symptoms or haemodynamic compromise.[16]

Q29: B. Flow murmur of pregnancy [evidence level 4].[15]

- Because of the increased blood volume and heart rate, flow murmurs are common.

Q30: D. Inherited cardiomyopathy [evidence level 4].

- Early sudden death is a feature of an inherited cardiomyopathy.[16]

Q31: E. There was a reduction from 10.12 to 9.02 deaths per 100 000 maternities [evidence level 2++].[2]

Q32: B. Cardiac disease at a rate of 2.18/100 000 maternities [evidence level 2++].[5]

- Two-thirds of maternal mortality is due to a medical or mental health condition, not pregnancy itself.

Q33: C. In the immediate postpartum period [evidence level 2++].[2]

- The relative risk of admission to a psychiatric hospital with a psychotic illness is extremely high in the first 30 days after childbirth.[2]
- Almost a quarter of women who died between six weeks and one year after the end of pregnancy died from psychiatric disorders.[2]
- A history of mental illness is an indicator of early postpartum high risk; this risk is highest for bipolar affective disorder and schizophrenia.

Q34: B. Arrange for urgent senior psychiatric assessment.[2]

- Urgent and red flag indications for prompt senior psychiatric assessment include recent significant change in mental state or emergence of new symptoms, new thoughts or acts of violent self-harm, new and persistent expressions of incompetency as a mother or estrangement from the infant.[2]

References

1. World Health Organization, UNICEF, UNFPA and The World Bank. *Trends in Maternal Mortality: 1990 to 2010. WHO, UNICEF, UNFPA and The World Bank Estimates.* [http://apps.who.int/iris/bitstream/10665/44874/1/9789241503631_eng.pdf]

2. Maternal, Newborn and Infant Clinical Outcome Review Programme. MBRRACE-UK. *Saving Lives, Improving Mothers' Care: Surveillance of Maternal Deaths in the UK 2012–2014.* December, 2016. [https://www.npeu.ox.ac.uk/downloads/files/mbrrace-uk/reports/MBRRACE-UK]

3. Royal College of Obstetricians and Gynaecologists. *Maternal Collapse in Pregnancy and the Puerperium.* February, 2011. [https://www.rcog.org.uk/en/guidelines-research-services/guidelines/gtg56]

4. Elkady AA, Keith L, Sinha P. Peri-mortem caesarean section delivery: a literature review and comprehensive overview. *Enliven Gynecol Obstet* 2015;2(2):005.

5. MBRRACE-UK. *Saving Lives, Improving Mothers' Care: Surveillance of Maternal Deaths in the UK 2009–2012.* December, 2014. [https://www.npeu.ox.ac.uk/downloads/files/mbrrace-uk/reports/MBRRACE-UK]

6. Knight M, Tuffnell P, Brocklehurst P, et al. Incidence and risk factors for amniotic-fluid embolism. *Obstet Gynecol* 2010;115:910–17.

7. Knight M, Berg C, Brocklehurst P, et al. Amniotic fluid embolism incidence, risk factors and outcomes: a review and recommendations. *BMC Pregnancy Childbirth* 2012;12:7.

8. Kaukonen KM, Bailey M, Pilcher D, Cooper J, Bellomo R. Systemic inflammatory response syndrome criteria in defining severe sepsis. *N Engl J Med* 2015;372:1629–38.

9. Royal College of Obstetricians and Gynaecologists. *Thrombosis and Embolism during Pregnancy and the Puerperium, Reducing the Risk.* April, 2015. [https://www.rcog.org.uk/en/guidelines-research-services/guidelines/gtg37a]

10. National Health Service. *Choices, Diagnosing Deep Vein Thrombosis.* [www.nhs.uk/Deep-vein-thrombosis]

11. British Committee for Standards in Haematology. *UK Guidelines on the Management of Iron Deficiency in Pregnancy.* July, 2011. [www.bcshguidelines.com/documents/UK]

12. Royal College of Obstetricians and Gynaecologists. *Postpartum Haemorrhage, Prevention and Management.* December, 2016. [https://www.rcog.org.uk/en/guidelines-research-services/guidelines/gtg52]

13. Kraus F, Redline RW, Gersell DJ, Nelson DM, Dicke JM. *Placental Pathology: Atlas of Nontumor Pathology 3.* American Registry of Pathology, 2004.

14. National Institute for Health and Clinical Excellence. *Epilepsies: Diagnosis and Management.* January, 2012. [https://www.nice.org.uk/guidance/cg137]

15. McAnulty JH. Arrhythmias in pregnancy. *Cardiol Clin* 2012;30(3):425–34.

16. Watkins H, Ashrafian H, Redwood C. Inherited cardiomyopathies. *N Engl J Med* 2011;364:1643–56.

Chapter 8

Infections in Pregnancy

PART 1

Questions

1.

A woman who came from a country in the developing world had just had an emergency Caesarean section for failure to progress. She was not sure if she had a past varicella zoster virus (VZV) infection. She has been tested and found to be non-immune. She requests postpartum vaccination.

What is your advice for breastfeeding?

A. Caesarean section delivery is a contraindication for postpartum vaccination.
B. It is safe to breastfeed.
C. She should formula-feed for the first four weeks.
D. She should not breastfeed because the vaccine is a live attenuated vaccine.
E. There is no benefit in vaccination because she has already delivered.

2.

A woman who is 26 weeks pregnant is referred by the general practitioner because of recent contact with a friend with chickenpox (varicella zoster). On testing, she is not immune to the infection.

What is your immediate plan of care?

A. Admit her to an isolation area under hospital care.
B. Inform the healthcare workers in the antenatal clinic of a potential exposure.
C. Offer one single dose of varicella zoster immunoglobulin (VZIG) as soon as possible.
D. Offer a two-dose course of VZIG.
E. Offer vaccination.

3.

The general practitioner phones you about a woman who is 24 weeks pregnant and has developed mild signs and symptoms of chickenpox in the last 24 hours. He wants to know what treatment he should offer her.

What advice will you give him?

A. Offer her oral administration of 800 mg acyclovir five times a day for seven days.
B. Offer oral acyclovir administration only if her condition worsens.
C. Start varicella vaccination.
D. Send her to the hospital to receive VZIG.
E. Start both antiviral therapy and VZIG.

4.

A woman who is 22 weeks pregnant is seen in the antenatal clinic. Her hepatitis-screening test shows IgM antibody to the hepatitis B core antigen (HBcAg).

What is your diagnosis?

A. Acute hepatitis B infection.
B. Chronic hepatitis B infection.
C. Recent hepatitis B vaccination.
D. She is recently vaccinated.
E. She is an inactive hepatitis B carrier.

5.

NICE guidelines *Antiviral Prophylaxis in Pregnant Women* advise offering tenofovir disoproxil fumarate (TDF) to hepatitis B-infected pregnant women, to reduce mother-to-child vertical transmission (MTCT).

At what gestational age should you advise starting this treatment?

A. Start treatment after confirming the pregnancy during the antenatal booking visit.
B. Start treatment around 20 weeks' pregnancy.
C. Start treatment around 32 weeks.
D. Start treatment from 28 weeks and continue until four to 12 weeks postpartum.
E. Start treatment when the woman requests it.

6.

A hepatitis B-positive woman has just been delivered. The midwife tells you the woman wants to discuss breastfeeding.

How will you counsel her?

A. Breastfeeding is contraindicated because the virus is present in the breast milk.
B. Breastfeeding is not contraindicated unless she is on antiviral therapy.
C. Breastfeeding should be started after 24 hours after immunoprophylaxis of the baby.
D. Formula-feeding is more protective to the child.
E. She can breastfeed, even if she is taking antiviral medications.

7.

An unbooked mother comes into early labour. On reviewing her notes, she was not screened for hepatitis B infection.

What is your advice for the immediate follow-up for the baby?

A. The mother should be tested and if found to be HBsAg positive, the child should receive vaccination within 24 hours.
B. No need to administer any vaccination as the mother may prove to be not infected.
C. She should receive the HBV vaccine within 72 hours of the birth.
D. She should receive both the HBV vaccine and hepatitis B immunoglobulin (HBIG) within seven days of the birth.
E. The newborn should be given immunoprophylaxis only if he/she is HBV negative.

8.

A woman who is 35 weeks pregnant is diagnosed with primary genital herpes. She received acyclovir treatment but was reluctant to accept Caesarean section delivery.

What are the risks of the baby developing neonatal herpes if she has a vaginal delivery?

A. 10%.
B. 17%.
C. 35%.
D. 41%.
E. 61%.

9.

A woman who is 35 weeks pregnant is complaining of painful vulval blisters. She was diagnosed with genital herpes when she was 25 weeks pregnant and received acyclovir treatment. She is not keen on Caesarean section delivery.

What is your first line of investigation to help her decide the mode of delivery?

A. Request a polymerase chain reaction (PCR) to confirm infection.
B. Take swabs from any vulval ulcers.
C. Test her for immunoglobulin G [IgG] antibodies to herpes simplex virus type 1 (HSV-1).
D. Test her for IgG antibodies to herpes simplex virus type 2 (HSV-2).
E. Test her for type-specific HSV-IgG antibodies to HSV-1 and HSV-2.

10.

For women who are diagnosed with suspected genital herpes in the primary care or obstetric services, what audit should you perform to ensure correct management?

A. Percentage of women referred to a genitourinary medicine specialist.
B. Percentage of women offered therapeutic oral acyclovir.
C. Percentage of women offered prophylactic oral acyclovir.
D. Percentage of women counselled about intravenous acyclovir during labour.
E. Percentage of women offered explanation of the management of genital herpes in pregnancy and the options and mode of delivery and human immunodeficiency virus (HIV).

11.

A woman who is 13 weeks pregnant is being counselled regarding HIV screening. She is keen to know the percentage of HIV-infected pregnant women in the United Kingdom.

What is the percentage of all HIV-positive women in the UK, who are identified because of antenatal screening in their current pregnancy?

A. 2.7%.
B. 3.0%.
C. 14%.
D. 16%.
E. 21%.

12.

A woman who is 13 weeks pregnant has screened positive to HIV infection. During counselling, you felt it was important to explain the declining rate of mother-to-child transmission (MTCT) because of interventions.

What is the current rate of MTCT of HIV infection?

A. <0.5%.
B. 1%–3%.
C. 3%–5%.
D. 5%–7%.
E. 7%–10%.

13.

A woman who is 26 weeks pregnant, and who has multiple sexual partners, is seen in the antenatal clinic. She had screened negative for HIV infection at her 13-week booking visit.

How would you re-counsel her to reduce possible MTCT?

A. Her child is at no risk as she has screened negative when she first booked.
B. Offer a prophylactic dose of antiretroviral therapy as she is at a higher risk of seroconversion.
C. Offer elective Caesarean section delivery to prevent MTCT.
D. Offer a repeat HIV screening.
E. Offer newborn screening for acquired HIV infection.

14.

A woman who is 14 weeks pregnant has screened positive for HIV infection. She agrees to start combined antiretroviral therapy (cART).

When would you test her viral load in order to monitor her adherence to treatment?

A. At the beginning of treatment and at delivery.
B. Four weeks after initiation of treatment.
C. At 36 weeks.
D. At 38 weeks as it is cost effective.
E. Two to four weeks after commencing cART, at the second and third trimester, at 36 weeks, and at delivery.

15.

A woman who is 11 weeks pregnant has screened positive for HIV infection.

How would you counsel her about her options for the best time to start cART?

A. She should start treatment at the end of the second trimester.
B. She should delay treatment until the 20-week anomaly scan.
C. She should start treatment around 26 weeks.

D. She should start treatment immediately.

E. She should start treatment after screening for Down syndrome.

16.

A full-term primigravida pregnant woman presented in established labour at 6-cm dilatation. Her previous screening showed she is HIV screen positive but did not have any treatment.

What is your immediate management?

A. Continue labour and treat the baby after delivery.

B. Carry out an immediate Caesarean section delivery.

C. Start oral combined antiretroviral therapy.

D. Start zidovudine infusion.

E. Treat with a stat dose of nevirapine 200 mg and commence fixed-dose zidovudine with lamivudine and raltegravir after delivery.

17.

An HIV screen-positive pregnant woman at 36 weeks is reviewed at the antenatal clinic. She was on cART and her viral load is <50 HIV-RNA copies/mL.

Justify your plan for her delivery.

A. Allow her to continue pregnancy until 42 weeks for a more effective duration of her cART.

B. Offer a planned Caesarean section birth to protect the baby against MTCT.

C. Offer induction of labour at 38 weeks as it reduces the risk of MTCT.

D. Offer induction of labour at 37 weeks to reduce the length of fetal exposure to her HIV infection.

E. There is no need for planned elective Caesarean section (PLCS) as she has a very low risk of MTCT.

18.

A 30-year-old woman has just come back from a tour of Brazil. She is 29 weeks pregnant. She has complained of a low-grade fever, and a maculopapular rash.

What is your next course of action?

A. Request serum transcription polymerase chain reaction (RT-PCR).

B. Start acyclovir treatment.

C. Start vaccination for the Zika virus.

D. Start dengue fever vaccine.

E. Start MMR vaccine.

ANSWERS

Q1: B. It is safe to breastfeed [evidence level 3].[1]

- The few small studies have not detected the varicella zoster virus (VZV) vaccine in breast milk.
- VZV vaccine is a live attenuated virus. Its protection (75%–95%) may last up to 20 years.
- Vaccinated non-pregnant women should be advised to avoid pregnancy for four weeks.
- The incidence of varicella zoster (chickenpox) in pregnancy in the UK is three in every 1000 women.

- VZV is an alpha herpes virus, occurring in the dorsal root and trigeminal ganglia. The virus persists for the life of the host and may reactivate at intervals.
- The virus causes two diseases, varicella (chickenpox) and herpes zoster (shingles).
  - **Chickenpox (VZV)** is the primary form and usually affects children. It is characterized by a vesicular pruritic rash that develops into crops of maculopapules, which crust over before healing. The incubation period is between one and three weeks. The disease is infectious 48 hours before the rash appears and continues to be infectious until the vesicles crust over, in about five days. Airborne transmission occurs via respiratory droplets or from shedding of infectious virions from vesicles on the skin.
  - **Herpes zoster (HZ)**, also called 'zoster' or 'shingles', occurs in adults and is reactivation of the virus from its latent state in the same person from a previous infection. Following the primary infection, the virus can be reactivated to cause a vesicular erythematous skin rash in a dermatomal distribution. Pain is a major feature. Pain usually appears before the appearance of the rash and disappears with the healing of the rash, although it may persist for longer periods.
  - Herpes zoster immunoglobulin (HZIG) is indicated only if there is a recent history of exposure. Testing for immunity is useful mainly for postpartum immunization, but immunization is not particularly effective in preventing the disease.
  - Vaccination is contraindicated during pregnancy because the vaccine is a live attenuated virus. It can potentially reactivate to cause zoster infection.[1]
  - A definite past history of infection indicates immunity.
  - The current UK National Screening Committee does not recommend universal screening for pregnant women.

Q2: C. Offer one single dose of varicella zoster immunoglobulin (VZIG) as soon as possible [grade of recommendation D].[1]

- VZIG prophylaxis is recommended for those who test seronegative within 7–10 days of exposure.
- The duration of protection is three weeks. If there is a second exposure after three weeks, repeat VZIG prophylaxis is recommended.
- Women with serious complications (respiratory symptoms, neurological symptoms such as photophobia, seizures or drowsiness, a haemorrhagic rash or bleeding, or a dense rash with or without mucosal lesions) should be referred to a hospital with intensive care access.
- **Fetal varicella zoster syndrome** (FVS) includes skin scarring in a dermatomal distribution; eye defects (microphthalmia, chorioretinitis or cataracts); hypoplasia of the limbs; and neurological abnormalities (microcephaly, cortical atrophy, mental retardation or dysfunction of bowel and bladder sphincters).
- FVS is more likely to occur if infection is contracted after 28 weeks of pregnancy [evidence level 2−].

Q3: A. Offer her oral administration of 800 mg acyclovir five times a day for seven days [evidence level 1−].[1]

- Acyclovir inhibits replication of the VZV if commenced within 24 hours of developing the rash.
- There is no increase in the risk of major fetal malformation with acyclovir exposure in pregnancy.
- VZIG is not a treatment for patients with clinical chickenpox. It is recommended for post-exposure prophylaxis.

- Maternal infection in the last four weeks of pregnancy may have a significant risk of varicella infection of the newborn (up to 50% of babies are infected and approximately 23% develop clinical varicella).
- If possible, a planned delivery should normally be avoided for at least seven days after the onset of the maternal rash to allow for passive transfer of antibodies from mother to child.[1]

Q4: A. Acute hepatitis B infection.[2]

- Hepatitis B is a highly infective, blood-borne DNA virus.
- Its prevalence is 1% in the UK.
- It is transmitted through blood and bodily secretions (blood transfusion, sexual contact, intravenous drug abuse and vertical transmission to the fetus).
- The virus has three antigens, s (surface) antigen (HBsAg), c (core) antigen (HBcAg) and e (envelope) antigen (HBeAg).
- Immunoglobulin M (IgM) indicates acute infection; it is produced by the immune system within 10 days of infection, but may persist for six months. Immunoglobulin G (IgG) indicates previous infection and possible immunity.
- **Acute infection** is characterized by the presence of HBsAg and anti-HBcAg).
- **Chronic infection** is characterized by IgG levels and the persistence of HBsAg without the antibody (anti-HBsAg).
- HBeAg without the presence of anti-HBeAg indicates a high degree of infectivity. The presence of anti-HBeAg indicates low infectivity.
- The presence of anti-HBsAg of >10–12 mIU/mL indicates recovery and immunity from infection or is an indication of successful vaccination.
- Without prophylaxes, the risk of vertical transmission is highest in HBsAg-positive and HBeAg-positive mothers and low for HBsAg-positive and HBeAg-negative mothers.
- Vertical transmission of infection to the fetus occurs at the time of delivery in 95% of cases. Transmission may also occur during pregnancy (5%).
- HBV-DNA level, or 'viral load', indicates viral replication. Higher HBV-DNA levels are usually associated with an increased risk of liver disease and hepatocellular carcinoma.
- Hepatitis B immunoglobulin (HBIG) provides passive immunity protection until the hepatitis B vaccine becomes effective.
- The DNA level typically falls in response to effective antiviral treatment.[2]

Q5: D. Start treatment from 28 weeks and continue until four to 12 weeks postpartum.[2]

- Antiviral therapy during the last trimester of pregnancy could decrease mother-to-child-transmission (MTCT) by reducing the level of hepatitis viral DNA at the time of delivery.
- Tenofovir disoproxil fumarate (TDF, category B medication) may also be the preferred antiviral for HBV infection in pregnancy. It is potent and is safe in relation to birth defects, and has a better resistance profile than lamivudine.[3]

Q6: B. Breastfeeding is not contraindicated unless she is on antiviral therapy [evidence level 1+].[3]

- Except for mothers taking antiviral medications, breastfeeding is not a contra-indication in infected mothers. The risk of transmission is low and is comparable between breast- and formula-fed infants.[3]

Q7: A. The mother should be tested and if found to be HBsAg-positive, the child should receive vaccination within 24 hours.[4]

- Pregnant women who are HBeAg-positive are particularly infectious, with 70%–90% risk of transmitting infection to the baby.
- In the UK, all women are screened during each pregnancy for hepatitis B.
- If an unbooked mother presents in labour, an urgent HBsAg test should be performed to ensure that vaccine can be given to babies born to positive mothers within 24 hours of birth.
- Babies with hepatitis B seropositive mothers should have the full primary course of hepatitis B vaccination to offer active immunization and most should also have HBIG to offer a passive immunization, within 24 hours of birth.[4]
- This post-exposure prophylaxis (PEP) programme can prevent up to 90% of vertical transmission. [4]

Q8: D. 41% [evidence level 2+].[5,6]

- Neonatal herpes is very rare in the UK. However, it has serious viral neonatal complications with a high morbidity and mortality. The treatment is mainly to treat the mother.
- Neonatal herpes may be caused by herpes simplex virus type 1 (HSV-1) or type 2 (HSV-2) affecting the mother.
- For vaginal delivery, the risk of neonatal herpes if there is a primary episode is 41%.
- In the newborn, the disease may be localized to skin or eye, or there may be local central nervous system encephalitis (80% mortality), or it may cause disseminated infection with multiple organ involvement.
- Most cases of neonatal herpes occur as a result of vertical transmission and direct contact with infected maternal secretions, mainly during labour events (the duration of rupture of membranes before delivery, the use of intrapartum invasive procedures such as fetal scalp electrodes or fetal blood sampling), preterm delivery and the mode of delivery.
- There is no clear evidence that daily suppressive acyclovir 400 mg three times daily will reduce the incidence of neonatal herpes. It may, however, reduce viral shedding at the time of delivery and may reduce the need for Caesarean section. It may be considered from 36 weeks' gestation.[6]

Q9: E. Test her for type-specific HSV-IgG antibodies to HSV-1 and HSV-2 [evidence level 2–].[7]

- Caesarean section is the recommended mode of delivery for all women developing first-episode genital herpes in the third trimester, particularly those developing symptoms within six weeks of expected delivery, as the risk of neonatal transmission of HSV during labour is very high at 41%.
- It may be difficult to differentiate clinically between primary and recurrent genital HSV infections.
- Recurrent genital herpes in the third trimester is not an indication for Caesarean section delivery to prevent neonatal transmission.
- Type-specific HSV antibody testing (IgG to HSV-1 and HSV-2) will help distinguish between primary and recurrent infection. The presence of antibodies of the same type as the HSV isolated from genital swabs would confirm this episode to be a recurrence rather than a primary infection.
- It takes two to three weeks for the results of this test. Based on the assumption that all first-episode lesions are primary genital herpes, Caesarean section should be the initial plan of delivery. This plan can be modified if HSV antibody test results subsequently confirm a recurrent rather than a primary infection.
- PCR is more accurate and offers a quicker result than biopsy of the ulcers.

Q10: A. Percentage of women referred to a genitourinary medicine specialist.[7]

Q11: D. 16% [evidence level 3].[8]

- In 2013, 16% of diagnosed HIV-positive women were identified because of antenatal screening in their current pregnancy.
- Incidence is the rate of newly diagnosed cases of a disease. The accuracy of incidence data depends upon the accuracy of diagnosis and reporting of the disease.
- Prevalence is the actual number of people alive who have the disease, either during a period (period prevalence) or on a particular date (point prevalence).

Q12: A. <0.5% [level 3].[9]

- The UK continues to have a very low rate (0.5%) of MTCT.
- Antiretroviral therapy, appropriate management of delivery and the avoidance of breastfeeding can reduce the risk of MTCT from 15%–25% to 1% or less.

Q13: D. Offer a repeat HIV screening.[10]

- Health professionals are encouraged to offer repeat tests to any woman at continuing high risk of infection to detect any seroconversion in order to plan for the necessary interventions to reduce MTCT.

Q14: E. Two to four weeks after commencing cART, at the second and third trimester, at 36 weeks, and at delivery [grade 1C].[10]

- Optimal HIV control is reflected by complete viral suppression with an undetectable viral load.[10]
- If a woman who has initiated combined antiretroviral therapy (cART) during pregnancy has not achieved a plasma viral load of <50 copies/mL at 36 weeks, she should be referred to a virologist.

Q15: D. She should start treatment immediately [evidence level 2a].[11]

- Data on the efficacy of cART in pregnancy are based on a three/four drug combination including zidovudine/lamivudine.
- Starting treatment at or before 28 weeks reduces the transmission rate of 1% or less.
- The British HIV adult prescribing guidelines now recommend tenofovir/emtricitabine or abacavir/lamivudine as first-line therapy on the basis of safety, tolerability and efficacy.
- A systematic review and meta-analysis (2014) of observational cohorts (2026 women) exposed to efavirenz during the first trimester found no increased risk of overall birth defects.[11]

Q16: C. Start oral combined antiretroviral therapy [grade 1B].[12]

- An immediate single dose of nevirapine crosses the placenta within two hours and maintains effective concentrations in the neonate for up to 10 days.
- An immediate start of cART (zidovudine with lamivudine and raltegravir) will also rapidly cross the placenta.
- Zidovudine infusion for the duration of labour in addition to cART will add further protection but alone is not the first-line management as it does not reduce MTCT significantly.[12]
- This regimen will reduce MTCT from 7.5% to 2.9% [evidence level 3].[12]

Q17: E. There is no need for planned elective Caesarean section (PLCS) as she has a very low risk of MTCT [evidence level 3].[12]

- In women on cART with a plasma viral load <50 HIV-RNA copies/mL, the MTCT rates are reduced (<0.5%) irrespective of the mode of delivery.
- Studies support recommending planned vaginal delivery for women on cART with these low plasma viral loads.
- Where the viral load is ≥400 HIV-RNA copies/mL at 36 weeks, PLCS is recommended.[12]
- In women with a viral load of <50 HIV-RNA copies/mL, it is unlikely that the type of instrument used for instrumental delivery will affect the MTCT.
- Where PLCS is indicated for the prevention of MTCT, surgery should be undertaken at between 38 and 39 weeks' gestation [grade 1C]
- If PLCS is indicated only for obstetric indications, and the plasma viral load is <50 copies/mL, surgery should be undertaken between 39 and 40 weeks.
- In the UK, all HIV-positive mothers, regardless of antiretroviral therapy, and infant post-exposure prophylaxis (PEP), should be advised to exclusively formula-feed.[11]

Q18: A. Request serum transcription polymerase chain reaction (RT-PCR).[13]

- Zika virus (ZIKV) is a viral infection transmitted by the *Aedes* mosquito, which is present throughout Africa, South and South East Asia, South and Central America, the Caribbean and the Pacific. The majority of those infected have few or no symptoms.
- If contracted in pregnancy, it may lead to microcephaly and brain defects.
- There is currently no evidence that ZIKV can be transmitted to babies through breast milk.
- The incubation period of ZIKV is usually from three to 12 days for most people.
- RT-PCR is the main diagnostic test. It detects the viral RNA, to identify the type of virus infection.
- Currently there is neither any specific antiviral treatment nor any vaccination for either the ZIKV or the dengue fever virus.

References

1. Royal College of Obstetricians & Gynaecologists. *Chickenpox in Pregnancy*. January, 2015. [https://www.rcog.org.uk/globalassets/documents/guidelines/gtg13]
2. National Institute for Health and Care Excellence. *Hepatitis B (Chronic), Diagnosis and Management*. June, 2013. [https://www.nice.org.uk/guidance/cg165]
3. Shi Z, Yan Y, Wang H, et al. Breastfeeding of newborns by mothers carrying hepatitis B virus. A meta-analysis and systematic review. *Arch Pediatr Adolesc Med* 2011;165:837–46.
4. Public Health England. *Infants Born to Hepatitis B-Infected Mothers: Immunization Policy*. [https://www.gov.uk/government/uploads/system/uploads/attach ment_data/file/]
5. Hollier LM, Wendell GD. Third trimester antiviral prophylaxis for preventing maternal genital herpes simplex virus (HSV) recurrences and neonatal infection. *Cochrane Database Syst Rev* 2008;(1):CD004946.
6. Brown Z. Preventing herpes simplex virus transmission to the neonate. *Herpes* 2004;11(3):175A–86A.
7. Royal College of Obstetricians and Gynaecologists and the British Association for Sexual Health and HIV (BASHH). *Management of Genital Herpes in Pregnancy*.

October, 2014. [https://www.rcog.org.uk/en/news/joint-rcogbashh-release-managing-genital-herpes-in-pregnancy–new-information-published]

8. Public Health England. *Antenatal Screening for Infectious Diseases in England: Summary Report for 2013.* Health protection report, HIV-STIs. *Infection reports* 8(43), November, 2014. [https://www.gov.uk/government/uploads]

9. National Screening Committee. *Infectious Diseases in Pregnancy Screening Programme Standards.* September, 2010. [https://www.gov.uk/government/uploads]

10. British HIV Association. *Guidelines for the Treatment of HIV-1-positive Adults with Antiretroviral Therapy 2012.* November, 2013. [www.bhiva.org/documents]

11. Lallemant M, Jourdain G, Ngo-Giang-Huong N, et al. A Phase III randomized, partially double-blind and placebo-controlled trial comparing the efficacy and safety of maternal and infant NVP vs infant only NVP, or maternal LPV/r, in addition to standard ZDV prophylaxis to prevent perinatal HIV transmission. 18th Conference on Retroviruses and Opportunistic Infections, Boston, MA. March, 2011. [Abstract 741].

12. Briand N, Warszawski J, Mandelbrot L, et al. Is intrapartum intravenous zidovudine for prevention of mother-to-child HIV-1 transmission still useful in the combination antiretroviral therapy era? *Clin Infect Dis* 2013; 57:903–14.

13. Royal College of Obstetricians and Gynaecologists, RCM, PHE, HPS. *Interim Clinical Guidelines Zika Virus Infection and Pregnancy.* November, 2016. [https://www.rcog.org.uk/en/news/interim-clinical-guidelines-on-zika-virus-infection-and-pregnancy]

PART 2

Questions

1.

A woman who is 12 weeks pregnant has a serum screening test showing a Venereal Disease Research Laboratory/rapid-plasma-reagin (VDRL/RPR) titre of >16.

This result indicates she has:

A. Active syphilis infection.
B. Acute on top of chronic syphilis infection.
C. Chronic syphilis infection.
D. Neurosyphilis infection.
E. Undergone effective treatment.

2.

A woman who is 14 weeks pregnant comes to the antenatal booking clinic after she has been diagnosed with a primary syphilis infection.

What will you tell her about the risk of transfer of the disease to her baby?

A. Around 10%.
B. Around 20%.
C. Around 40%–50%.
D. Around 70%.
E. The germ that caused her infection does not cross the afterbirth and will not reach the baby.

3.

A woman who is 33 weeks pregnant is diagnosed with a syphilis infection.

What is your first-line treatment option?

A. A single dose of benzathine benzyl penicillin G 2.4 MU.
B. A single dose of benzathine benzyl penicillin G 2.4 MU followed by a second dose after one week.
C. Oral dose of third-generation cephalosporin.
D. Oral doxycycline therapy for 10 days.
E. Procaine penicillin intramuscular injection 750 mg daily for 10 days.

4.

A woman who is 15 weeks pregnant comes to see you and wants to know why she was not screened for group beta-streptococcus infection (GBS). She has read that it is a frequent cause of severe infection in newborn babies.

What is the incidence of early onset neonatal group B-streptococcal (EOGBS) disease in the UK?

A. 0.01/1000 live births.
B. 0.05/1000 live births.
C. 0.5/1000 live births.
D. 5/1000 live births.
E. 6/1000 live births.

5.

On reviewing the notes of a woman who is 16 weeks pregnant, you notice she was a GBS carrier diagnosed from a vaginal swab in her previous pregnancy.

What treatment options would you recommend?

A. Offer intrapartum antibiotic prophylaxis (IAP) if she is induced.
B. Start oral penicillin for two weeks near term.
C. Start oral penicillin for two weeks and intrapartum antibiotic prophylaxis (IAP) during labour.
D. Start intrapartum antibiotic prophylaxis during labour.
E. There is no need for current or intrapartum treatment.

6.

A woman who is 27 weeks pregnant complains of dysuria and loin pains. Urine cultures indicated GBS growth greater than 105 CFU (colony-forming units)/mL. She received the appropriate treatment.

What is your further management?

A. If the urine infection has cleared, there is no need for IAP.
B. She should receive IAP.
C. She should receive appropriate treatment and IAP if her vaginal swab shows GBS-carrier state at 38 weeks.
D. Treat the urine infection and offer IAP if she was a carrier in a previous pregnancy.
E. Treat her urine infection and offer IAP if she has premature labour.

7.

A woman who is 22 weeks pregnant has a vaginal swab because of symptomatic vaginal discharge. The swab shows heavy growth of GBS. She has received the appropriate treatment.

What is your further management?

A. Repeat a second course of treatment at 38 weeks.
B. She should be screened for any recurrent infection every four weeks.
C. She should receive IAP.
D. Screen the newborn for any evidence of infection.
E. There is no need for any further management.

8.

A woman who is 22 weeks pregnant comes to the emergency department complaining of flu-like symptoms. She is pyrexial with no other clinical signs.

What is the most relevant information in her history that makes you suspect malaria infection?

A. History of night shivering.
B. History of contact with another pregnant woman who had parvovirus infection.
C. Travel to an endemic area.
D. She is not immune to rubella and did not receive pre-pregnancy vaccination.
E. She has recently been in contact with pets.

9.

A woman who is 16 weeks pregnant is referred by the general practitioner because of pyrexia and flu-like symptoms. You noticed a yellowish tinge to her conjunctiva; she says she has been to sub-Saharan Africa. You suspected malaria infection.

How will you confirm the diagnosis?

A. Microscopic examination of blood films for parasites.
B. PCR of the placental blood to detect parasite DNA.
C. Placental histology.
D. Rapid diagnostic test to detect specific parasite antigen (detect soluble HRP2 or pLDH).
E. Rapid diagnostic test to detect specific parasite enzyme.

10.

A woman who is 11 weeks pregnant is admitted with uncomplicated *Plasmodium falciparum* malaria infection.

What management options would you offer?

A. Artemisinin combination therapy for 14 days, which is highly effective and prevents relapse.
B. No treatment until she is well into her second trimester.
C. A seven-day repeat course of oral clindamycin, which is simple monotherapy and is an effective treatment.
D. Start oral quinine 600 mg eight hourly and oral clindamycin 450 mg eight hourly for seven days.
E. Start combination therapy of oral clindamycin and doxycycline.

11.

A woman who is 17 weeks pregnant comes for advice, as she has to travel to Nigeria. She is worried about malaria infection.

What chemoprophylaxis medication would you prescribe?

A. Atovaquone with proguanil (malarone).
B. Chloroquine.

C. Chloroquine and proguanil.
D. Doxycycline.
E. Mefloquine.

12.

A woman who is 13 weeks pregnant comes to see you at the early pregnancy assessment unit. She works at a childcare facility and has heard that contact with children is a common cause for cytomegalovirus (CMV) infection.

How will you counsel her about prevention?

A. Avoid all contact with young children until she is beyond the first trimester.
B. Follow the advice about hygienic measures to prevent infection.
C. Have a serial ultrasound examination from 20 weeks to confirm fetal normality.
D. Leave work immediately.
E. Recommend termination of pregnancy as she may have already been infected.

13.

A woman who is 16 weeks pregnant has a urine culture showing an *Escherichia coli* bacteria concentration of 10^5 CFU/mL. She is completely asymptomatic and was reluctant to receive antibiotic treatment.

What will you say to her?

A. Antibiotic treatment is effective in reducing the risk of renal complications.
B. She needs a renal ultrasound to see if she has developed renal complications to justify treatment.
C. She can wait to see if she develops any symptoms.
D. She must have treatment if a repeat urine test in two weeks shows infection.
E. Treatment is mandatory if serial growth scans show fetal growth restriction.

14.

The general practitioner calls you to ask about the best test to confirm asymptomatic bacteriuria (ASB) in an asymptomatic 14-week pregnant woman who had a previous urinary tract infection preceding this pregnancy.

What is the most reliable test?

A. Reagent strip test.
B. Reagent strip test and urine microscopy.
C. Rapid enzymatic screening test (detection of catalase activity).
D. Urine microscopy.
E. Urine culture.

15.

A woman who is 16 weeks pregnant presents at the booking clinic complaining of dysuria, frequency, urgency and suprapubic pain. She also noticed her urine is slightly blood stained. On examination, you observed a urethral discharge. Urine culture did not show significant bacteriuria.

What is the most likely diagnosis?

A. Acute cystitis.
B. Acute pyelonephritis.
C. Gonococcal urethritis.
D. Interstitial cystitis.
E. No gonococcal urethritis.

16.

A woman who is 30 weeks pregnant has a recurrent urinary tract infection (UTI).

What would you recommend for prevention of recurrence until the end of pregnancy?

A. A daily suppressive dose of 50 mg nitrofurantoin.
B. A daily suppressive dose of 250 mg cephalexin.
C. Drink two litres of water daily.
D. Take cranberry supplements.
E. Twice daily trimethoprim.

17.

A 32-year-old woman who is 17 weeks pregnant complains of recent polyarthralgia, affecting the hands, wrists, ankles and knees. On history taking, she admits to being in recent contact with a child who developed a non-vesicular rash.

What is your provisional diagnosis?

A. CMV infection.
B. Epstein–Barr virus infection.
C. Human parvovirus infection.
D. Rubella infection.
E. Measles infection.

18.

A woman who is 32 weeks pregnant had a proven B19 infection and has developed fetal hydrops at 36 weeks.

What is your management?

A. Administer steroids for lung maturity and deliver.
B. Arrange for an immediate middle cerebral artery peak systolic velocity (MCA-PSV) to detect fetal anaemia.
C. Arrange for intrauterine transfusion according to the severity of the hydrops.
D. Continue ultrasound monitoring and deliver at 38 weeks for better fetal maturity.
E. Deliver if the MCA-PSV was more than 1.5 MoM.

19.

A woman who is 26 weeks pregnant with confirmed B19 infection and non-immune hydrops fetalis (NIHF) is being followed up for any further developments in the fetus. The MCA-PSV is >1.5 MoM.

What is your management?

A. Arrange for cordocentesis and intrauterine blood transfusion (IUT).
B. Arrange for a liquor sample and B19 DNA PCR to confirm fetal infection.
C. Continue monitoring until the MCA-PSV is doubled before considering IUT.
D. Continue monitoring to see if there may be spontaneous resolution of the hydrops.
E. No need for IUT if the fetal blood sample demonstrates raised reticulocyte count, indicating spontaneous recovery.

20.

A woman who is 13 weeks pregnant gives a history of contact with a German measles-infected child. She thinks she had rubella when young but did not receive any vaccination.

How will you handle this situation?

A. Assure her as she had the infection in the past and must have developed immunity.
B. Arrange for an urgent ultrasound scan in the fetal medicine unit.
C. Counsel for termination of pregnancy.
D. Offer a vaccination course.
E. Perform IgM and IgG immunoglobulin test.

21.

A woman who is 15 weeks pregnant gives a history of recent contact with an infected child. Her blood test was negative for both IgM and IgG rubella antibodies.

What advice will you offer?

A. Assure her if you can confirm that she had the rubella infection when she was young.
B. Assure her not to worry as she is after the first trimester with no risk of fetal involvement.
C. Arrange for an urgent departmental ultrasound scan.
D. Further serum test required one month after contact.
E. Refer her to the abortion clinic.

22.

A woman who is 25 weeks pregnant is referred by her general practitioner with a confirmed measles infection. She has already been given human normal immuno-globulin (HNIG) post-exposure prophylaxis.

What are your plans for the rest of her antenatal care and management?

A. Arrange for a repeat dose of HNIG.
B. Follow her up with fortnightly ultrasound scans to detect any fetal congenital anomalies.
C. Plan for an amniocentesis to exclude fetal infection.
D. She should carry on with her usual antenatal care.
E. She should consider termination of pregnancy.

ANSWERS

Q1: A. Active syphilis infection [evidence level 3].[1]

Screening and testing for syphilitic infections

- Non-treponemal Venereal Disease Research Laboratory/rapid-plasma-reagin (VDRL/RPR) antibody test. It disappears in an adequately treated person after about three years.
- Or a more specific treponemal antibody test, the fluorescent treponemal antibody absorption (FTA-ABS) test, which lasts for life. The treponemal antibody test does not differentiate between acute and old, chronic infection.[1]
  - Diagnosis is confirmed by dark ground microscopy to look for the syphilis *Treponema pallidum* in a sample of fluid or tissue from an open sore.
  - Response to treatment produces a four-fold or greater titre decrease in the VDRL/RPR within three to six months after treatment.[1]

Q2: C. Around 40%–50%.[2]

- Pregnancies complicated by syphilis may cause intrauterine growth restriction, non-immune hydrops fetalis, stillbirth, preterm delivery and spontaneous abortion in up to 50% of pregnancies.[2]

Q3: B. A single dose of benzathine penicillin G 2.4 MU followed by a second dose after one week.[1]

- The above regimen is effective in most cases, after testing for allergy or desensitization.
- A second course is recommended if maternal treatment is initiated in the third trimester.[1]

Alternative second line therapy includes:[1]
- Oral amoxicillin 500 mg six hourly plus oral probenecid 500 mg six hourly for 14 days.
- Intramuscular ceftriaxone 500 mg for 10 days.
- Oral erythromycin 500 mg six hourly for 14 days.
- Oral azithromycin 500 mg daily for 10 days.
- **All babies should be evaluated at birth and treated with penicillin.**

Q4: C. 0.5/1000 live births.[3,4]

- In the UK, screening for early onset group beta-streptococcus (EOGBS) is not recommended [evidence level 2+].[3,4]
- Screening carries a significant burden without any appreciable impact on mortality and long-term morbidity caused by group beta-streptococcus (GBS).[4]

Q5: E. There is no need for current or intrapartum treatment [evidence level 3].[4]

Q6: B. She should receive intrapartum antibiotic prophylaxis (IAP) [evidence level 2+].[4]

- Women with GBS bacteriuria are at a higher risk (10.2%) of chorioamnionitis.
- GBS bacteriuria is also associated with neonatal disease, consequently IAP is recommended.[4]

Q7: C. She should receive IAP [evidence level 3].[4]

Recommended IAP treatment regimens[4]
- Intravenous benzylpenicillin 3 g be given as soon as possible after the onset of labour and 1.5 g four hourly until delivery.
- Clindamycin 900 mg should be given intravenously eight hourly to those allergic to benzylpenicillin.
- An alternative agent vancomycin.

Q8: C. Travel to an endemic area.[5]

- History of travel to endemic areas will lead clinicians to consider targeted investigations according to the region visited and hence avoid delayed diagnoses and treatment.
- No symptoms or signs can predict malaria accurately. Most of the symptoms are non-specific.

Q9: A. Microscopic examination of blood films for parasites.[5]

- The infecting species are *Plasmodia falciparum*, *P. vivax*, *P. malariae*, *P. knowlesi*, and *P. ovale*, of which *P. falciparum* is the most dangerous and is the main cause of the vast majority of deaths worldwide.

- Microscopic examination of blood films for parasites is the gold standard for a definite diagnosis of malaria infection.
- A blood film has the advantage of quantifying the number of infected red blood cells (parasitaemia) and of confirming the infecting species and the stage of the parasites.[5]
- Results of blood films and rapid diagnostic tests can be available in one hour.
- In the UK, malaria in pregnancy must be reported to the public health authorities and the Health Protection Agency.[5]

Q10: D. Start oral quinine 600 mg eight hourly and oral clindamycin 450 mg eight hourly for seven days.[5]

- The reported prevalence of congenital malaria varies from 8% to 33%.[5]
- Malaria in pregnancy may cause severe anaemia, renal or liver failure, hypoglycaemia, sudden drop of BP and even death.[5]
- Fetal complications: fetal mortality, miscarriage, stillbirth, fetal growth restriction, low birthweight and premature birth, which are best prevented by prompt treatment.
- Quinine has significant maternal side effects (tinnitus, headache, nausea, diarrhoea, altered auditory acuity and blurred vision) which may lead to non-compliance and failure of treatment. Hospitalization improves compliance with better cure results.[5]
- Even in severe malaria, the role of early Caesarean section for the viable fetus is unproven.
- There has not been any evidence of congenital defects in babies born to mothers who received antimalarial treatment.

Q11: E. Mefloquine [evidence level 2−].[5]

- Mefloquine is the first choice; it is highly effective against drug-resistant *P. falciparum*.[5]
- Different studies have not shown any strong association for mefloquine with stillbirths or miscarriages in the second and third trimesters.[5]
- Doxycycline is contraindicated in pregnancy and other regimens offer relatively poor protection against drug-resistant *P. falciparum*.

Q12: B. Follow the advice about hygienic measures to prevent infection.[6,7]

- Cytomegalovirus (CMV) is a double-stranded DNA herpes virus.
- CMV infection remains for life. Most CMV infections do not produce any signs or symptoms.
- Contact with the saliva or urine of young children is a major cause of CMV infection among pregnant women. It can spread by breastfeeding.
- Advice includes washing hands often, with soap and water for 15–20 seconds, especially after changing diapers, feeding a young child, wiping a young child's nose or handling children's toys.
- She should not share foods or drinks with young children.
- Wearing gloves offers added protection.[6,7]
- In the UK, it is estimated that one to two babies in every 200 will be born with congenital CMV.[7]
- Children who develop serious consequences of congenital CMV may have loss of hearing or vision, be developmentally or intellectually handicapped, have small head size or have cerebral palsy.
- There is no treatment or vaccination for CMV infection.
- Recent CMV infection can be diagnosed if the IgM level is elevated or if there is a four-fold increase in previously tested IgG titres.[6]

Q13: A. Antibiotic treatment is effective in reducing the risk of renal complications [evidence level 1−].[8]

- A 2015 Cochrane review of 14 randomized trials (2000 women) found evidence that antibiotic treatment in asymptomatic bacteriuria (ASB) is effective in reducing the incidence (28%–47%) of pyelonephritis [evidence levels 1a, 2b].
- A systematic review comparing single-dose versus a four- to seven-day course of antibiotic treatment for ASB did not show a difference in the prevention of preterm birth or pyelonephritis between the two regimens. Longer duration of treatment was associated with increased reports of adverse effects.[8]
- Ten to thirty per cent of women with bacteriuria in the first trimester develop an upper urinary tract infection (UTI) in the second or third trimester.

Q14: E. Urine culture [evidence level 2a].[9]

- Urine culture has a higher sensitivity and specificity than all other tests.
- Urine culture offers the added advantage of a quantified assessment of the concentration of bacteria and reliable identification of the organism with antibiotic sensitivity to guide effective therapy.
- Ordering urine culture at the first antenatal visit will allow for timely efficient treatment and follow-up.

Q15: C. Gonococcal urethritis.[10]

- The main distinguishing clinical issues between urethritis and cystitis are the presence of urethral discharge and insignificant bacteriuria in urine cultures.
- History of multiple partners raises strong suspicion about gonococcal infection.

Q16: B. A daily suppressive dose of 250 mg cephalexin.[11]

- Most authorities recommend a daily dose of an antibiotic until delivery.
- Nitrofurantoin should not be given after 36 weeks. There is no evidence to support trimethoprim use for treatment of UTI infection.

Q17: C. Human parvovirus infection [evidence level 2b].[12]

- Arthropathy is the most common symptom (80%) of parvovirus B19 infection in adults. In children, it is characterized by the facial rash (*Erythema infectiosum*, slapped cheek or 'fifth disease').[12]
- Parvovirus B19 IgM appears within two to three days of acute infection (10–12 days after inoculation) and may persist for up to six months. Parvovirus B19 IgG appears a few days after IgM appears and usually remains positive for life.
- Characteristic rubella rash begins on the face and spreads to the trunk and extremities. It will usually resolve within three days.
- In Epstein–Barr infection, infectious mononucleosis (IM) is a common presentation in young adults.
- IM is characterized by generalized lymphadenopathy, fever and sore throat.
- Measles signs and symptoms include disseminated rash, coryza, conjunctivitis, pneumonia, otitis media and or encephalitis. It is usually uncommon in pregnancy.

Q18: A. Administer steroids for lung maturity and deliver [evidence level 3].[13]

- At this advanced age of gestation, preterm delivery and postpartum management of the newborn represents less risk for the fetus than continued gestation or intrauterine interventions.

Long-term neonatal outcome

- Most children born to parvovirus B19 infected mothers do not appear to suffer long-term sequelae. Severe anaemia may be an independent risk factor for long-term neurological sequelae.[13]

Q19: A. Arrange for cordocentesis and intrauterine blood transfusion (IUT).[14]

- Hydrops is a symptom of fetal anaemia, cardiac decompensation and imminent death.
- Middle cerebral artery peak systolic velocity (MCA-PSV) is a reliable, highly sensitive, non-invasive means for predicting fetal anaemia.
- Timely IUT to correct fetal anaemia significantly reduces the risk of fetal death.
- Proven parvovirus infection or non-immune fetal hydrops should be followed with weekly MCA-PSV measurements, and schedule an IUT when the MCA-PSV exceeds 1.5 MoM.
- For option (B), B19 DNA in the amniotic fluid is only a diagnostic modality and is not a treatment option for hydrops and fetal anaemia.
- IUT is indicated if the cordocentesis fetal blood sample shows anaemia (haemoglobin below 8 gm/dL).
- A fetal blood sample should be taken during IUT to perform a measurement of B19V DNA, haemoglobin, platelet and reticulocyte counts.
- IUT has a fetal loss risk of 6% for intravascular transfusion to 30% without intravascular transfusion.

Q20: E. Perform IgM and IgG immunoglobulin test.[15]

- Currently in the UK, the incidence of rubella infection has fallen dramatically because of the vaccination programme.
- The fetal risks for infection are 90% at 11 weeks, 55% at 11–16 weeks and 45% (minimal risk of deafness) if infection is contracted between 16 weeks and 20 weeks.
- There is usually no increased risk of an adverse fetal outcome if infection is contacted after 20 weeks.
- A past history of exposure is not sure evidence of immunity and an immunity blood test should be requested.

Q21: D. Further serum test required one month after contact.[15]

- The incubation periods for rubella infections are 14 to 21 days while the infectivity period is seven days before appearance of the rash and continues until 10 days after the development of the rash.
- Immunity blood tests are required one month after the first negative test to confirm if the woman is acutely infected, susceptible or immune.
- The most common fetal congenital rubella syndrome (CRS) complications include cataracts, heart defects, hearing impairment, and developmental delay. Other less specific signs of CRS include purpura, hepatosplenomegaly, jaundice, microcephaly, meningoencephalitis and radiolucent bone disease.[15]
- A normal scan may assure parents, but cannot absolutely exclude infection.
- Rubella vaccination is contraindicated in pregnancy and if given outside pregnancy, the woman is advised to avoid pregnancy for the next three months.
- PCR is a specific 24-hour test result. It will definitely exclude a rubella infection.

Q22: D. She should carry on with her usual antenatal care [evidence level 3].[16]

- There is no treatment for measles, and it does not cause congenital anomalies. There is no need for any extra antenatal-specific measures. There is no need to expose her to the risks of amniocentesis (1% fetal loss) because findings will not affect her management.

- In the UK, measles infection in pregnancy is relatively uncommon because of the MMR (against measles, mumps, rubella and chickenpox) vaccination programme.
- Human normal immunoglobulin (HNIG) (0.25 mL/kg IM) immediately after exposure attenuates the illness. There is no evidence that it prevents intrauterine death or preterm delivery. [16]
- The rash of rubella (German measles) is pink or light red, spotted, and lasts up to three days. It begins on the face and then spreads downwards to the rest of the body.
- Other symptoms may include one to two days of a mild fever, swollen lymph nodes and joint swelling.
- The rash of regular measles is a full-body red or reddish-brown bumpy rash, which lasts for several days. However, the first symptom is usually a hacking cough, runny nose and high fever.

Neonates born to measles infected mothers
- Administration of HNIG immediately after birth or postnatal exposure is recommended for neonates born to mothers in whom the rash appears six days before to six days after birth.

References

1. Kingston M, French P, Goh B, et al. UK National Guidelines on the management of syphilis, 2008. *Intern J STD AIDS* 2008;19:729–40.
2. Values M, Kirk D, Ramsey P. Syphilis in pregnancy: a review. *Prim Care Update Ob/Gyns* 2000;7:26–30.
3. Ohlsson A, Shah VS. Intrapartum antibiotics for known maternal group B streptococcal colonization. *Cochrane Database Syst Rev* 2009;(3):CD007467.
4. Royal College of Obstetricians and Gynaecologists. *The Prevention of Early-onset Neonatal Group B Streptococcal Disease*. July, 2012. [https://www.rcog.org.uk/globalassets/documents/guidelines/gtg_36.pdf]
5. Royal College of Obstetricians and Gynaecologists. *Malaria in Pregnancy, Diagnosis and Treatment*. April, 2010. [https://www.rcog.org.uk/en/guidelines-research-services/guidelines/gtg54b]
6. Centers for Disease Control and Prevention. *Cytomegalovirus (CMV) and Pregnancy*. [https://www.cdc.gov/pregnancy]
7. Great Ormond Street Hospital for Children. *Congenital Cytomegalovirus Infection*. July, 2011. [www.gosh.nhs.uk/medical-information/search-medical-conditions]
8. Smaill FM, Vazquez JC. Antibiotics for asymptomatic bacteriuria in pregnancy. [Cochrane Database Syst Rev 2015]. *Cochrane Database Syst Rev* 2007;(2): CD000490.
9. Scottish Intercollegiate Guidelines, Network. *Management of Suspected Urinary Tract Infection in Adults. A National Clinical Guideline*. July, 2012. [www.sign.ac.uk/pdf/sign88]
10. McCormick T, Ashe RG, Kearney PM. Urinary tract infection in pregnancy. *Obstet Gynaecol* 2008;10:156–62.
11. National Institute for Health and Care Excellence. *Urinary Tract Infection (Lower) – Women*. Clinical Knowledge Summaries.July, 2015. [https://cks.nice.org.uk/urinary-tract-infection-lower-women]
12. Institute of Obstetricians and Gynaecologists, Royal College of Physicians of Ireland. *Parvovirus B19 Exposure/Infection During Pregnancy*. Clinical Practical Guideline No. 31. September, 2017. [www.hse.ie/eng/about/Who/clinical/nat clinprog/obsandgynaeprogramme/parvovirus.pdf]

13. Enders M, Weidner A, Zoellner I, Searle K, Enders G. Fetal morbidity and mortality after acute human parvovirus B19 infection in pregnancy: prospective evaluation of 1018 cases. *Prenat Diagn* 2004;24:513–18.

14. Shourbagy SE, Elsakhawy M. Prediction of fetal anemia by middle cerebral artery Doppler. *Middle East Fertil Soc J* 2012:17,275–82.

15. National Health Service. *Choices, Rubella – Diagnosis*. [www.nhs.uk/Conditions/Rubella/Diagnosis.aspx]

16. Manikkavasagan G, Ramsay M. The rationale for the use of measles post-exposure prophylaxis in pregnant women: a review. *J Obstet Gynaecol* 2009;29 (7):572–5.

Chapter 9

Substance Abuse and Domestic Abuse

Tamara Kubba

QUESTIONS

1.

A 19-year-old books her pregnancy at 18 weeks' gestation. Her anomaly ultrasound scan is normal. She has attended maternity triage on five occasions in the last six weeks complaining of abdominal pain. On each occasion, she was discharged home with analgesia. She presents to maternity triage at 28 weeks' gestation complaining of abdominal pain. Examination is unremarkable and all investigations are normal.

Which of the following management options is the most appropriate?

A. Admit for cardiotocography (CTG) monitoring.
B. Arrange an appointment in the consultant antenatal clinic.
C. Arrange an ultrasound scan.
D. Discharge home with analgesia.
E. Refer to the safeguarding team.

2.

A 24-year-old woman attends the antenatal clinic at 13 weeks' gestation. In her previous pregnancy, she had an elective Caesarean section for breech presentation at 39 weeks. She reports that she found the recovery after the Caesarean section difficult as she was discharged to a women's refuge because her previous partner had been physically abusive.

What proportion of women experience domestic abuse in pregnancy?

A. 5%.
B. 10%.
C. 15%.
D. 20%.
E. 25%.

3.

A 33-year-old woman attends the gynaecology outpatient clinic with a six-month history of pelvic pain and dyspareunia. She reports having had chlamydia in the past. On examination you notice bruises of various colours on the medial aspect of her thighs.

What is the most appropriate next step?

A. Arrange a transvaginal ultrasound scan.
B. Ask about domestic abuse.
C. Check her clotting profile.
D. Refer for psychosexual counselling.
E. Take triple swabs.

4.

A 25-year-old woman attends the antenatal clinic, with her partner, at 32 weeks' gestation. She appears anxious and makes very little eye contact. You notice her partner gives you her maternity book and he is answering the majority of the questions on her behalf.

What is the most appropriate next management step?

A. Book another antenatal clinic appointment for 34 weeks.
B. Call hospital security.
C. Call the police.
D. Make a safeguarding referral.
E. Speak to the woman on her own.

5.

A 32-year-old hedge fund manager is admitted at 34 weeks' gestation with signs suggestive of a placental abruption. A few hours following admission, she has a spontaneous vaginal delivery of an 1100 g female infant.

What is the most likely cause of her preterm delivery?

A. Alcohol abuse.
B. Amphetamine use.
C. Benzodiazepine use.
D. Cannabis use.
E. Cocaine use.

6.

An unemployed 22-year-old has a spontaneous vaginal delivery of a male infant at 38 weeks' gestation. She is breastfeeding; however, the baby is not gaining weight. The health visitor notices that the baby has a thin upper lip and small palpebral fissures.

What is the most likely diagnosis?

A. Crack cocaine use.
B. Fetal alcohol syndrome.
C. Noonan syndrome.
D. Trisomy 21.
E. Verloes–David syndrome.

7.

A 19-year-old has a Caesarean section for failure to progress at 37 weeks' gestation. It was noted previously that it was difficult to secure intravenous access, because her veins are difficult to cannulate. While she was in recovery, her baby started to have seizures and was taken to the neonatal unit.

What is the most likely cause for the neonatal seizures?

A. Bacterial meningitis.
B. Hypoglycaemia.
C. Hypoxic ischaemic encephalopathy.
D. Intraventricular haemorrhage.
E. Neonatal abstinence syndrome.

8.

An 18-year-old books her pregnancy at 26 weeks' gestation. She is a smoker and lives in a hostel. At her first ultrasound scan, the fetus is found to have gastroschisis and a cleft lip and palate.

What is the most likely cause of these fetal abnormalities?

A. Amphetamine use.
B. Cannabis use.
C. Crack cocaine use.
D. Benzodiazepine use.
E. Heroin use.

9.

A 35-year-old woman books her pregnancy at 11 weeks' gestation. She had a forceps delivery two years previously and developed postpartum psychosis on day 3 post-partum. She has been discharged from the community mental health team and is not currently on any psychiatric medication.

What is her risk of developing postpartum psychosis in this pregnancy?

A. 10%.
B. 25%.
C. 40%.
D. 50%.
E. 75%.

10.

A 27-year-old woman is brought in to the maternity triage on day 5 postpartum by her husband. She is visibly detached and unkempt. She claims that her baby is not hers and refuses to look at the baby.

What is the most appropriate next management step?

A. Admit to a general psychiatric ward.
B. Admit to a mother-and-baby unit.
C. Admit to the postnatal ward.
D. Make a safeguarding referral.
E. Prescribe an antidepressant.

11.

A 35-year-old woman attends the antenatal clinic at 30 weeks' gestation. She reports feeling anxious about the pregnancy and is especially anxious about contracting an infection. She is washing her hands multiple times a day and has stopped using public transport.

What is the most appropriate initial treatment?

A. Anxiolytic therapy.
B. Cognitive behavioural therapy.
C. Group therapy.
D. Non-directive counselling.
E. Psychodynamic psychotherapy.

12.

From the MBRRACE-UK report published in 2015, almost a quarter of women who died between six weeks and one year after pregnancy died of mental health-related causes.

Of those women who committed suicide, what was the most common method of death?

A. Drowning.
B. Hanging.
C. Jumping from a height.
D. Overdose.
E. Stabbing.

ANSWERS

Q1: E. Refer to the safeguarding team.[1]

- Frequent attendances with non-specific symptoms or symptoms with no clear diagnosis should alert healthcare professionals to the possibility of domestic abuse, therefore a safeguarding referral is the most appropriate management option.[1–3] Obstetric victims of domestic abuse are more likely to book late or have a concealed pregnancy, have an unintended pregnancy, be a teenager, have bleeding in early pregnancy, have a problem with drugs or alcohol, have repeated attendances with no clear diagnosis, be socially isolated, suffer depression/anxiety/self-harm, experience preterm labour, have low-birthweight babies and unexplained stillbirth.[1]
- The safeguard team can be doctors, social workers, psychiatrists, etc. Their aim is to keep the individual safe and prevent further abuse from occurring.

Q2: E. 25%.[1]

- At least one in four women will experience domestic abuse at some point in their lives.
- 30% of this abuse starts in pregnancy and gets worse during the antenatal or postnatal period.

Q3: B. Ask about domestic abuse.[1]

- All women should be asked about domestic abuse in a women's health setting. A more focused domestic abuse/social history should be taken if there are any suspicions of domestic abuse.[1]
- From a gynaecological perspective, women who experience domestic abuse may present with any of the following: pelvic pain, dyspareunia, vaginal discharge, genitourinary symptoms/recurrent urinary tract infections, pelvic inflammatory disease, sterilization requests, psychiatric problems, alcohol or other substance misuse, self-harm and/or vaginal bleeding or sexually transmitted infections.

Q4: E. Speak to the woman on her own.[1]

- All women should have at least one consultation on their own in pregnancy.[1]
- If domestic abuse is suspected, then the next appropriate management step is to talk to the patient on her own. After this has been done, it may be appropriate to take further steps, such as making a safeguarding referral.[1]

Q5: E. Cocaine use [evidence level 1+].[2]

- Cocaine (and crack cocaine) use can cause placental abruption (occurs around the time of use), intrauterine growth restriction, low-birthweight babies and/or preterm delivery.
- These effects of cocaine use are thought to be mediated by its vasoconstrictive effects on the placenta.[2]

Q6: B. Fetal alcohol syndrome [evidence level 1+].[3]

- Fetal alcohol syndrome can cause cardiac and skeletal abnormalities, microcephaly, intrauterine growth restriction, failure to thrive, characteristic facial abnormalities such as short palpebral fissures and a short upturned nose, central nervous system problems leading to learning difficulties and neurological abnormalities.[3]

Q7: E. Neonatal abstinence syndrome.[4]

- Opiates freely cross the placenta and enter the fetal circulation.
- Symptoms of neonatal withdrawal or neonatal abstinence syndrome (in 40%–80% of infants born to heroin users) include irritability/jitteriness, seizures, poor feeding, high-pitched shrill cry, irregular sleep patterns, respiratory distress.[4]

Q8: A. Amphetamine use.[5]

- Studies have shown that the use of amphetamines increase the risk of cardiac defects, gastroschisis, intestinal atresia and cleft lip and palate.

Q9: D. 50%.[6]

- The Perinatal Community Mental Health team should review all women with a history of postpartum psychosis prior to discharge from hospital.
- The perinatal team (community psychiatric nurses, a specialist consultant perinatal psychiatrist and the administrative support) provides a community service to support women experiencing mental health difficulties related to pregnancy, childbirth and early motherhood.
- The incidence of postpartum psychosis is 1–2/1000 births.
- Risk factors for developing postpartum psychosis include a previous episode of postpartum psychosis (~50%), bipolar disorder (at least 25%), schizoaffective disorder, discontinuation of mood stabilizer, family history of bipolar disorder, mother or sister who has had postpartum psychosis, primiparity, sleep deprivation and shorter gestation period.[6]

Q10: B. Admit to a mother-and-baby unit.[6]

- Admission to a mother-and-baby unit should always be considered where a woman has any of the following: rapidly changing mental state, suicidal ideation, pervasive guilt or hopelessness, significant estrangement from the infant, new or persistent beliefs of inadequacy as a mother, evidence of psychosis.[6]

- The mother–and-baby unit cares for mothers who experience severe mental health difficulties during and after pregnancy. The staff include mental health nurses, social therapists and life-skills recovery workers, a psychologist and an occupational therapist.

Q11: B. Cognitive behavioural therapy.[7]

- This patient is suffering from an obsessive compulsive disorder. The first-line treatment for mild to moderate anxiety disorders is cognitive behavioural therapy.[7]

Q12: B. Hanging.[7]

- A feature unique to pregnancy-related suicide is the violence involved; 82% of the total suicide deaths were by violent means and over 50% of these deaths were caused by hanging.[7]
- Mental health services should have a low threshold for initial and ongoing assessment for women with suicidal thoughts in pregnancy or the postpartum period.[1]

References

1. National Institute for Health and Care Excellence. *Domestic Violence and Abuse.* February, 2016. [https://www.nice.org.uk/guidance/qs116]
2. Gouin K, Murphy K, Shah PS. Knowledge Synthesis Group on determinants of low birth weight and preterm births. Effects of cocaine use during pregnancy on low birthweight and preterm birth: systematic review and meta-analyses. *Am J Obstet Gynecol* 2011;204:340.e1–12.
3. Henderson J, Gray R, Brocklehurst P. Systematic review of effects of low-moderate prenatal alcohol exposure on pregnancy outcome. *Brit J Obstet Gynaecol* 2007;114:243–52.
4. Dryden C, Young D, Hepburn M, Mactier H. Maternal methadone use in pregnancy: factors associated with the development of neonatal abstinence syndrome and implications for healthcare resources. *Brit J Obstet Gynaecol* 2009;116:665–71.
5. Werler MM, Sheehan JE, Mitchell AA. Association of vasoconstrictive exposures with risks of gastroschisis and small intestinal atresia. *Epidemiol* 2003;14:349–54.
6. Di Florio A, Smith S, Jones I. Postpartum psychosis. *Obstet Gynaecol* 2013;15:145–50.
7. National Institute for Health and Care Excellence. *Antenatal and Postnatal Mental Health, Clinical Management and Service Guidance.* June, 2015. [https://www.nice.org.uk/guidance/cg192]

Chapter 10

Teenage Pregnancy

Ahmed M Khalil

QUESTIONS

1.

A 14-year-old girl comes to the labour ward in early labour at 2 am. She is 38 weeks pregnant with a single viable fetus. She had regular uneventful antenatal care. Her serial growth scans are all normal. She had stopped smoking during this pregnancy and her sexually transmitted disease screening is negative.

What would you recommend in her delivery?

A. Avoid epidural anaesthesia at all costs.
B. Advise tocolysis to try to stop labour until 39 weeks.
C. Continuous electronic fetal monitoring.
D. Recommend emergency Caesarean section.
E. Routine care of labour.

2.

In the antenatal clinic, the midwife tells you about your next patient. She is one of a group of five schoolgirls who decided to get pregnant. They are all under-achieving in school. They do not attend all their clinic appointments.

What should you do in this situation?

A. Advise them to terminate the pregnancy.
B. Do not give any further appointments if they do not attend.
C. Do nothing extra.
D. Send a letter to the school manager to criticize this event.
E. Try to encourage them to attend the clinics and arrange a school visit to give information to other girls.

3.

A 15-year-old girl comes to the antenatal clinic. She is 11 weeks pregnant. She comes from a broken family. She claims it was an unintended pregnancy; she does not want to terminate the pregnancy but is not sure what to do with the child when it is born.

What options will you offer her?

A. Insist she should have a termination of pregnancy.
B. She can offer the child for adoption.
C. She can leave the child to her divorced mother.
D. She can leave the child to the social healthcare services.
E. She can leave the child to any of her relatives.

4.

You work as an ST 5 in an inner city hospital. You are asked to discuss the high incidence of teenage pregnancy with the local school administration to see how it may be possible to prevent and reduce teenage pregnancy.

What is the primary prevention management that you may propose?

A. Advise arrangement of a series of presentations for sexual education of the school girls.
B. Advise that the administration will dismiss any girl who becomes pregnant.
C. Advise a school survey for those who have unprotected sex and refer them to a contraception clinic.
D. School administration should talk to parents about preventing their children from having sex.
E. Set up a contraception clinic in the school.

5.

You are working as a year ST 5 in an inner city hospital. You are asked to propose an effective family planning method for the teenage girls.

What will you propose?

A. A combination of both the condom and an oral combined contraception.
B. Condom.
C. Emergency contraception.
D. Etonogestrel-releasing implant and the condom.
E. Intrauterine device.

ANSWERS

Q1: E. Routine care of labour.[1]

- The United States has the world's highest teenage pregnancy rate (43/1000 girls aged 15–17 years).
- The United Kingdom has the highest rate of teenage pregnancy in Western Europe (41.5/1000 girls aged 15–17 years).
- Teenage pregnancy is associated with a range of adverse outcomes (premature delivery, infants being small for gestational age, low birthweight and increased neonatal mortality, anaemia and pregnancy-induced hypertension), especially in the 13–16-year age group.
- These risks are likely to reflect a complex interplay between sociodemographic variables, gynaecological immaturity and the growth and nutritional status of the mother.
- Where age is the only risk factor, management is usually the same as for other labouring women.
- In very young adolescents, there is an increased likelihood of obstructed labour because of a small, immature pelvis.[1]

- Teenage pregnancy may be associated with increased prevalence of domestic abuse, alcohol and substance misuse and smoking.
- Teenage pregnant young girls have a higher incidence of postpartum depression and problems with breastfeeding. They need postpartum extra care of support.
- In the long term, the offspring of adolescents have poorer cognitive development, lower educational attainment, more frequent criminal activity and a higher risk of abuse, neglect and behavioural problems during childhood.
- It is unknown whether the poor outcomes of teenage pregnancy are partly attributable to the biological challenges presented by young maternal age or if they are solely the consequence of sociodemographic variables, which undoubtedly increase the risk of adverse outcomes.[1]
- There is no evidence of increased risk of early pregnancy miscarriage.[1]

Q2: E. Try to encourage them to attend clinic and arrange a school visit to give information to other girls.[1]

- Although teen pregnancy is often viewed as unplanned and unwanted, statistical evidence shows it may be more by design and will than just an inadvertent event (the majority choose to continue and over 25% will become pregnant again during their teenage years).
- It is important to recognize that teenage pregnancy can be a positive life choice for some young women.
- Girls who score below average on educational achievement measures at ages seven and 16 years have a significantly increased risk of becoming teenage parents.
- Adolescents should be encouraged to attend clinics for antenatal care from an early stage, as attendance is frequently poor. This is an opportunity to offer advice on nutrition and adverse habits such as smoking and alcohol use.
- Social support is important and many teenagers may benefit from an early referral to a specialist midwife or social worker. Information regarding antenatal care and labour should be provided in a format that is accessible and easily understood.[1]

Q3: B. She can offer the child for adoption.

- Termination of pregnancy and adoption are the two options for a teenage girl who does not want to keep the child.[1]

Q4: A. Advise arrangement of a series of presentations for sexual education of the school girls.

- Sexual education is the main primary prevention policy. The availability of contraception and contraception advice is a secondary prevention policy.[1]

Q5: D. Etonogestrel-releasing implant and the condom.

- Young women should be informed about all methods of contraception, highlighting the benefits of the long reversible methods, which have lower failure rates with typical use and are more cost effective than combined oral contraceptives or condoms if used for one year or longer. They require low compliance and have a lower discontinuation rate.[1]
- **The implant long-acting reversible contraception** method may be more appropriate for teenagers. It offers a three-year contraceptive protection without the need to remember to take pills daily. With a failure rate of 0.1% over three years, the insertion technique is simple and acceptable to young women, being virtually pain free after a local anaesthetic injection. It is important to

counsel the women about the irregular uterine bleeding, which if troublesome, may be treated with mefenamic acid or ethinyloestradiol,

- Condoms prevent sexually transmitted infection but teenagers are relatively poor users of barrier contraceptives.[1] The correct and consistent use of condoms should be advised to reduce the risk of transmission of sexually transmitted infections (STIs).[2]
- The 'double Dutch' method (the use of a contraceptive method and a barrier method) should be encouraged in this age group to offer both an effective contraception and protection against STIs.
- It may be difficult to insert a coil into a nulliparous uterus and there is no protection against sexually transmitted diseases. There is a small increase in risk of pelvic infection in the 20 days after IUCD insertion.[1]
- Rates of teenage pregnancy in the UK have halved in the past two decades and are now at their lowest levels since record-keeping began in the late 1960s.
- There is a 51% drop in conceptions over a 16-year period.
- Teenage pregnant girls are more prone to suffer anaemia, eclampsia, puerperal endometritis and postnatal depression. With pregnancy, they have a serious social problem damaging their mental and physical health, limiting their education and career progress, and increasing their risk of living in poverty and social isolation.[2]
- Children of teenage mothers are much more likely to become teenage parents themselves and experience a range of negative outcomes in later life.
- If a pregnant teenager chooses abortion, she is exposed to medical and emotional adverse effects, while continuing pregnancy carries the above higher risk of maternal and fetal disadvantages.
- Babies born to teenage mothers have higher rates of perinatal mortality, low birth weight, sudden infant death syndrome and substance dependence.[3]

References

1. Sedgh G, Finer LB, Bankole A, Eilers MA, Singh S. Adolescent pregnancy, birth, and abortion rates across countries: levels and recent trends. *J Adolesc Health* 2015;56(2):223–30.
2. Faculty of Sexual and Reproductive Healthcare. *Contraceptive Choices for Young People*. 2010. [file:///C:/Users/pc/Downloads/cec-ceu-guidance-young-people-mar-2010%20(2).pdf]
3. Patient: Trusted Medical Information and Support. *Contraception and Young People*. January, 2017. [www.patient.info/doctor/contraception-and-young-people].

Chapter 11

Contraception

QUESTIONS

1.

A 23-year-old woman is using male and female barrier contraception to prevent sexually transmitted infections (STIs). She wants to know if there is further protection if a spermicide is included.

What will you tell her regarding spermicidal creams and STIs?

A. Does not offer added protection.
B. Does not offer any protection against HIV.
C. Offers added protection.
D. Offers specific protection against HIV.
E. Protects against some types of sexually transmitted infections.

2.

A 26-year-old woman consults you. She was at a hen party and may have had unprotected sex. She wants to make sure she did not acquire any sexually transmitted infections. She wants to know when she should be tested.

What will you tell her?

A. After two weeks.
B. After four weeks.
C. After eight weeks.
D. After 14 weeks.
E. Immediately.

3.

A 39-year-old woman consults you about the risk of venous thrombosis if she uses a combined hormonal contraceptive. She shows you a brand, which contains 35 μg ethinylestradiol and levonorgestrel norethisterone progestogen.

How will you counsel her?

A. She should change to an intrauterine contraceptive device.
B. She should change to another oral contraceptive, which contains one of the new progestogens.
C. Her current pill has the lowest risk of blood clotting.
D. Her current pill has the highest risk of blood clotting.
E. Use it for one year only.

4.

A 36-year-old woman consults you about her contraception. She is seeking a method with the lowest risk of thrombosis. She has a family history of venous thromboembolism (VTE) in a first-degree relative aged under 45 years. She is not keen on any intrauterine devices.

How will you counsel her?

A. All methods have a risk of VTE.
B. If she herself has no personal history of any clotting, then all methods have the same risk.
C. If she has a family history of VTE, she should have a thrombophilia screen first.
D. It is safe to use any progestogen-only method.
E. Permanent long-acting contraception is her only option.

5.

A woman who weighs 100 kg wants to start the combined transdermal patch (CTP) for contraception.

What is your advice?

A. Efficacy may be decreased because of her weight; she should use additional precautions or an alternative method should be advised.
B. It is as effective as the oral combined pill.
C. It is not effective because of her weight.
D. It is as effective as any other hormonal method, if she can guarantee compliance with the correct method of use.
E. She would be better using a non-hormonal contraceptive.

6.

A 28-year-old woman consults you about combined hormonal contraception (CHC). Her mother died of breast cancer at the age of 55 years. She is healthy but has a problem with painful periods.

What will you tell her?

A. Combined hormonal contraception is contraindicated because of her family history.
B. She can use it for only one year where the risk decreases after one year of use.
C. She is at no risk and it will help her period pains.
D. She can use it, but with breast screening every six months.
E. She cannot use it if she has breastfed before.

7.

On a Saturday morning, an 18-year-old girl who is on an enzyme-inducing drug comes to the accident and emergency department requesting advice as she had unprotected sexual intercourse on the 18th day of her cycle. She does not wish to become pregnant. She did not accept your advice for an intrauterine device (IUD) fitting.

What alternatives can you offer her?

A. Copper IUD is the only available option for women on enzyme-inducing medications.
B. Offer hormonal emergency contraception and advise her to stop the enzyme-inducing drugs until she has her next period.
C. Offer a single 30 mg dose of progesterone receptor modulator, ulipristal acetate (UPA) (ellaOne®).
D. Offer a single 3 mg dose of levonorgestel (LNG) (two Levonelle® tablets).
E. There is no need if the single unprotected intercourse occurred in the infertile days of her cycle.

8.

A 17-year-old girl comes to the accident and emergency department. She had unprotected intercourse four days previously. She was not very keen on an intrauterine device (IUD).

What other alternatives do you wish to offer?

A. Double-dose Levonelle tablet.
B. Single dose of 30 mg micronized ulipristal acetate (ellaOne®).
C. IUD can offer her long-term reversible contraception.
D. Single-dose 150 mg Levonelle tablet.
E. Two combined oral contraceptive tablets.

9.

A 35-year-old woman comes for a suitable family planning method. She is obese (BMI ≥ 35 kg/m^2), with a family history of endometrial cancer.

What are her options?

A. Either the copper intrauterine device (IUD) or the levonorgestrel (LNG) IUD is a suitable option.
B. The copper IUD is a suitable option because it has a protective effect against endometrial cancer.
C. The condom is her only safe method.
D. The levonorgestrel IUD has a protective effect against endometrial cancer.
E. The combined oral contraception method has a proven protective role against endometrial cancer.

10.

An 18-year-old woman asks about contraception. She has acne and complains of heavy bleeding.

How will you help her to choose?

A. She can have the low-dose 13.5 mg levonorgestrel intrauterine device (IUD) to avoid acne exacerbation.
B. She can use the higher-dose 52 mg levonorgestrel for better control of her heavy bleeding.
C. She is better with a copper IUD because it has no hormones.
D. She can use a product with cyproterone acetate (CPA/EE).
E. She can try the progesterone-only pill.

11.

The general practitioner calls you to ask about one of his patients who is on progesterone-only contraception. She will be started on an enzyme-inducing drug. He says this new medication is expected to be taken long term.

What will you tell him?

A. Continue with her current progesterone-only contraceptive but double the dose.
B. She should change to another long-term reversible contraceptive.
C. She can use the new progestogen desogestrel because it may be more effective.
D. She can request tubal ligation.
E. She can start on combined oral contraception.

12.

A woman with sickle cell disease is seeking a long-acting reversible contraception method. She is asking if there is any method that may also help reduce her risk of sickle cell crisis and pain.

What well you tell her?

A. Contraception is contraindicated in sickle cell disease patients.
B. No method will help reduce her risk.
C. She can use only barrier contraception.
D. She is best with long-acting irreversible contraception.
E. The long-acting injectable contraceptive may help reduce her crisis pain.

13.

A woman with systemic lupus erythematosus comes to see you regarding safer contraception. From her notes, you see she has positive antiphospholipid antibodies.

According to the UK medical eligibility criteria (UKMEC), which contraceptive would you offer?

A. Combined hormonal contraception.
B. Long-acting injectable contraception.
C. The progesterone implant.
D. The progesterone-only pill.
E. The copper intrauterine device.

14.

A healthy 47-year-old woman comes for contraception counselling. She was under the impression that the combined hormonal contraception (CHC) method is contraindicated at her age.

How will you counsel her?

A. Age alone is not a contraindication to any method.
B. Agree with her that combined hormonal contraception is contraindicated.
C. She can use it for only one year to avoid complications.
D. Tell her that the transdermal patch is the safest method because it is not metabolized by the liver.
E. Tell her that the vaginal ring is more suitable.

15.

A healthy 33-year-old woman is on the combined hormonal contraceptive (CHC). She is involved in a road traffic accident and requires surgery with prolonged immobilization. The orthopaedic surgeon is asking for advice.

Based on our knowledge of the UKMEC, what is your advice?

A. She can continue if she is not under any specific thrombotic risk, e.g. family or past history.
B. She can continue the method if her treatment is for only three months.
C. She can continue until she finishes the current pack.
D. She should change to the progesterone-only pill, as it is category 2.
E. She fulfills medical eligibility criteria 4.

16.

A 33-year-old woman is on the levonorgestrel intrauterine system. She has recently suffered from a cerebral transient ischaemic attack. She is now improving. The general practitioner asks for your advice as she still requires effective contraception.

What will you tell him?

A. Counsel her for sterilization.
B. Continue the same method if it was category 1 when first used.
C. Discontinue the method, as it is now a category 3.
D. Discontinue the method and offer a more suitable option.
E. She can use only barrier contraception.

17.

A 28-year-old woman who is on the combined hormonal contraceptive comes to see you because she has recently developed migraine without aura. She has thus far been happy with her current method of contraception.

What is your contraceptive advice?

A. She can continue because she has no aura.
B. She can continue if she has no risk factors for cerebrovascular accidents.
C. She can continue if she agrees to take low-dose aspirin.
D. She should discontinue, as the method is now category 3.
E. She can continue if she does not have a family history of cerebrovascular accidents.

18.

You are counselling a 30-year-old woman with hypertrophic cardiomyopathy regarding contraception. You explain that according to UKMEC, intrauterine (IUD) contraception is her best option.

What is your advice for prophylactic antibiotics?

A. A doxycycline dose for 10 days.
B. Azithromycin 1 gm stat dose.
C. A broad-spectrum antibiotic before IUD insertion and oral cephalosporin for five days.
D. A prophylactic dose for three days before IUD application.
E. There is no need to administer prophylactic antibiotics.

19.

Your consultant has successfully carried out a hysteroscopic tubal occlusion (Essure ESS305 microinsert. © Bayer). You are asked to review the patient before discharge.

What is the most important advice to give the patient prior to discharge?

A. She should come for a review after her next period.
B. She should seek medical advice if she misses her next period.
C. She should come for an X-ray after her next period to confirm proper placement of the occlusion device.
D. She should avoid intercourse until she has her next period.
E. She should use a reliable method of contraception for three months and until proper placement of the device is confirmed.

ANSWERS

Q1: A. Does not offer added protection.[1]

Q2: A. After two weeks.[2]

- Sexually transmitted infection (STI) screening tests are those for chlamydia, gonorrhoea, syphilis and HIV.
- Immediate testing will only identify current infection.
- An STI screen two weeks after exposure allows detection of infections acquired at the time of potential risk exposure.
- Individuals at a specific risk of HIV infections should have a repeat test at four weeks and 12 months from exposure.[2]

Q3: C. Her current pill has the lowest risk of blood clotting [evidence level 1+].[3]

- The risk of venous thromboembolis (VTE) is influenced by progestogen type.
- Combined hormonal contraceptives containing levonorgestrel, norethisterone or norgestimate, have the lowest risk (5–7/10 000 women) compared with those containing drospirenone, desogestrel or gestodene (9–12/10 000 women).[3]
- Compared to non-users, the risk of VTE with use of combined hormonal contraceptives is approximately doubled but the absolute risk is still very low.[3]

Examples of progestogens according to their classified 'generation'
- First generation: norethisterone acetate.
- Second generation: levonorgestrel.
- Third generation: desogestrel, gestodene, norgestimate.
- Fourth generation: drospirenone, dienogest, nomegestrol acetate.[3]

Q4: D. It is safe to use any progestogen-only method.[4,5]

- A thrombophilia screen is not recommended routinely for women considering hormonal contraception.[4]
- There is no evidence that progestogen-only methods increase the risk of venous thromboembolism [evidence level 3].[4]
- Because of her family history, the combined oral contraceptive is category 3 (the risk outweighs the advantage).[5]
- Even with her family history, according to the UK medical eligibility criteria (UKMEC) for progestogen-only methods or the copper intrauterine device, she comes under category 1 (there is no restriction)[5]

For women on anticoagulation
- The combined oral contraception is category 4 (unacceptable risk).[5]
- Progestogen-only methods are category 2 (the benefits outweigh the risk).[5]

Q5: A. Efficacy may be decreased because of her weight; she should use additional precautions or an alternative method should be advised [evidence level 3].[6]

- The Summary of Product Characteristics (SPC) for the combined transdermal patch (CTP) specifies that contraceptive efficacy may be decreased in women weighing ≥90 kg, therefore additional precautions or an alternative method should be advised.[6]

Q6: C. She is at no risk and it will help her period pains [evidence level 1−].[7]

- Current evidence from systematic reviews does not show an increased risk of breast cancer in women with a family history.
- UKMEC classifies her under category 1 (no restriction).[5]
- The combined hormonal contraceptive will offer her a long-term protection against ovarian cancer [evidence level 2+].[7]

Non-contraceptive benefits of CHC
- Improves and treats menstrual disorders (irregular periods, dysmenorrhea, premenstrual tension syndrome and menorrhagia).
- Reduces the risk of ovarian, endometrial and colorectal cancer.
- May improve acne and improve bone health.

Q7: D. Offer a single 3 mg dose of LNG (two Levonelle® tablets).[8]

- Enzyme-inducing drugs have the potential to decrease the contraceptive efficacy of levonelle.[2]
- Its use in this dose is outside product license.
- The use of lamotrigine with CHC is a UKMEC category 3 (risks outweigh the benefits).[5]
- The clinical effectiveness unit does not advise the use of the progesterone receptor modulator ulipristal acetate (UPA) (ellaOne®) for women on enzyme-inducing drugs.

Q8: B. Single dose of 30 mg micronized ulipristal acetate (ellaOne®) [evidence level 2+].[8]

- The 30 mg selective progesterone receptor modulator tablet ulipristal acetate (ellaOne®) is the only licenced oral emergency contraception that can be used between 72 and 120 hours after unprotected intercourse.[8]
- Ulipristal acetate is more effective than levonorgestrel in women who are categorized as overweight or obese [evidence level 2+, grade 1 recommendation].[8]

Q9: A. Either the copper intrauterine device (IUD) or the levonorgestrel (LNG) IUD is a suitable option.[9]

- Both copper and LNG IUDs have a protective effect against endometrial cancer [evidence level 1− and 2++].[9]
- Meta-analysis, systematic reviews and cohort studies have shown that the LNG IUD causes regression of endometrial hyperplasia and that the copper IUD has a protective effect against endometrial cancer.[9]
- A ≥35 kg/m^2 BMI is UKMEC for use of the combined oral contraceptive, which is category 3 (risk outweighs benefit).

Q10: D. She can use a product with cyproterone acetate (CPA/EE) [evidence level 1−].[10]

- A product with cyproterone acetate might result in better acne outcomes than one with desogestrel.
- CPA/EE may be prescribed as an oral contraceptive, although it is outside the product license.

Q11: B. She should change to another long-term reversible contraceptive [grade C recommendation].[11]

- Enzyme-inducing cytochrome P450 drugs may decrease the efficacy of progesterone-only contraception.

Q12: E. The long-acting injectable contraceptive may help reduce her crisis pain [evidence level 2++/grade of recommendation B].[12]

Q13: E. The copper intrauterine device.[5]

- The copper IUD is the only category 1 (safe to use) method; CHC is category 4 (unsafe), and all other options are category 3 (risks outweigh the benefits).

Sexually transmitted infection screening for IUD applications
- Women at increased risk should be tested prior to or at the time of insertion; however, it is not necessary to delay insertion until results are returned [evidence level 2−).[13] IUDs can be inserted immediately after a termination of pregnancy, but there are increased expulsion rates.[13]

Risk factors to screening for sexually transmitted infections (STIs)
- Risk factors include being sexually active and aged <25 years, having had a new sexual partner in the last three months, having had more than one sexual partner in the last year, having a regular sexual partner who has other sexual partners, having a history of STIs or attending as a previous contact of STI, alcohol/substance abuse.[13]

Q14: A. Age alone is not a contraindication to any method.[14]

Q15: E. She fulfills medical eligibility criteria 4.[5]

- Because of her expected long immobilization, she is under a grave risk of thromboembolism if she continues using the method. She may not consider stopping on her own, therefore attention should be drawn to the fact that she has to stop.

Q16: D. Discontinue the method and offer a more suitable option.

- Because of the new condition, the method has become a category 3 and she should discontinue it and be offered a category 1 contraception (barrier or a copper intrauterine device).[5]
- Option (A) is not the best as she has other options and should be counselled for all suitable options.[5]

Q17: D. She should discontinue, as the method is now category 3 [evidence level 2+, grade B recommendation].[5]

- An increased risk of both ischaemic stroke and ischaemic heart disease have been reported in women with headache who take the combined oral contraceptive.

Q18: E. There is no need to administer prophylactic antibiotics [evidence level 2–].[15]

- Cardiomyopathy increases the risk of bacterial endocarditis. However, there is insufficient evidence that the administration of prophylactic antibiotics reduces the incidence of infective endocarditis.[15]

Q19: E. She should use a reliable method of contraception for three months and until proper placement of the device is confirmed.[16]

- An X-ray after three months is required to confirm the proper placement of the device.

References

1. World Health Organization. *WHO/CONRAD Technical Consultation on Nonoxynol-9.* October, 2001. [http://whqlibdoc.who.int/hq/2003/WHO_RHR_03.08.pdf]
2. Radcliffe K, Edwards S. *BASHH Statement on HIV Window Period.* October, 2014. [https://www.bashh.org]
3. de Bastos M, Stegeman BH, Rosendaal FR, et al. Combined oral contraceptives: venous thrombosis. *Cochrane Database Syst Rev* 2014;19(5):194.
4. Faculty of Sexual and Reproductive Healthcare. *Venous Thromboembolism (VTE) and Hormonal Contraception.* November, 2014. [www.fsrh.org]
5. Faculty of Sexual and Reproductive Healthcare. *UK Medical Eligibility Criteria for Contraceptive Use.* May, 2016. [www.fsrh.org]
6. Janssen-Cilag Ltd. *Evra Transdermal Patch. Summary of Product Characteristics.* May, 2016. [https://www.medicines.org.org/emc/medicine]
7. Gaffield ME, Culwell KR, Ravi A. Oral contraceptives and family history of breast cancer. *Contraception* 2009;80:372–80.
8. Faculty of Sexual and Reproductive Healthcare Clinical Effectiveness Unit. *Emergency Contraception.* August, 2011. [www.fsrh.org/pdfs/CEUguidance/Contraception]
9. Gallos ID, Shehmar M, Thangaratinam S, et al. Oral progestogens vs levonorgestrel-releasing intrauterine system for endometrial hyperplasia: a systematic review and meta-analysis. *Am J Obstet Gynecol* 2010;203:547–10.
10. Arowojolu AO, Gallo MF, Lopez LM, Grimes DA, Garner SE. Combined oral contraceptive pills for treatment of acne. *Cochrane Database Syst Rev* 2007;(1): CD004425.
11. Faculty of Sexual and Reproductive Healthcare Clinical Effectiveness Unit. *Progestogen-only Pills.* March, 2015. [www.fsrh.org/pdfs/CEU/ProgestogenOnly Pills.pdf]
12. Faculty of Sexual and Reproductive Healthcare Clinical Effectiveness Unit. *Progestogen-only Injectable Contraception.* December, 2014. [www.Users/pc/Down loads/cec-ceu-guidance-injectables-dec-2014.pdf]
13. Society of Obstetricians and Gynaecologists of Canada. *Best Practices to Minimize Risk of Infection with Intrauterine Device Insertion.* March, 2014. [www.sogc.org/ wp-content/uploads]
14. Faculty of Sexual and Reproductive Health Care Clinical Effectiveness Unit. *Contraception for Women Aged Over 40 Years.* July, 2010. [www.fsrh.org/pdfs/ ContraceptionOver40July10.pdf]
15. Faculty of Sexual and Reproductive Health Clinical Effectiveness Unit. *Antibiotic Prophylaxis for Intrauterine Contraceptive Use in Women at Risk of Bacterial Endocarditis.* July, 2008. [www.fsrh.org/pdfs]
16. Bayer. *Could Essure® Be Right for Me?* 2014. [www.essure.com/what-is-essure]

Chapter 12

Paediatric and Adolescent Gynaecology

QUESTIONS

1.

A seven-year-old girl is brought to the clinic because she has been having regular monthly bleeds for the last four months. You suspect gonadotropin-dependent precocious puberty. What is the gold standard to confirm your diagnosis?

A. Accelerated growth velocity of more than 6 cm/year.
B. Advanced bone age.
C. A pearl-shaped uterine length >35 mm with an endometrial line.
D. Brain MRI to exclude intracranial pathology.
E. Luteinizing hormone (LH) peak after gonadotropin-releasing hormone (GnRH) stimulation.

2.

A six-year-old girl is referred to the clinic because she showed signs of precocious puberty (thelarchy, adrenarche and menarche). She was otherwise healthy and asymptomatic.

What is the incidence of this condition in girls?

A. 1 in 1000–2000.
B. 1 in 3000–5000.
C. 1 in 5000–10 000.
D. 1 in 10 000–20 000.
E. 1 in 20 000–50 000.

3.

A 12-year-old girl is referred because she has had regular vaginal bleeding for the last four months, although her breasts had not developed beyond a small breast bud and she had no visible pubic hair. She is otherwise asymptomatic with a normal growth velocity.

The most likely diagnosis is:

A. A normal variant.
B. An abnormal variant.
C. Central precocious puberty.
D. Oestrogen-secreting ovarian tumour.
E. Pseudo-precocious puberty.

4.

A five-year-old girl presents with a history of accelerated growth, menarche and signs of sexual development. Examination revealed light to dark brown spots, predominantly noticeable on one side of the body without crossing the midline.

What is your differential diagnosis?

A. Central precocious puberty.
B. Cushing syndrome.
C. Exogenous oestrogen exposure.
D. Iatrogenic excessive use of cortisol treatment.
E. McCune–Albright syndrome.

5.

A five-year-old girl is referred because of Tanner classification stage 3 breast development, pubic hair growth and irregular uterine bleeding. She also complained of the occasional right-sided abdominal pain.

Based on her history, what is your first line of investigation?

A. Abdominal MRI.
B. Gonadotropin challenge test.
C. Pelvic ultrasound.
D. Serum oestrogen.
E. Tumour markers.

6.

A mother presents with her seven-year-old daughter. The girl has developed noticeable pubic and axillary hair growth. The daughter is otherwise asymptomatic with no history of vaginal bleeding. On examination, pubic hair was easily noticeable, but the area covered is smaller than in most adults without spread to the medial side of the thighs. Her breasts had not developed beyond a small bud. Physical examination did not reveal any abnormality with a normal linear growth pattern.

What is your provisional diagnosis?

A. Central precocious puberty.
B. Cushing syndrome.
C. Pseudopuberty.
D. Physiological premature adrenarchy.
E. Virilizing ovarian tumours.

7.

A mother comes to see you with her six and a half-year-old child. The child has had an advanced growth spurt with thelarchy and adrenarchy to Tanner classification stage 4, and with regular uterine bleeding for the last five months. Her bone age report showed she is three years more advanced than her chronological age. A pelvic ultrasound showed a pear-shaped uterus and with a 4 mm endometrial thickening and normal ovaries. She was otherwise asymptomatic with no signs of any illnesses or disorders.

What is your diagnosis?

A. Central precocious puberty (CPP).
B. Hyperthyroidism.
C. McCune–Albright syndrome.
D. Oestrogen-secreting ovarian tumours.
E. Pseudopuberty.

8.

A 6-year-old girl presents to the outpatient clinic with a diagnosis of central precocious puberty. Her bone age/height ratio was less than 1.2.

What management do you offer her to attain a normal adult height?

A. A combination of gonadotrophin-releasing hormone antagonist and growth hormone.
B. Aromatase inhibitors.
C. Gonadotrophin releasing hormone antagonist.
D. No pharmacotherapy is required.
E. Oral progestogens.

9.

A 6-year-old girl comes with her mother because she has been bleeding vaginally for the last week.

What is the most common cause of this complaint?

A. Foreign body.
B. Precocious puberty.
C. Sexual abuse.
D. Uretheral prolapse.
E. Vulvovaginitis.

10.

During your labour ward on call, the midwife asks you to see a newborn baby; she is unable to assign the sex of the baby because of abnormal-looking external genitals. On examination, you realized the baby has ambiguous genitalia.

What is the incidence of ambiguous genitalia and uncertain sex?

A. 1 in 500 newborn babies.
B. 1 in 1000 newborn babies.
C. 1 in 2000 newborn babies.
D. 1 in 3000 newborn babies.
E. 1 in 4500 newborn babies.

11.

You delivered a baby with complete fusion of the labioscrotal folds, absent scrotal gonads and clitoromegaly. You provisionally diagnosed congenital adrenal hyperplasia (CAH).

When do you expect to observe clinical signs of a salt-losing form of the disease?

A. Between the fourth and the 14th day.
B. In the first three days.

C. Immediately after birth.
D. Only discovered incidentally after blood tests.
E. When the child reaches adulthood.

12.

You are asked by the midwife to review a baby she has just delivered because she was not able to identify the sex of the baby. Your examination reveals ambiguous genitalia.

What is your first urgent investigation?

A. Blood karyotyping.
B. Magnetic resonance imaging.
C. Serum cortisol and or 17-hydroxyprogesterone.
D. Testosterone response to human chorionic gonadotrophin (hCG).
E. Ultrasound for internal organ anatomy.

13.

A 14-week pregnant woman attends your antenatal clinic. She is worried because she has a relative who delivered an ambiguous genitalia child. She is wondering if there are any NHS screening tests carried out at delivery to make an early diagnosis.

What will you tell her about the current recommendations in the UK Screening Policy for Congenital Adrenal Hyperplasia (CAH)?

A. Adrenocorticotropic hormone (ACTH)-stimulation test is the accepted screening test because it is valuable in cases of mild forms of CAH with normal basal adrenal steroids.
B. Basal plasma 17-hydroxyprogesterone (17-OHPG) immunoassay is an accurate screening test.
C. Excess serum androgen is a valuable screening test for clinical hyperandrogenism.
D. Genotype analysis of the 21-OH gene.
E. The current UK National Screening Committee (UKNSC) does not recommend screening for CAH as part of the newborn bloodspot screening programme.

14.

A mother brings her five-year-old girl to the clinic. She noticed early excess pubic and body hair with clitoromegaly. She also noticed that her girl is taller than her peers. You suspect a mild non-classical form of CAH.

What is the most sensitive investigation to diagnose mild forms of CAH?

A. Adrenocorticotrophic hormone (ACTH)-stimulation test.
B. Basal plasma 17-hydroxy progesterone (17-OHPG).
C. Molecular gene analyses.
D. Testosterone, DHEA-S, androstenedione.
E. Urinary steroid profile.

15.

The parents of a baby girl with ambiguous genitalia are requesting your advice for immediate cosmetic surgery to correct her ambiguous genitalia.

You counsel them that it should be carried out:

A. After initiation of breastfeeding.
B. In the neonatal period, if there is an imminent threat to the child's health.

C. In the neonatal period to overcome parental distress.
D. In the neonatal period to reinforce early gender assignment.
E. Not in the immediate neonatal period.

16.

The general practitioner calls you to ask about the best test to measure the adequacy of glucocorticoid treatment for a two-year-old baby with CAH.

What will you tell him?

A. Measure 17-hydroxyprogesterone (17-OHP) every month.
B. Measure hydroxyprogesterone every three months.
C. Measure 17-hydroxyprogesterone (17-OHP), androstenedione and testosterone every three months.
D. Measure plasma renin and electrolytes.
E. Measure plasma cortisol.

17.

A fifteen and a half-year-old girl presents to the outpatient department complaining of absent menstruation. On examination, she has well-developed breasts but no pubic or axillary hair. Ultrasound reveals absent ovaries, no uterus and no upper vagina.

What is your provisional diagnosis?

A. Complete androgen insensitivity syndrome.
B. Congenital adrenal hyperplasia.
C. Mild androgen insensitivity syndrome.
D. Partial androgen insensitivity syndrome.
E. True hermaphroditism.

18.

A twenty-eight-year-old woman who has just delivered a baby with complete androgen insensitivity (AIS) comes to ask you about her risk in a future pregnancy of having a child with the same condition.

You tell her that there is:

A. A 50% likelihood of an affected male offspring and a healthy female carrier.
B. A 25% likelihood of an affected male carrier.
C. A 25% likelihood of an affected female sibling.
D. A 50% likelihood of an affected male sibling and no likelihood of female carriers.
E. A 50% likelihood of affected female carriers.

19.

The mother of a three-year-old child with complete androgen insensitivity syndrome and undescended gonads comes to the clinic asking about removal of the undescended testicles. She has heard there is a risk that they would become malignant.

How will you counsel her with regard to timing of orchiectomy?

A. Advise early removal to prevent osteoporosis.
B. Advise removed after puberty
C. Advise testosterone replacement therapy if necessary, if the gonads are removed before puberty.
D. Suggest removal before puberty if the undescended testes are physically or aesthetically uncomfortable and/or if inguinal herniorrhaphy is necessary.
E. Tell her malignancy is more common before puberty.

20.

A mother of a three-year-old child with incomplete androgen sensitivity syndrome brings the child to the clinic. She asks about the best time for cosmetic vaginal surgery. On examination, you notice mild clitoromegaly, some fusion of the labia and undescended testes.

How will you counsel her?

A. Surgery should be carried out immediately.
B. Surgery should be delayed until the child is more mature, e.g. at the age of five years.
C. Surgery should be carried out immediately before puberty.
D. Surgery should be carried out at puberty.
E. Surgery should be carried out in adulthood.

21.

A 15-year-old girl is referred by her general practitioner because she has not yet menstruated. The general practitioner's letter states that she has been diagnosed as Turner syndrome.

What is the percentage of this condition in the female population at birth?

A. 1 in 1000–1 in 2000.
B. 1 in 2500–1 in 3000.
C. 1 in 3500–1 in 5000.
D. 1 in 7000–1 in 10 000.
E. 1 in 15 000–1 in 20 000.

22.

A 36-year-old Hispanic woman who previously had a child affected by Turner syndrome consults you because she is considering another pregnancy. She is worried about recurrence of this condition.

What advice will you give her regarding the inheritance of Turner syndrome?

A. Turner syndrome is an inherited disease passed from the mother to her offspring.
B. Turner syndrome is an inherited disease passed from the father to the baby.
C. Turner syndrome is a paternal inherited disorder.
D. Turner syndrome is usually not passed from mother to child.
E. Turner syndrome is more common in Hispanic women.

23.

A 39-year-old woman came to see you when she was 13 weeks pregnant. The triple screening test showed abnormal levels of human chorionic gonadotropin, unconjugated oestriol and alpha-fetoprotein. The ultrasound scan showed severe lymph oedema, a cystic hygroma and a horse shoe kidney.

Based on these findings, what is your provisional diagnosis?

A. Down syndrome.
B. Edward syndrome.
C. Klinefelter syndrome.
D. Patau syndrome.
E. Turner syndrome.

24.

A woman brings in her 10-year-old-girl complaining of short stature. A standard karyotyping has confirmed your clinical diagnoses of Turner syndrome.

What management options will you offer?

A. A combination of oestrogen and growth hormone.
B. Continuous non-cyclical progestogens.
C. Oestrogen therapy.
D. Recombinant growth hormone and progesterone therapy.
E. Recombinant growth hormone.

ANSWERS

Q1: E. Luteinizing hormone (LH) peak after gonadotropin-releasing hormone (GnRH) stimulation.[1]

- Precocious puberty is the development of pubertal maturation before the age of eight years in girls.
- Central precocious puberty (CPP) is due to premature activation of the hypothalamic–pituitary–ovarian axis. The pulsatile secretion of GnRH leads to increase in the LH levels and, to a lesser degree, of follicle stimulating hormone (FSH).
- The premature appearance of clinical pubertal symptoms of breast development (thelarchy) and pubic and axillary hair (adrenarchy) does not always indicate precocious puberty. It may be a variant of a slowly progressive pubertal development.[1]
- The gold standard for the diagnosis of CPP remains the rise of LH in response to GnRH stimulation.
- The test distinguishes centrally mediated from gonadotrophin-independent precocious puberty.[1]
- The standard test included measuring LH and FSH levels 30–60 min after stimulation with GnRH at 100 mcg or with a GnRH analogue.
- Brain MRI is carried out to exclude intracranial reasons for precocious puberty.
- Central nervous system (CNS) abnormalities associated with precocious puberty include tumors (eg, astrocytomas, gliomas, germ-cell tumours secreting human chorionic gonadotropin (hCG)), hypothalamic hamartomas, acquired CNS insult (inflammation or infection), surgery, trauma or radiation.
- A family history of precocious puberty was found in 25% of cases. A positive family history is relevant and helps to decrease the likelihood of an organic cause [evidence level 3].

Q2: C. 1 in 5000–10 000.[1,2]

Q3: A. A normal variant [evidence level 2b].

- The development of regular menstruation before breast and pubic hair development can occur in normal girls who do not have clinical evidence of any hormonal imbalance.
- As she is over the age of eight years, she does not comply with the definition of precocious puberty.
- The incidence of oestrogen-producing ovarian tumours in young adolescents is only 5%. Oestrogen-secreting ovarian tumours cause breast development and irregular uterine bleeding rather than a regular menstrual bleed.
- Marshall and Tanner[2] studied the variations in the pattern of pubertal changes in girls. Breast and pubic hair development was divided into five stages: stage 1,

prepubertal; stage 2, early development of subareolar breast bud and small amounts of pubic and axillary hair; stage 3, increase in size of palpable breast tissue and areolae, increased amount of dark pubic hair and of axillary hair; stage 4, further increase in breast size and areolae that protrude above breast level and of adult pubic hair; the last stage 5 is the adult stage, with full-contour adult breast size and pubic hair with extension to the upper thigh.

- Stages 2, 3 and 4 occur between the ages of 11 and 12, while stage 5 is usually completed by the age of 14–15 years of age.[7]

Q4: E. McCune–Albright syndrome.[3]

- **McCune–Albright syndrome** (MAS) is a gonadotropin-independent precocious pseudopuberty, due to somatic mutation in the *GNAS1* gene.
  - It is characterized by *café-au-lait* skin pigmentation ranging from light brown to dark brown in colour, often displaying a segmental distribution, and frequently on one side of the body without crossing the midline. It is associated with precocious puberty and bony fibrous dysplasia affecting long bones, the pelvis, skull and fascial bones. It is rare, with an estimated prevalence that is between 1/100 000 and 1/1 000 000.
  - Oestrogen receptor antagonist binds to oestrogen receptors and inhibits the action of oestrogen (e.g. raloxifene and tamoxifen). Treatment is well tolerated and is moderately effective in decreasing vaginal bleeding and rates of skeletal maturation in girls with MAS.
- **Cushing syndrome** is due to endogenous (adrenal glands) or exogenous prolonged exposure to cortisol. Signs include high BP, abdominal obesity but with thin arms and legs, reddish stretch marks, a round red face, a fat lump between the shoulders, weak muscles, weak bones, acne and fragile skin that heals poorly and irregular menstruation. It is not associated with accelerated growth.
  - Treatment by medications to reduce the cortisol levels (e.g. cabergoline can normalize adrenocorticotropic hormone (ACTH) and cortisol production). Surgery may be indicated for pituitary tumours or may be adrenalectomy.

Q5: C. Pelvic ultrasound [evidence level 3].[4]

- Because of her pubertal growth before the age of eight years, she may have central or precocious pseudopuberty or oestrogen-secreting tumours of the ovary.
- The first-line diagnostic test to differentiate central from precocious pseudopuberty is the LH peak after GnRH stimulation, but as she is complaining of the occasional right-sided abdominal pain, her signs and symptoms may be due to steroid-secreting ovarian tumours. Pelvic ultrasonography is mandatory if precocious pseudopuberty is suspected in girls because an ovarian tumour or cyst may be detected. Pelvic ultrasound is least expensive and offers instantaneous results.
- The most likely ovarian tumour in this case is granulosa cell tumour (GCT) (5%).
- In oestrogen-secreting ovarian cysts or granulosa cell tumours, oestradiol levels often exceed 100 pg/mL.
- **The aetiology of precocious pseudopuberty** includes congenital adrenal hyperplasia (CAH), human chorionic gonadotropin (hCG)-secreting tumours, tumours of the adrenal gland, ovary or testis, McCune–Albright syndrome (MAS), aromatase excess syndromes or iatrogenic pseudopuberty due to exposure to exogenous oestrogens.

Q6: D. Physiological premature adrenarchy [evidence level 2b].[5]

- Central precocious puberty and pseudopuberty also include thelarchy and menarche along with accelerated growth, which this girl did not have besides the adrenarchy. She has no signs or symptoms of Cushing syndrome.
- Virilizing ovarian tumours cause other signs of virilization (increased facial hair, acne, deepening of the voice and clitoromegaly).
- As she was otherwise completely normal without accelerated growth or signs of virilization, her symptoms are due to a normal variant of pubertal development owing to idiopathic premature adrenal androgen secretion.[5]
- In the Marshall and Tanner study, around 10% of the girls had adult secondary sexual characteristics before they began to menstruate and 2% had pubic hair growth to stage 4, while the breast had developed only to stage 2.[2]

Q7: A. Central precocious puberty (CPP) [evidence level 3].[4,6]

- This girl did not have any signs of any syndromes, which confidently excludes pseudopuberty. Her pelvic ultrasound showed a postpubertal uterine growth with no ovarian cysts.
- Girls with CPP show a marked increase in growth velocity beyond the average 5–6 cm yearly increase in height. The bone age is more than two years in advance of the chronological age.[4]
- Bone age measures how far the child has advanced in the development of the skeleton. A single X-ray of the left wrist, hand and fingers estimates bone age. There is small radiation exposure.
- Bone age is estimated according to the Greulich–Pyle bone age scale.[6]
- Hyperthyroidism has been reported to accelerate growth in normal children and in patients with Turner syndrome. It is, however, not associated with pubertal changes.[4]

Q8: D. No pharmacotherapy is required [evidence level 3].[7]

- If the ratio of bone age to height age is <1.2 and remains so, normal height potential is likely to be maintained, and no pharmacotherapy is indicated.[7]
- GnRH agonists are the medical treatment of choice for rapidly progressive complete precocious puberty.[7]
- The main treatment to achieve a normal final height is GnRH agonist.
- The mean duration of treatment is between three and five years.[7]
- The addition of growth hormone for two to three years during the conventional treatment with GnRH analogue improves final adult height [evidence level 2b].[7]
- GnRH analogue treatment is safe for the reproductive system, bone mineral density and BMI and helps to achieve the target height.[7]

Q9: E. Vulvovaginitis.[8]

- Vulvovaginitis is generally considered to be the most common gynaecological problem in prepubertal girls.[8]
- Different causes of vulvovaginitis (yeast, bacteria, viruses and parasites, bubble baths, soaps, sprays and perfumes or lack of cleanliness) are the most common cause of vaginal bleeding during the prepubertal period.
- Sexual abuse is not found to be a common contributing factor for the development of vulvovaginitis.[8]
- In prepubertal girls, low oestrogen levels cause thinning and dryness of the vulval and vaginal skin, leading to irritation and itching. Intense itching may cause bleeding.

Q10: E. 1 in 4500 newborn babies [evidence level 2+].[9]

Q11: A. Between the fourth and the 14th day [evidence level 2+].[10]

- Salt loss and hyperkalaemia in congenital adrenal hyperplasia (CAH) may not be apparent at birth and will not usually occur until between the fourth and 14th day.[10]

Congenital adrenal hyperplasia (CAH): an autosomal recessive condition
- Human adrenal glands synthesize three main classes of hormones: mineralo-corticoids, glucocorticoids and sex steroids.
- CAH is a heterogeneous group of inherited disorders due to 21-hydroxylase (21-OH) enzyme deficiency.[10] This results in deficiency of glucocorticoid characterized by impaired adrenal cortisol biosynthesis, impaired mineralocorticoid (aldosterone) and androgen excess.
- The aldosterone mineralocorticoid causes increased sodium loss and potassium retention while excess androgen causes the different androgenic effects.

The clinical forms of CAH are classified as:
- The classical form (the severe form), which presents in the neonatal period.
- The non-classical form (the mild or late-onset form), which presents in adolescence or adulthood.
- The asymptomatic cryptic form.
- **The classic severe form** is sub-classified as the salt-wasting (SW) (75%) or the simple-virilizing (SV) form (25%). The salt-losing form (SW) is characterized by aldosterone deficiency resulting in reduced sodium (<125 mmol/L) and rising potassium levels. In the SW form, neonates present at age one to four weeks with failure to thrive, recurrent vomiting, dehydration, hypotension, hyponatremia, hyperkalemia, and shock. If hyperkalemia is not treated, it will lead to circulatory collapse and death.
- Females with the severe virilizing form are born with signs of ambiguous genitalia ranging from complete or partial fusion of the labioscrotal folds, clitoromegaly, or both.
- **In the non-classical mild or late form**, signs and symptoms usually appear after five years of age. Androgen excess causes premature development of pubic and axillary hair, accelerated growth but with short final height (because of early epiphyseal fusion). Adult females may have delayed or irregular menstruation and infertility and may develop virilzation (hirsutism, acne and temporal baldness).
- The differential diagnosis of non-classical CAH includes polycystic ovary syndrome (PCOS), Cushing syndrome, hyperprolactinemia, thyroid dysfunction and androgen-secreting tumours.
- Salt-wasting form should be anticipated in a baby with ambiguous genitalia until CAH has been excluded. The state of hydration and BP should be assessed.
- The urine should be checked for protein as a screen for any associated renal anomaly.

Treatment of CAH
- Glucocorticoids to replace cortisone deficiency (hydrocortisone, dexamethasone, prednisolone and prednisone).
- Intravenous or oral sodium chloride in the salt-losing forms.
- Mineralocorticoids (fludrocortisone acetate) to promote sodium retention in exchange for potassium or hydrogen ions and thus maintain intravascular and extracellular volume.

Q12: A. Blood karyotyping [evidence level 2+].[10]

- Genetic sex will define subsequent investigations and management and will help in differential diagnosis, consequently an urgent karyotyping is the primary investigation.
- It should be carried out in day 1.
- A full karyotype is still required to confirm or exclude mosaicism.[10]
- Magnetic resonance imaging is useful to identify undescended gonads and any associated renal abnormalities but it will not identify genetic sex.

Q13: E. The current UK National Screening Committee (UKNSC) does not recommend screening for CAH as part of the newborn bloodspot screening programme.[11]

- A systemic review for screening studies has shown that the screening tests are less likely to identify mild conditions of the disorder in preterm babies.
- Screening test results may not be available in time to prevent death from the severe salt-wasting form of the disease.

Q14: A. Adrenocorticotrophic hormone (ACTH)-stimulation test [evidence level 3].[10]

- All of these investigations can help to diagnose CAH. Basal plasma 17-OHPG is the primary test, but it is not sensitive enough in mild forms of CAH.
- The ACTH-stimulation test is the preferred test to evaluate adrenal gland function in mild forms of CAH with normal basal adrenal steroids. CAH is considered if basal 17-OHPG levels are elevated and/or ACTH-stimulated 17-OHPG is >260 ng/dL (7.87 nmol/L) above the basal level.[10]

Q15: B. In the neonatal period, if there is an imminent threat to the child's health [evidence level 3].[12]

- Cosmetic genital surgeries are rarely indicated in the immediate neonatal period unless there is an imminent threat to the child's health, e.g. creating a new urinary opening or removing malignant tissue.[12]
- Surgery is more effective if it is delayed until after puberty to involve the patients in the decision making and to make sure surgery will match the developed chosen gender identity rather than the initial assigned gender.[12]
- Delaying surgery until after puberty will also avoid the need for repeated surgeries.
- Gender assignment is a complex interaction between genes, environment and social circumstances. It is more of a social and legal process than a medical or surgical intervention, or chromosomal or phenotypic sex.[12]

Q16: C. Measure 17-hydroxyprogesterone (17-OHP), androstenedione and testosterone every three months [evidence level 2+].[13]

- Electrolytes and plasma renin assess the mineralocorticoid treatment.
- 17-OPH, androstenedione and testosterone assess the glucocorticoid treatment.

Q17: A. Complete androgen insensitivity syndrome.[14]

- In androgen insensitivity syndrome (AIS) (sometimes known as testicular feminization syndrome), there is complete or partial failure of external genitals to respond to androgens.[14]
- There are mutations in the androgen receptor gene with insensitivity of internal and external male genitals to androgens.

- AIS is an X-linked disease with variable defects in virilization of a 46,XY individual.
  - Affected individuals are a 46,XY male karyotype.
  - AIS individuals have a well-developed testis but underdevelopment of the epididemis, vas deferens and seminal vesicles, the scrotum and the penis.[14]
- The testis may be found in any position, mostly in the inguinal region or anywhere from the abdomen to the scrotum/labia majora [evidence level 2−].[14]
  - All forms of androgen insensitivity are associated with infertility.
  - AIS does not affect female XX fetuses.

Based on the phenotype, AIS is classified into three clinical subgroups:
- **Complete androgen insensitivity syndrome** (CAIS).
  - In complete CAIS, the male XY fetus is born with female or ambiguous genitalia.
  - Treatment includes gonadectomy and oestrogen replacement therapy.
- **Mild androgen insensitivity syndrome** (MAIS), when the external genitalia are that of a normal male.
  - They may present with isolated infertility (oligospermia or azoospermia), mild gynaecomastia in young adulthood, decreased secondary terminal hair, high-pitched voice or minor hypospadias.
  - They have normal external male genitalia (penis, scrotum and urethra) and normal Wolffian structures (the epididymides, vasa deferentia and seminal vesicles). The prostate is also normal.
  - Treatment of MAIS includes surgical correction of mild gynaecomastia, minor hypospadias repair and testosterone supplementation.
- **Partial androgen insensitivity syndrome** (PAIS), when the external genitalia are partially but not fully masculinized.
  - Main treatment is testosterone and/or dihydrotestosterone (DHT).

True hermaphroditism is a very rare condition with both ovaries and testicular tissue in the same individual.

Q18: A. A 50% likelihood of an affected male offspring and a healthy female carrier.[14]

- The mother is usually a healthy carrier.
- The affected XY infants receive the X-linked androgen receptor mutation from their carrier mothers.

Q19: D. Suggest removal before puberty if the undescended testes are physically or aesthetically uncomfortable and/or if inguinal herniorrhaphy is necessary [evidence level 4].[15]

- Experts recommend removal of the undescended testes after puberty, if the undescended testes are physically or aesthetically uncomfortable and/or if inguinal herniorrhaphy is necessary.[15]
- Early removal before puberty will expose the patient to lack of oestrogen with less feminization, risk of osteoporosis and delayed puberty.
- If the gonads are removed before puberty, oestrogen administration is required.
- There is no indication to administer progesterone because there is no uterus.[15]
- The gonadal malignancy risk (5%) seldom occurs before puberty.[15]

Q20: D. Surgery should be carried out at puberty.[15]

- Cosmetic reconstructive genital surgery is best delayed until puberty, when the individual is mature enough to decide on gender assignment and to avoid recurrent surgery.[15]

Q21: B. 1 in 2500–1 in 3000.[16]

- Turner syndrome babies are born with swelling of the hands and feet, redundant nuchal skin with a webbed neck, a broad chest, a low hairline and low-set ears.
- **Turner syndrome** is due to absence of the Y-chromosome (monosomy 45,XO); 30%–50% of Turner syndrome babies have typical 45,XO monosomy and are diagnosed at birth because of the classic features as given here.
- One third of Turner syndrome patients have a cardiac malformation (e.g. coarctation of the aorta or a bicuspid aortic valve).
- Babies with **Klinefelter syndrome** are XXY males, but do not show any clinical signs until they reach early adulthood.[16]
- Babies born with trisomy 18 (**Edward syndrome**) have some or all of: kidney malformations, structural heart defects (e.g. ventricular septal defect, atrial septal defect, patent ductus arteriosus), omphalocele and oesophageal atresia.[16]

Q22: D. Turner syndrome is usually not passed from mother to child.[16]

- Generally, Turner syndrome is not passed on from mother to child. In most cases, Turner syndrome is a sporadic event. The risk of recurrence is not increased for subsequent pregnancies.[16]

Q23: E. Turner syndrome [evidence level 3].[17]

- The prenatal diagnosis of Turner syndrome is suspected when there is elevation of the triple test components, serum alpha-fetoprotein (SAFP), unconjugated oestriol (UE_3) and elevated human chorionic gonadotropin (BhCG) together with ultrasound signs of generalized oedema and renal tract abnormalities.[17]
- **Down syndrome** is not usually associated with renal congenital anomalies and the triple test shows a low SAFP and UE_3 but elevated BhCG.
- In **Edward syndrome** (trisomy 18), the most common prenatal ultrasound characteristic is cardiac anomalies, followed by central nervous system anomalies such as microcephaly and head shape abnormalities. The most common intracranial anomaly is the presence of choroid plexus cysts. The triple test shows low levels of all three components (SAFP, UE_3 and BhCG) [evidence level 3].[6,7]
- **Klinefelter syndrome** does not show any ultrasound evidence of hydrops or other markers of structural or chromosomal abnormalities and is usually diagnosed clinically during late childhood or early adulthood.[8]
- **Patau syndrome** is characterized by a chromosomal abnormality (trisomy 13), where some or all the body cells contain extra genetic material from chromosome 13. It is usually diagnosed clinically after birth. There are no specific ultrasound features and the biochemical screening is not reliable as the results show different and variable levels.[17]
- In all these conditions, the final diagnosis depends on invasive testing and karyotyping (chorionic villous sampling or amniocentesis).

Q24: E. Recombinant growth hormone [evidence level 2+].[18]

- The treatment of Turner syndrome includes growth hormone to achieve a normal final height, oestrogen to prevent oesteoporoses and induce regular menstruation, and progesterone to protect against endometrial hyperplasia and uterine adenocarcinoma.

References

1. Chalumeau M, Chemaitilly W, Trivin C, et al. Central precocious puberty in girls: an evidence-based diagnosis tree to predict central nervous system abnormalities. *Pediatrics* 2002;109(1):61–7.
2. Marshall WA, Tanner JM. Variations in pattern of pubertal changes in girls. *Arch Dis Childh* 1969;44:291.
3. Sims EK, Garnett S, Guzman F, et al. Fulvestrant treatment of precocious puberty in girls with McCune-Albright syndrome. *Int J Pediatr Endocrinol* 2012;2012(1):26.
4. Sekkate S, Kairouani M, Serji B, et al. Ovarian granulosa cell tumors: a retrospective study of 27 cases and a review of the literature. *World J Surg Oncol* 2013;11:142.
5. Oberfield SE, Sopher AB, Gerken AT. Approach to the girl with early onset of pubic hair. *J Clin Endocrinol Metab* 2011;96(6):1610–22.
6. Greulich WW, Pyle SI. *Radiographic Atlas of Skeletal Development of the Hand and Wrist*, 2nd edn. Stanford, CA: Stanford University Press, 1959.
7. Leger J, Reynaud R, Czernichow P. Do all girls with apparent idiopathic precocious puberty require gonadotropin-releasing hormone agonist treatment? *J Pediatr* 2000;137:819–25.
8. McCormack WM. Vulvovaginitis and cervicitis. In: Mandell GL, Bennett JE, Dolin R, eds. *Principles and Practice of Infectious Diseases*, 7th edn. Philadelphia, PA: Elsevier Churchill Livingstone, 2009; Ch. 107.
9. The Intersex Society of North America. *How Common is Intersex?* [www.isna.org/faq/frequency]
10. Ogilvy-Stuart AL, Brain CE. Early assessment of ambiguous genitalia. *Arch Dis Child* 2004;89:401–7.
11. Wilson G. *Screening for Congenital Adrenal Congenital Hyperplasia, External Review Against Programme Appraisal Criteria for the UK National Screening Committee.* Ver. 2.0. June, 2015. [www.legacy.screening.nhs.uk/adrenalhyperplasia]
12. Dessens A, Slijper F, Drop S. Gender dysphoria and gender change in chromosomal females with congenital adrenal hyperplasia. *Arch Sex Behav* 2005;34(4):389–97.
13. Schaeffer TL, Tryggestad JB, Mallappa A, et al. An evidence-based model of multidisciplinary care for patients and families affected by classical congenital adrenal hyperplasia due to 21-hydroxylase deficiency. *Int J Pediatr Endocrinol.* 2010;2010:692439.
14. Galani A, Kitsiou-Tzeli S, Sofokleous C, Kanavakis E, Kalpini-Mavrou A. Androgen insensitivity syndrome: clinical features and molecular defects. *Hormones (Athens)* 2008;7(3):217–29.
15. Dacou-Voutetakis C. A multidisciplinary approach to the management of children with complex genital anomalies. *Nat Clin Pract Endocrinol Metab* 2007;3:668–9.
16. Gardner RJ, Sutherland GR. *Chromosome Abnormalities and Genetic Counselling*, 3rd edn. New York, NY: Oxford University Press, 2004; pp. 199–200.
17. Sybert VP, McCauley E. Turner's syndrome. *N Engl J Med* 2004;351:1227–38.
18. Quigley CA, Crowe BJ, Anglin DG, Chipman JJ. Growth hormone and low dose estrogen in Turner syndrome: results of a United States multi-center trial to near-final height. *J Clin Endocrinol Metab* 2002;87:2033–41.

Chapter 13

Genital Infections and Pelvic Inflammatory Disease

Ahmed M Khalil

QUESTIONS

1.

A 21-year-old woman comes to the accident and emergency unit complaining of bilateral lower abdominal pain and fever. On examination, her temperature is 38.2°C with bilateral adnexal tenderness.

What is your first line of investigation?

A. Endocervical swab for gonorrhoea and chlamydia.
B. HIV antibody test.
C. Pelvic ultrasound.
D. Pregnancy test.
E. Total leucocyte count.

2.

A 21-year-old woman comes to the outpatient clinic requesting testing for gonorrhoea as she read a poster about gonorrhoea infection. She has had three sexual partners in the last year but uses condoms for contraception.

What tests should you offer her?

A. Gonorrhoea only.
B. Gonorrhoea and chlamydia.
C. Gonorrhoea, chlamydia, HIV and syphilis.
D. Gonorrhoea, chlamydia, HIV and human papilloma virus (HPV).
E. Gonorrhoea, chlamydia, HIV and hepatitis C virus (HCV).

3.

A 23-year-old woman presents complaining of vaginal discharge. She has had recurrent episodes of vulvovaginal candidiasis. You prescribe an induction and maintenance regimen for six months. She is worried about use of contraception as she had a copper intrauterine device (IUD) inserted two months earlier.

What advice would you offer her?

A. Should remove the IUD.
B. Should remove the copper IUD and insert the Mirena coil.
C. Switch to a suitable oral contraceptive.
D. Should continue with this method.
E. Use the condom as an additional method to prevent recurrence of infection.

4.

A 21-year-old woman comes to the genitourinary medicine clinic complaining of vaginal discharge. Vaginal high-swab results show that she has bacterial vaginosis. She asks you about treatment of her sexual partner.

Which infection needs treatment of an asymptomatic sexual partner?

A. Bacterial vaginosis.
B. Candidiasis.
C. Human papilloma virus.
D. Herpes simplex virus.
E. *Trichomonas vaginalis.*

5.

A 21-year-old woman comes to the accident and emergency unit complaining of bilateral lower abdominal pain. On examination, her temperature is 38.5°C with bilateral adnexal tenderness. She tested negative for gonorrhoea and chlamydia the previous week.

What is the management for this woman?

A. Reassure and discharge her.
B. Reassure, give pain killers and ask to repeat gonorrhoea and chlamydia testing in one week.
C. Repeat tests for gonorrhoea and chlamydia, and start treatment according to the results.
D. Start empirical IV antibiotic treatment.
E. Start empirical oral antibiotic treatment.

6.

A 26-year-old woman comes to the accident and emergency unit complaining of abnormal vaginal bleeding, including post-coital and intermenstrual bleeding and menorrhagia. Her temperature is 38°C. On bimanual vaginal examination, there is adnexal tenderness and cervical motion tenderness. A pregnancy test is negative. You diagnosed a pelvic inflammatory disease (PID). The patient tells you that she has been abroad and had unprotected sex.

What is the recommended regimen for this patient?

A. Azithromycin 1 g per week orally for two weeks plus ceftriaxone 500 mg intramuscular stat dose.
B. Ciprofloxacin 200 mg twice a day (BD) plus oral doxycycline 100 mg BD for seven days.
C. Levoflaxacin 500 mg once daily (OD) plus oral metronidazole 400 mg BD for 14 days.
D. Moxifloxacin 400 mg OD oral for 14 days.
E. Ofloxacin 400 mg twice daily oral *plus* oral metronidazole 400 mg twice daily for 14 days.

7.

A 25-year-old woman comes to the outpatient clinic for follow-up after a diagnosis of PID three weeks previously. Results of swabs were negative for chlamydia and gonorrhoea. You explained the significance of PID and its sequelae. She stated that the symptoms resolved and she had her antibiotics regularly.

What else should you check at this visit?

A. Reassure and do nothing.
B. Review again in four to six weeks.
C. Repeat swaps for chlamydia and gonorrhoea.
D. Repeat bloods and C-reactive protein.
E. Screening and treatment of sexual contacts.

8.

A 24-year-old woman comes to the genitourinary medicine clinic complaining of small multiple groups of painful vulval ulcers. On examination, the base of the ulcer was erythematous and inguinal lymph nodes were painful.

What is the most likely diagnosis?

A. Chancroid.
B. Granuloma inguinale.
C. Herpes simplex virus (HSV).
D. Lymphogranuloma venereum.
E. Syphilis.

9.

A 24-year-old woman comes to the genitourinary medicine clinic complaining of multiple painful ulcers on the vulval area. On examination, the ulcers are sharply circumscribed with a yellow exudate in the base. There are also painful inguinal lymph nodes on the left side.

What is the most likely causative organism?

A. *Calymmatobacterium granulomatis.*
B. *Chlamydia trachomatis.*
C. *Haemophilus ducreyi.*
D. HSV-type 2.
E. *Treponema pallidum.*

10.

During diagnostic laparoscopy on a 28-year-old female for chronic pelvic pain, you noticed inflammation of the liver capsule and adjacent peritoneum.

What is the most likely causative organism?

A. *Calymmatobacterium granulomatis.*
B. *Chlamydia trachomatis.*
C. *Haemophilus ducreyi.*
D. HSV-type 2.
E. *Treponema pallidum.*

11.

A young woman presents to the genitourinary medicine clinic. After a swab was taken from the endocervix, microscopic examination reveals a Gram-positive diplococcus.

What organism looks like this under a microscope?

A. *Actinomyces israeli.*
B. *Chlamydia trachomatis.*
C. *Haemophilus ducreyi.*
D. *Neisseria gonorrhoea.*
E. *Trichomonas vaginalis.*

12.

A 20-year-old pregnant woman presented to the genitourinary medicine clinic with anogenital warts. She is diagnosed with human papillomavirus (HPV) infection-type 11.

What are her treatment options?

A. 5-fluorouracil.
B. Cryotherapy.
C. Imiquimod.
D. Podophylline.
E. Trichloracetic acid.

13.

A 20-year-old pregnant woman presented to the genitourinary medicine clinic two weeks previously and was found to have a chlamydia infection. She received azithromycin 1 g as a single dose. You arranged for contact tracing.

What is the next step?

A. Follow-up after six months.
B. Full STI screen.
C. Nothing to be done.
D. Test of cure during this visit.
E. Test of cure after five weeks.

14.

You made a diagnosis of moderate PID in a young 24-year-old woman who presented to the accident and emergency unit with lower abdominal pain and pyrexia. You prescribe a combination of a single intramuscular injection of cefoxitin and oral doxycycline and antipyretics. She is worried about her future fertility as a result of her PID.

Where is she best treated to preserve her fertility?

A. As an inpatient.
B. As an outpatient.
C. In the accident and emergency unit until her temperature normalizes.
D. In a fever hospital.
E. In an isolation ward.

ANSWERS

Q1: D. Pregnancy test.[1]

- In women of childbearing age, ectopic pregnancy should be excluded if they come in complaining of lower abdominal pain, in order to start the proper antibiotic treatment and/or arrange for management of any pregnancy complications.

- Pregnancy in association with pelvic inflammatory disease (PID) is an indication for hospital admission and intravenous antibiotic therapy.[1]
- Acute salpingitis during pregnancy occurs more commonly in the first trimester.
- Diagnosis may be difficult if the obstetrician is not aware that pelvic inflammatory disease can occur during pregnancy.
- Salpingitis during pregnancy is amenable to antibiotic therapy and surgery may not be necessary, sparing the risks of general anaesthesia and surgery. Antibiotic therapy is started without delay.
- Surgery is indicated if there is no response to treatment or if there is a collecting pelvis abscess.

Q2: C. Gonorrhoea, chlamydia, human immunodeficiency virus (HIV) and syphilis.

- Women assessed as being at risk of a sexually transmitted infection (STI) or who request testing should be offered appropriate tests for chlamydia, gonorrhoea, syphilis and HIV.[2]

Q3: D. Should continue with this method.[1]

- Copper IUDs do not influence vulvovaginal candidiasis (VVC).
- Copper-bearing IUDs should be changed in women complaining of recurrent bacterial vaginosis (BV) infection.[2]
- For recurrent VVC, oral fluconazole (150 mg or 200 mg dose) weekly for six months is the first-line regimen. Intermittent topical treatments may be considered.[2]
- There is no need for routine screening or treatment of sexual partners in the management of candidiasis.[2]

Q4: E. *Trichomonas vaginalis.*[3,4]

- Current sexual partners of women diagnosed with *Trichomonas vaginalis* (TV) should be offered a full sexual health screen and should be treated for TV irrespective of the results of their tests.
- Concurrent treatment of all sexual partners is essential for symptomatic relief, microbiological cure, and to prevent reinfections or transfer to a new partner.
- Sexual partners are advised to abstain from intercourse until they and their sexual partners have been cured.[3]
- Oral nitroimidazole drugs (e.g. metronidazole) are effective in treating trichomoniasis.
- In the management of BV, testing and treatment of male sexual partners is not indicated.
- In herpes simplex virus (HSV), symptomatic sexual partners should receive the same treatment. Asymptomatic sexual partners should be offered type-specific serological testing for HSV infection.[3,4]

Q5: D. Start empirical IV antibiotic treatment[5] [evidence level 3].

- Symptoms of PID include lower abdominal pain that is typically bilateral, deep dyspareunia, abnormal vaginal bleeding (post-coital, intermenstrual and/or menorrhagia) and/or abnormal vaginal or cervical discharge that is often purulent.
- Signs of PID include lower abdominal pain, adnexal tenderness and cervical motion tenderness on bimanual vaginal examination and fever (>38°C).

- Empirical antibiotic treatment, should be considered in any young (<25 years) sexually active woman who has recent onset bilateral lower abdominal pain associated with local tenderness on bimanual vaginal examination and in whom pregnancy has been excluded.
- Intravenous therapy is recommended for patients with more severe clinical disease, e.g. pyrexia >38°C, clinical signs of a tubo-ovarian abscess, signs of pelvic peritonitis.
- Because of the lack of definitive diagnostic criteria, a low threshold for empirical treatment of PID is recommended.

Q6: A. Azithromycin 1 g per week orally for two weeks plus ceftriaxone 500 mg intramuscular stat dose.[5]

- Metronidazole is included in some regimens to improve coverage for anaerobic bacteria. Anaerobes are of relatively greater importance in patients with severe PID.
- Ofloxacin and moxifloxacin should be avoided in patients who are at high risk of gonococcal PID because of increasing quinolone resistance in the UK (e.g. when the patient's partner has gonorrhea, in clinically severe disease or following sexual contact abroad).
- Quinolones should also be avoided as first-line empirical treatment for PID in areas where >5% of PID is caused by quinolone-resistant *Neisseria gonorrhea*.
- Levofloxacin is the L-isomer of ofloxacin and has the advantage of once-daily dosing (500 mg OD for 14 days). It may be used as a more convenient alternative to ofloxacin.
- Oral cephalosporin (e.g. cefixime) is not recommended because there is no clinical trial evidence to support its use and tissue levels are likely to be lower, which might have an impact on efficacy.[5]

Q7: E. Screening and treatment of sexual contacts [grade C recommendation].[5]

Review schedule for patients with PID
- Review at 72 hours to check for substantial improvement in clinical symptoms and signs (grade C (IV)). Failure of improvement indicates the need for further investigation, parenteral therapy and/or surgical intervention.
- Further review two to four weeks (grade C (IV)) after therapy to ensure compliance with oral antibiotics, adequate clinical response, screening and treatment of sexual contacts and repeat pregnancy test, if clinically indicated.
  - Repeat testing for gonorrhoea or chlamydia after two to four weeks is appropriate if there are persisting symptoms, poor compliance with antibiotics or if tracing of sexual contacts indicate the possibility of persisting or recurrent infection.[5]

Q8: C. Herpes simplex virus (HSV).[6]

- In HSV, the aetiological agent is HSV-type 2 in most cases; HSV-type 1 is less common.
- Classic ulcer characteristics include multiple small grouped ulcers with an erythematous base. Occasionally, single lesions/fissures can be seen. Ulcers are usually painful or pruritic.
- Vesicles can open, forming shallow ulcers or erosions.
- Incubation period is two to seven days.

Q9: C. *Haemophilus ducreyi.*[7]

- Chancroid aetiological agent is fastidious Gram-negative streptobacillus *Haemophilus ducreyi.*
- Chancroid (also known as soft chancre and ulcus molle) is a bacterial STI.
- The classic ulcer is markedly painful, sharply circumscribed or irregular with ragged undermined edges, not indurated but the base may have a grey or yellow exudate and multiple ulcers.
- Incubation period is three to ten days.
- Adenopathy: 50% with inguinal adenopathy, often painful, usually unilateral and may suppurate.

Q10: B. *Chlamydia trachomatis.*[8]

- The Fitz–Hugh–Curtis syndrome comprises right upper quadrant pain associated with peri-hepatitis, which occurs in some women with PID.
- There is insufficient clinical trial evidence to make specific recommendations for treatment beyond those for an uncomplicated PID.

Q11: D. *Neisseria gonorrhoea.*[9]

- *Neisseria gonorrhoea* is a Gram-negative diplococcus that can infect the mucous membranes of the urethra, endocervix, rectum, pharynx and conjunctiva by direct inoculation of infected secretions.
- Less than 50% of women are symptomatic, usually with non-specific vaginal discharge and lower abdominal discomfort.
- Pharyngeal infection is asymptomatic in >90% of both men and women, and can be contracted from an infected partner by unprotected oral sex.

Q12: B. Cryotherapy.[10]

- The topical use of podophylline paint on vulval and perianal warts, trichloracetic acid (TCA) on vaginal and cervical warts and cryotherapy with liquid nitrogen are widely used.
- Diathermy, laser treatment and excision of more extensive genital warts under local or even general anaesthia may be considered in more severe or resistant cases.
- The options for the treatment of anogenital warts during pregnancy are limited by potential teratogenicity of some modalities such as podophylline. TCA and imiquimod can be used safely, as well as ablative techniques such as cryotherapy.
- Treatment of the warts may reduce transmission of the human papillomavirus (HPV) to the fetus during vaginal delivery.[10]

Q13: B. Full STI screen.[11]

- Contact tracing ('look back') policy in the NHS recommends contact tracing and a full STI screening (hepatitis B, syphilis and HIV) for all sexual partners dating back six months for asymptomatic patients.
- Two-thirds of sexual partners are likely to become infected following sexual intercourse with an asymptomatic chlamydia-positive partner.
- Nucleic acid amplification test (NAAT) is a highly sensitive molecular technique to detect a virus or a bacterium. It detects low levels of viral RNA or DNA. It has the ability to detect the infectious agent during the incubation period. Results can be ready in three days.

- A test-of-cure (repeat NAAT) is not recommended unless the patient is pregnant, has been non-compliant to treatment or been re-exposed.
- You should wait for six weeks with azithromycin treatment for a test-of-cure as NAAT can give false-positive results for up to five weeks following successful treatment.

Q14: B. As an outpatient [evidence level 2+].[12]

- In women with moderate PID, there is no difference in long-term fertility outcomes between women who were treated as inpatients and those treated as outpatients.
- Admission for parenteral therapy, observation, further investigation and/or possible surgical intervention should be considered in the following situations: surgical emergency cannot be excluded, lack of response to oral therapy, clinically severe disease, presence of a tubo-ovarian abscess, or intolerance to oral therapy.
- Current male partners of women with PID should be screened for gonorrhoea and chlamydia.
- Tracing of contacts within a six-month period of onset of symptoms is recommended.

References

1. Centres for Diseases Control and Prevention. *Sexually Transmitted Diseases, Treatment Guidelines*. June, 2015. [https://www.cdc.gov/std/tg2015/pid.htm]
2. Faculty of Sexual and Reproductive Healthcare Clinical Effectiveness Unit. *Management of Vaginal Discharge in non-Genitourinary Medicine Settings*. February, 2012. [www.fsrh.org/pages]
3. Centres for Disease Control and Prevention. *Sexually Transmitted Diseases Guidelines. Genital HSV Infection*. June, 2015. [https://www.cdc.gov/std/tg2015/herpes.htm].
4. Centres for Disease Control and Prevention. *Sexually Transmitted Diseases Guidelines. Trichomoniasis*. June, 2015. [https://www.cdc.gov/std/tg2015/trichomoniasis.htm]
5. Agency for Health Care Research and Quality. *UK National Guideline for the Management of Pelvic Inflammatory Disease*. June, 2011. [https://www.guideline.gov/content.aspx?id=36068]
6. British Association for Sexual Health and HIV Clinical Effectiveness Group. *National Guideline for the Management of Genital Herpes*. June, 2015. [https://www.stratog.rcog.org.uk/files/rcog- orp/elearn]
7. Rapini RP, Bolognia JL, Jorizzo JL. *Dermatology: 2-Volume Set*. St. Louis, MO: Mosby, 2007.
8. Scottish Intercollegiate Guidelines Network. *Management of Genital Chlamydia trachomatis Infection. A National Clinical Guideline*. March, 2009. [www.sign.ac.uk/pdf/sign109.pdf]
9. British Association of Sexual Health and HIV Clinical Effectiveness Group. *United Kingdom National Guideline for Gonorrhoea Testing*. July, 2012. [https://www.bashh.org/documents/4490.pdf]
10. Lacey CJ, Woodhall SC, Wikstrom A, Ross J. 2012 European guideline for the management of anogenital warts. *J Eur Acad Dermatol Venereol* 2013;27(3):e263–70.
11. British Association of Sexual Health and HIV. *UK National Guideline for the Management of Genital Tract Infection with Chlamydia trachomatis*. April, 2006. [https://www.bashh.org/documents/65.pdf]
12. Ness RB, Soper DE, Holley RL, et al. Effectiveness of inpatient and outpatient treatment strategies for women with pelvic inflammatory disease: results from the Pelvic Inflammatory Disease Evaluation and Clinical Health (PEACH) Randomized Trial. *Am J Obstet Gynecol* 2002;186(5):929–37.

Chapter 14

Minimal Access Gynaecological Surgery

Nahed Shaltoot

QUESTIONS

1.

You are demonstrating a laparoscopic myomectomy procedure to your minimal access surgery module trainee.

What is the most serious complication?

A. Adhesions.
B. High recurrence rate.
C. Hysterectomy.
D. Incomplete removal.
E. Severe blood loss.

2.

You are demonstrating laparoscopic hysterectomy (LH) to one of your trainees.

What is the most common surgical complication with this procedure compared to abdominal hysterectomy (AH)?

A. Bladder injury.
B. Bowel injury.
C. Minor intraoperative haemorrhage.
D. Major intraoperative haemorrhage.
E. Ureteric injury.

3.

You are demonstrating laparoscopic hysterectomy (LH) to one of your trainees.

What is the most common surgical complication with this procedure compared to vaginal hysterectomy (VH)?

A. Bladder injury.
B. Bowel injury.

C. Minor vessel injury.
D. There was no difference.
E. Ureteric injury.

4.

While reviewing the outpatient cases, your junior colleague wants to discuss the management of ovarian cyst in a woman who is 35 years old.

What is the cyst size at which laparoscopic management should be a cost-effective procedure?

A. >40 mm.
B. >50 mm.
C. >60 mm.
D. >70 mm.
E. >80 mm.

5.

You are performing an outpatient hysteroscopy while investigating postmenopausal bleeding.

What is the most common cause of failure to obtain a good view of the cavity?

A. Difficult entry.
B. Failure to distend the uterus.
C. Faulty equipment.
D. Excessive bleeding.
E. Inefficient cervical preparation.

6.

A 29-year-old woman comes for her scheduled antenatal care appointment. She is 36 weeks pregnant. She had a hysteroscopic resection of a uterine septum because of recurrent pregnancy loss. All her antenatal visits have been normal.

What is your plan for her delivery?

A. Allow for continuation of pregnancy and await spontaneous labour.
B. Caesarean section at 39 weeks for fear of rupture of the uterus if allowed vaginal delivery.
C. Caesarean section at 38 weeks after a course of steroids.
D. Offer a choice of vaginal versus Caesarean section delivery.
E. Induce at 37 weeks.

7.

You are planning a laparoscopic adhesiolysis procedure for a 28-year- old woman who had secondary infertility, previous pelvic inflammatory disease (PID) and two Caesarean section procedures.

Which one of the following anti-adhesion agents would you like to use to prevent adhesion formation?

A. Chemically modified sodium hyaluronate/carboxymethylcellulose.
B. Hyaluronic acid derivatives.
C. Hydro-floatation agents.
D. Polytetrafluoroethylene barrier.
E. Solid barrier agents derived from oxidized regenerated cellulose.

8.

A 24–year-old primigravida woman presented for a dating scan, which showed a 6-cm right ovarian cyst. A follow-up scan at 15 weeks confirms an increase in size up to 14 cm, with radiological and laboratory features suggestive of benign disease. The pregnancy is otherwise progressing normally.

Which one of the following options is the most appropriate management?

A. Cyst drainage.
B. Laparoscopic cystectomy.
C. Laparotomy and cystectomy/oophorectomy.
D. Laparoscopic right oophorectomy.
E. Two-weekly ultrasound follow-up.

9.

A 36-year-old Afro-Caribbean woman with a subserosal fibroid (5 x 7 cm) is coun-selled for a laparoscopic myomectomy using a morcellator. She would like to know about the associated adverse outcomes.

What is the most common complication?

A. Death.
B. Disseminated sarcoma.
C. Infertility.
D. Peritoneal myomatosis.
E. Visceral injuries.

10.

You are starting your hysteroscopy training module and are shown different diameter hysteroscopes.

Which one would you recommend for outpatient hysteroscopy?

A. 1.7 mm with a 2.7 mm sheath.
B. 2.7 mm with a 3–3.5 mm sheath.
C. 3 mm with a 4 mm sheath.
D. 4 mm with an 8 mm sheath.
E. 4 mm with foroblique 30°.

11.

While performing a diagnostic laparoscopy, blood was dripping into the pelvis soon after inserting the lateral secondary trocar, quickly filling the operative field.

Which blood vessel is more likely to be injured?

A. Deep inferior epigastric artery.
B. Deep inferior epigastric vein.
C. External iliac artery.
D. Superior epigastric artery.
E. Superficial inferior epigastric artery.

12.

A 26-year-old woman is admitted for diagnostic laparoscopy for assessment of chronic pelvic pain.

What is the estimated risk of death associated with this procedure?

A. 1/500.
B. 1/1000.
C. 1/2000.
D. 1/10 000.
E. 1/15 000.

13.

A 42-year-old complains of cyclical cramping with or without menses. She had an endometrial ablation and tubal sterilization two years previously. Review of the operative findings showed an uncomplicated procedure. MRI imaging during times of symptomatic cramping showed blood trapped in the uterine cornua and swollen tubes. The diagnosis of post-ablation tubal sterilization syndrome was made (PATSS).

What is the risk of PATSS after endometrial ablation?

A. 1%–5%.
B. 6%–10%.
C. 11%–15%.
D. 16%–20%.
E. 21%–25%.

14.

A 68-year-old woman presented with vaginal spotting on three occasions. She was not sexually active before her menopause. She suffers from depressive anxiety disorders. An ultrasound scan shows a thickened irregular endometrium of 10 mm.

What is the most suitable management?

A. Hysterectomy.
B. Hysteroscopy and polypectomy under general anaesthesia.
C. Outpatient hysteroscopy and polypectomy under conscious sedation.
D. Outpatient hysteroscopy after cervical preparations with misoprostol vaginally or orally.
E. Outpatient vaginoscopic hysteroscopy.

15.

A 46-year-old woman is attending the outpatient hysteroscopy clinic for the removal of a 2-cm endometrial polyp. You decided to use electrosurgery for removal of the polyp.

Which distention media should be used?

A. Carbon dioxide.
B. Dextran 70.
C. Glycine.
D. Normal saline.
E. Mannitol solution.

ANSWERS

Q1: E. Severe blood loss [evidence level 2+].[1]

- In a prospective study of 2050 laparoscopic myomectomies, the most serious events were haemorrhages (14 cases, 0.68%), requiring blood transfusions in three cases (0.14%).

‌

Q2: D. Major intraoperative haemorrhage [evidence level 2−].[2]

- In a non-randomized controlled study of 37 048 women, the incidence of major operative haemorrhage was significantly higher (4.4%, 51/1154) for laparoscopic techniques (LH) than for abdominal hysterectomy (AH) (2.0%, 218/11 122).

Q3: D. There was no difference [evidence level 1+].[2]

Q4: D. >70 mm.[3]

- Asymptomatic simple cysts of 30–50 mm in diameter do not require follow-up, cysts of 50–70 mm in diameter require follow-up, and cysts >70 mm in diameter should be considered for either further imaging (MRI) or surgical intervention.[3]
- Laparoscopic management is cost effective because of earlier discharge and return to work.[3]

Q5: A. Difficult entry.[4]

- Difficult entry accounted for 50% of complications.[4]
- A systematic review of over 26 000 cases found that failures in the outpatient setting were attributed to either technical problems (cervical stenosis, anatomical factors and structural abnormalities) or patient factors (pain, vasovagal episodes or intolerance).
- The most frequent complications of operative hysteroscopy include haemorrhage, 2.4%; uterine perforation, 1%; cervical laceration, 1%–11%; excessive fluid, <1%.
- Excessive fluid absorption may cause absorption with or without hyponatraemia, hypo-osmolality, hyperglycinaemia and volume overload, including pulmonary oedema.
- Uterine synechiae after hysteroscopic metroplasty were reported in 2% of cases.
- Routine cervical preparation before outpatient hysteroscopy should not be used in the absence of any evidence of benefit in terms of reduction of pain, rates of failure or uterine trauma [grade of recommendation A].[4]

Q6: D. Offer a choice of vaginal versus Caesarean section delivery.[5]

- In the absence of consensus of opinion and or guidelines, the patient should be counselled for vaginal delivery versus Caesarean section.
- In a series of 69 cases, there were 31 (67.4%) term pregnancies, five (10.8%) ended in preterm delivery, six (13%) ended in spontaneous abortion. The modality of term pregnancy deliveries was Caesarean section in 48% of the cases and vaginal delivery in the remaining 52%.[5]
- Vaginal delivery seems safe, but rare serious complications like rupture of the uterus have to be considered.

Q7: B. Hyaluronic acid derivatives [evidence level 1+].[6]

- Meticulous surgical technique is an adequate means of preventing adhesions (minimizing tissue trauma, achieving optimal haemostasis, minimizing the risk of infection, and avoiding contaminants and the use of foreign materials when possible [evidence level 2−].[6]
- Meta-analysis of four randomized controlled trials investigated laparoscopic myomectomy, and laparotomy for benign conditions demonstrated a

significant reduction in the proportion of adhesions (odds ratio (OR) 0.31) with the use of hyaluronic acid derivatives.

- There is little evidence to support the use of pharmacological and hydro-floatation agents, including icodextrin, in gynaecological surgery.[6]

Q8: B. Laparoscopic cystectomy.[7]

- If the tumour is >6 cm in diameter, it is better to operate and remove during pregnancy, as it may present as an emergency cyst accident or interfere with the birth of the baby.
- There are no randomized controlled trials to compare benefits and harm of using laparoscopic surgery for benign tumours of the ovary during pregnancy on maternal and fetal health.

Q9: D. Peritoneal myomatosis.[8]

- Peritoneal myomatosis causes fibrosis of tissues and affects organ function. If left untreated, it will result in compression of organs and will destroy the function of the colon, small intestine, stomach or other organs.
- The disease is lethal if untreated, with death by cachexia, bowel obstruction, or other types of complications.
- An earlier systematic review of morcellator-related injuries found 14 non-trivial visceral injuries and three patient deaths.[9]

Q10: B. 2.7 mm with a 3–3.5 mm sheath.[9]

Q11: A. Deep inferior epigastric artery.[10]

- Bleeding from puncture of the deep inferior epigastric artery is more serious. The artery is at risk during the insertion of secondary trocars.
- The deep epigastric arteries can be seen just lateral to the lateral obliterated hypogastric arteries.
- The immediate or delayed appearance of a large abdominal wall haematoma indicates injury to the deep inferior epigastric artery.

Q12: D. 1/10 000.[11]

- Laparoscopy for chronic pelvic pain carries significant risks with an estimated risk of death of approximately 1 in 10 000, and a risk of injury to bowel, bladder or blood vessel of approximately 2.4 in 1000, of which two-thirds will require laparotomy.

Q13: B. 6%–10%.[12]

- Post-ablation tubal sterilization syndrome (PATSS) was first reported in 1993, in patients presenting with unilateral or bilateral pelvic pain and vaginal spotting and who had previously undergone tubal sterilization and endometrial ablation. It has also been reported with newer ablation devices.
- The incidence of PATSS is approximately 6%–8% and usually develops two to three years after endometrial ablation.
- Usually the confirmatory diagnosis is made surgically; however, MRI imaging during times of symptomatic cramping may be useful in looking for blood trapped in the uterine cornua. Ultrasound scanning has not been reliably sensitive at diagnosing PATSS.
- The definitive treatment of PATSS is hysterectomy.

Q14: E. Outpatient vaginoscopic hysteroscopy.[9]

- Vaginoscopy (direct insertion of the hysteroscope without the use of a vaginal speculum) should be the standard technique for outpatient hysteroscopy, especially where successful insertion of a vaginal speculum is anticipated to be difficult.
- Conscious sedation for outpatient hysteroscopy confers no advantage in terms of pain control and the woman's satisfaction over local anaesthesia.
- Life-threatening complications can result from the use of conscious sedation. Appropriate monitoring and staff skills are mandatory if procedures are to be undertaken using conscious sedation.

Q15: D. Normal saline.[9]

- For routine outpatient hysteroscopy, the choice of a distension medium between carbon dioxide and normal saline should be left to the discretion of the operator, as neither is superior in reducing pain. Uterine distension with normal saline appears to reduce the incidence of vasovagal episodes.
- Uterine distension with normal saline allows improved image quality and outpatient diagnostic hysteroscopy to be completed more quickly compared to the use of carbon dioxide.
- Operative outpatient hysteroscopy, using bipolar electrosurgery, requires the use of normal saline to act as both the distension and conducting medium.

References

1. Sizzi O, Rossetti A, Malzoni M, et al. Italian multicenter study on complications of laparoscopic myomectomy. *J Minim Invasive Gynecol* 2007;14 (4):453–62.
2. National Institute of Clinical Excellence. *Laparoscopic Techniques for Hysterectomy.* November, 2007. [https://www.nice.org.uk/guidance /ipg239/chapter/2-The-procedure]
3. Royal College of Obstetrics and Gynaecology. *Management of Suspected Ovarian Masses in Premenopausal Women.* December, 2011. [https://www.rcog.org.uk/ globalassets/documents/guidelines/gtg62.pdf]
4. National Institute of Clinical Excellence Interventional Procedure Guidance. *Hysteroscopic Metroplasty of a Uterine Septum for Primary Infertility.* January, 2015. https://www.nice.org.uk/guidance/ipg509/chapter/1]
5. Saygili-Yilmaz E, Yildiz S, Erman-Akar M, Akyuz G, Yilmaz Z. Reproductive outcome of septate uterus after hysteroscopic metroplasty. *Arch Gynecol Obstet* 2003;268(4):289–92.
6. Royal College of Obstetricians and Gynaecologists. *The Use of Adhesion Prevention Agents in Obstetrics and Gynaecology.* June, 2013. [https://www.rcog.org.uk/en/ guidelines-research-services/guidelines/sip39]
7. Bunyavejchevin S, Phupong V. Laparoscopic surgery for presumed benign ovarian tumor during pregnancy. *Cochrane Database Syst Rev* 2013;(1):CD005459. [www.evidence.nhs.uk/Search] =ovarian+cyst]
8. Royal College of Obstetricians and Gynaecologists. *Laparoscopic Myomectomy Using a Morcellator* (Query Bank). March, 2009. [https://www.rcog.org.uk/en/ guidelines-research-services/guidelines]
9. Royal College of Obstetricians and Gynaecologists and the British Society of Gynaecologic Endoscopy. *Best Practice in Outpatient Hysteroscopy.* March, 2011. [https://www.rcog.org.uk/globalassets/documents/guidelines/gtg59]

10. Wong C, Merkur H. Inferior epigastric artery: surface anatomy, prevention and management of injury. *Aust N Z J Obstet Gynaecol* 2016;56:137–41.
11. Royal College of Obstetricians and Gynaecologists. *The Initial Management of Chronic Pelvic Pain*. May, 2012. [https://www.rcog.org.uk/globalassets/documents/guidelines/41.pdf]
12. Sharp HT. Endometrial ablation: postoperative complications. *Am J Obstet Gynecol* 2012;207(4):242–7. [www.musaeduca.cl/site/lib/revistas/ablation]

Chapter 15

Gynaecological Oncology

PART 1

Questions

1.

A 28-year-old woman presents to the antenatal clinic at 14 weeks pregnant with mild lower abdominal pain and frequency in micturition. An ultrasound scan notes a solid adnexal mass. Her serum lactate dehydrogenase (LDH) and human chorionic gonadotropin (hCG) levels are raised.

Which of the following tumours is the most likely cause of her symptoms?

A. Dysgerminoma.
B. Endodermal sinus tumour.
C. Germ cell tumour.
D. Immature teratoma.
E. Mature teratoma.

2.

A 21-year-old woman presents with an abdominal mass and constipation. She also has lower abdominal pain. At laparotomy, the tumour appeared solid, fleshy and pink. Unilateral salphingo-oophorectomy was performed. The histology showed T-cell lymphoid infiltration of the fibrous stroma. Which of the following is the most likely diagnosis?

A. Dysgerminoma.
B. Endodermal sinus tumour.
C. Embryonal carcinoma.
D. Granulosa cell tumour.
E. Serous cyst adenocarcinoma.

3.

A cyst is sent for histologic investigation and the report shows an insular pattern of round uniform cells with 80% neurosecretory granules. This patient also has 5-hydroxyindoleacetic acid (5-HIAA) in her urine sample.

Which of the following cysts is the most likely diagnosis?

A. Clear cell tumour.
B. Dermoid cyst.
C. Immature teratoma.
D. Ovarian carcinoid.
E. Struma ovarii.

4.

An 18-year-old girl presents with a large abdominal mass with abdominal pain. She claims the mass has increased in size within the last three months. A laparotomy and unilateral salphingo-oophorectomy is performed. The histology report shows a meso-dermal core with a central capillary (Schiller–Duval body).

Which ovarian tumour is this most likely to be?

A. Chorioarcinoma of the ovary.
B. Dysgerminoma.
C. Embryonal carcinoma.
D. Endodermal sinus tumour.
E. Serous adenocarcinoma.

5.

An 8-year-old girl presents with symptoms and signs of precocious puberty. Which of the following tumours should not be included in the differential diagnosis?

A. Choriocarcinoma of the ovary.
B. Embryonal carcinoma.
C. Endodermal sinus tumour.
D. Granulosa cell tumour.
E. Polyembryoma.

6.

You are reading the histology report of a patient who had a laparotomy for an abdominal mass. A biopsy was taken as the mass was deemed to be inoperable. The histology report showed a tumour with an appearance of mucin-filled epithelial glandular cells ('signet-ring' cells).

Which of the following organs is the most likely origin of the primary cancer?

A. Breast.
B. Biliary tract.
C. Colon.
D. Ovary.
E. Stomach.

7.

Your ST1 asks you about a 42-year-old patient with a 5-cm right-sided ovarian cyst. The patient has occasional right iliac fossa pain. She would like to know the overall chance of a symptomatic ovarian cyst in a premenopausal female being malignant.

Which of the following statements is most accurate?

A. 1:1000.
B. 3:1000.
C. 5:1000.
D. 7:1000
E. 9:1000

8.

You are reading an ultrasound scan report concerning a patient with left-sided pelvic pain. The report reads 'a 6 x 5 x 5-cm left adnexal mass possibly ovarian in origin'.

In adnexal masses, what is the incidence of a non-ovarian origin?

A. 1%.
B. 5%.
C. 10%.
D. 15%.
E. 20%.

9.

A 38-year-old woman presents with an ultrasound scan report showing a unilocular anechoic left ovarian cyst measuring 5.6 x 5.2 x 5 cm. The CA-125 is 25.

What is the risk of malignancy index?

A. 0.
B. 5.
C. 25.
D. 125.
E. 225.

10.

A 67-year-old patient developed a recurrence of ovarian cancer two months after completing her last dose of platinum chemotherapy.

How would you define her response to platinum chemotherapy?

A. Platinum-partially sensitive disease.
B. Platinum-refractory disease.
C. Platinum-resistant disease.
D. Platinum-sensitive disease.
E. Platinum-zero sensitive disease.

11.

A 54-year-old patient is found to have advanced stage III disease.

What is the best management?

A. Cytoreductive surgery.
B. Neo-adjuvant chemotherapy and interval debulking surgery.
C. Primary debulking followed by adjuvant chemotherapy.
D. Palliative therapy.
E. Radiotherapy.

12.

A 64-year-old woman developed resistance to platinum chemotherapy after undergoing surgery for grade III ovarian cancer.

What are her chances of responding to second-line chemotherapy in this case?

A. <10%.
B. 10%–20%.
C. 21%–30%.
D. 40%–75%.
E. 76%–90%.

13.

A 51-year-old woman had a total hysterectomy, bilateral salpingo-oophorectomy and surgical staging for stage IC ovarian cancer. The pathologist's report confirmed clear cell histology.

What is your care plan for her?

A. Adjuvant chemotherapy.
B. Clinical follow-up and further imaging if she develops symptoms.
C. Neo-adjuvant chemotherapy and interval debulking.
D. Yearly follow-up with the test for cancer antigen (CA-125).
E. Yearly follow-up with the CA-125 test and pelvic ultrasound.

ANSWERS

Q1: A. Dysgerminoma [evidence level 2++].[1]

- The positive rate of lactate dehydrogenase (LDH) for malignant germ cell tumours of the ovary is 94.5%.[1]

Q2: A. Dysgerminoma.[2,3]

- A dysgerminoma is a tumour of the ovary that is composed of primitive, undifferentiated germ cells.
- 97% are benign proliferations (mature teratomas); the remaining 3% are malignant.
- Dysgerminoma constitutes <1% of ovarian malignancies; it is bilateral in 15%.
- The five-year survival rate is 95%.
- 15%–20% of tumours will recur.
- Chemotherapy including platinum is successful in almost all of the tumours.[2]

Management of ovarian masses in pregnancy
- Surgery in the first trimester carries an abortion risk approaching 30%.
- 2% of masses presenting in pregnancy are malignant.
- The ideal time for surgical intervention is 16–18 weeks' gestation.
- The five-year patient survival rate for dysgerminoma removal in pregnancy is 90%. Fetal mortality approaches 25%.
- For dermoid cysts during pregnancy, most references recommend surgery, preferably in the second trimester, if they grow beyond 6 cm in diameter, particularly if they are bilateral (10%)[evidence level 2−].[4]
- Methotrexate and cisplatin adjuvant chemotherapy can be used during pregnancy with success in the second and third trimesters. Chlorambucil has been used as early as the first trimester.

- **Struma ovarii** is a rare ovarian tumour (approximately 1%). Thyroid tissue comprises more than 50% of the overall mass. The vast majority are benign.
  - It may present with abdominal pain, a palpable abdominal mass and/or abnormal vaginal bleeding or thyroid hyperfunction in 5%–8% of patients.
  - Cancer antigen (CA-125) may be elevated but is not specific.
  - Surgical resection of the ovary is sufficient to treat benign unilateral disease.
  - Postoperatively adjuvant therapy with radioablative iodine-131 is recommended.

Q3: D. Ovarian carcinoid [evidence level 3].[4]

- Ovarian carcinoid tumours are uncommon and considered to be of germ cell origin.
- The estimated annual incidence of approximately 3/100 000/year.
- Primary ovarian carcinoids should be treated as ovarian tumours of low malignant potential.
- A 24-hour excretion of 5-hydroxyindoleacetic acid (5-HIAA) >25 mg provides strong evidence for the diagnosis of carcinoid syndrome.[4]

Q4: D. Endometrial sinus tumour.[5]

- Endometrial sinus tumour, also known as yolk sac tumour (YST), is a germ cell group of cancers. They are usually malignant.
- Treatments typically involve some combination of surgery and chemotherapy.
- Schiller–Duvall bodies are present in only 50%–75% of these tumours.
- With a combination of surgical treatment and adjuvant cisplatin-based chemotherapy, the survival rate in YSTs is >90%.[5]

Q5: C. Endodermal sinus tumour.[6,7]

- Endodermal sinus tumours secrete alpha-fetoprotein and not oestrogen.
- **Embryonal carcinoma** secretes human chorionc gonadotrophin (hCG) and is associated with precocious puberty.[6]
- **Polyembryoma** is an aggressive type of tumour that develops from germ cells. It may be associated with precocious puberty.
- **Granulosa cell tumours** (GCT) secrete oestrogen, a possible cause of precocious puberty.[6,7]
  - The incidence of GCT in juveniles is 5%. Tumour markers are oestradiol, inhibin and anti-Müllerian hormone. Cancer antigen 125 (CA-125) is not correlated to the tumour progression. Management is surgical removal of the tumour and adjuvant chemotherapy to prevent tumour recurrence.
  - The currently available specific tumour marker for GCT is serum inhibin. Inhibin is a peptide hormone normally produced by granulosa cells of the ovary.
  - Inhibin levels are undetectable in the postmenopausal woman, due to depletion of ovarian follicles; in GCT, inhibin levels are elevated even in postmenopausal women.[7]

Q6: E. Stomach.[8]

- Primary signet-ring cell carcinomas of the ovary are extremely rare.
- Mostly, the primary tumours arise from the gastrointestinal tract, stomach, pancreas, biliary tract, appendix or colorectum.
- If an ovarian signet-ring cell carcinoma is diagnosed, it is still important to examine the intestinal tract to exclude or confirm if it is the primary or secondary cancer and for proper surgical and chemotherapy management.[8]

Q7: A. 1:1000.[9]

- Up to 10% of women will have some form of surgery during their lifetime because of an ovarian mass.
- The overall incidence of a symptomatic ovarian cyst in a premenopausal female being malignant is approximately 1:1000, increasing to 3:1000 at the age of 50 years.[9]

Q8: C. 10%.[10]

- Common non-ovarian adnexal masses may be a pedunculated uterine fibroid, lymphocele, paraovarian cysts, hydrosalpinx, extraovarian endometrioma, lymphangioma or an ectopic pregnancy.[10]

Q9: A. 0 [evidence 1+].[9]

- The risk of malignancy index (RMI) is calculated according to the ultrasound scan score (U) characteristics, the menopausal status (M) and the serum CA-125 level (IU/mL) as follows:

$$RMI = U \times M \times (CA\text{-}125).$$

- The ultrasound result is scored as 1 point for each of the following characteristics: multilocular cysts, solid areas, metastases, ascites and bilateral lesions. Therefore, U = 0 for an ultrasound score of 0, U = 1 for an ultrasound score of 1, U = 3 for an ultrasound score of 2–5.
- The menopausal status is scored as 1 = premenopausal and 3 = postmenopausal.
- A low RMI of <25 still carries a malignancy risk of 3% and does not exclude malignancy in all cases.
- RMI 25–250 indicates risk of 20%; RMI <250 indicates risk of 75%.
- Ovarian cystectomy is not recommended for the management of ovarian cysts in postmenopausal women; bilateral oophorectomy should be the chosen line of management.[10]

Q10: C. Platinum-resistant disease.[11]

- **Platinum-resistant disease:** patients who develop recurrent disease within six months of completing their last dose of platinum.
- **Platinum-refractory disease:** patients who develop resistance while receiving chemotherapy.
- **Platinum-sensitive disease:** patients who develop recurrence beyond six months after completing their last dose of platinum.

Q11: B. Neo-adjuvant chemotherapy and interval debulking surgery [evidence level 2++].[12]

- Several randomized trials have shown that patients who received neo-adjuvant chemotherapy followed by interval debulking surgery had significantly lower adverse effects and mortality rates than patients undergoing primary debulking surgery. Carboplatin and paclitaxel have become the 'backbone' of treatment of advanced ovarian cancer.
- The survival for early stage cancer is 90%, dropping to <30% for stages III and IV.
- The standard-of-care for patients with advanced ovarian cancer consists of primary maximal debulking surgery and platinum-based chemotherapy.

- Several studies have shown a significant improvement in recurrence-free survival (76% versus 65%, P=0.001) and overall survival with the use of adjuvant chemotherapy.

Q12: A. <10%.[12]

- Ovarian cancer is one of the most sensitive to primary anti-neoplastic platinum-based and paclitaxel-based chemotherapy, with an expected response in over 80% of cases.
- However, a majority of women with advanced ovarian cancer will ultimately relapse and develop drug-resistant disease, necessitating a need for the use of second-line chemotherapy.
- A progressive rise in serum CA-125 may indicate recurrence.
- Second-line chemotherapy may include cisplatin, carboplatin or paclitaxel, as single agents or in combination, or new non-platinum-based agents, e.g. gemcitabine or pegylated liposomal doxorubicin.[12]

Q13: A. Adjuvant chemotherapy.[13]

- Adjuvant chemotherapy for stage IC clear cell carcinoma is effective in suppressing disease recurrence.
- Carboplatin and paclitaxel have become the 'backbone' of treatment of advanced ovarian cancer.
- The standard-of-care for patients with advanced ovarian cancer consists of primary maximal debulking surgery and platinum-based chemotherapy.
- Several studies have shown a significant improvement in recurrence-free survival (76% versus 65%, P=0.001) and overall survival with the use of adjuvant chemotherapy.

References

1. Patel PS, Sharma VM, Raval GN, et al. Serum lactate dehydrogenase levels in malignant germ cell tumors of ovary. *Intern J Gynecol Cancer* 1996;6:328–32.
2. *Ovarian Dysgerminomas.* [www.csh.org.tw/dr.tcj/educartion/f/web/Dysgermi noma/index.htm]
3. Kim D, Cho HC, Park JW, et al. Struma ovarii and peritoneal strumosis with thyrotoxicosis. *Thyroid* 2009;19(3):305–8.
4. Cafà EV, Angioli R, Scollo P. Ovarian carcinoid tumor with nodal metastases: case report. *J Cancer Sci Ther* 2010;2:120–1.
5. Duval M. Le placenta des rongeurs. *Journal de l'anatomie et de la physiologie normales et pathologiques de l'homme et des animaux, Paris,* 1891;27:24–73, 344–95, 513–612.
6. Kurman RJ, Norris HJ. Embryonal carcinoma of the ovary: a clinicopathologic entity distinct from endodermal sinus tumor resembling embryonal carcinoma of the adult testis. *Cancer* 1976;38(6):2420–33.
7. Robertson DM, Stephenson T, Pruysers E. Characterization of inhibin forms and their measurement by an inhibin alpha-subunit ELISA in serum from postmenopausal women with ovarian cancer. *J Clin Endocrinol Metab* 2002;87(2):816–24.
8. Pernot S, Voron T, Perkins G, et al. Signet-ring cell carcinoma of the stomach: impact on prognosis and specific therapeutic challenge. *World J Gastroenterol* 2015;21(40):11428–38.
9. Royal College of Obstetricians and Gynaecologists. *Management of Suspected Ovarian Masses in Premenopausal Women.* December, 2011. [https://www.rcog.org.uk/globalassets/documents/guidelines/gtg62.pdf]
10. Biggs WS, Marks ST. Diagnosis and management of adnexal masses. *Am Fam Physician* 2016;93(8):676–81.

11. Reed NS, Sadozye AH. Update on chemotherapy in gynaecological cancers. *Obstet Gynaecol* 2016;18(3):182–8.
12. Sato S, Itamochi H. Neoadjuvant chemotherapy in advanced ovarian cancer: latest results and place in therapy. *Ther Adv Med Oncol* 2014; 6(6): 293–304.
13. Raja FA, Chopra N, Ledermann JA. Optimal first-line treatment in ovarian cancer. *Ann Oncol* 2012;23(10):188–27.

PART 2
Questions

1.

A 38-year-old woman attends for her cervical screening appointment. You have tried to do the smear but you failed because of severe cervical stenosis resulting from traumatic surgery six years previously. In her notes, it was documented that the same thing happened in her last two appointments. Her first two smear results were normal.

What will you do next?

A. Offer cervical biopsy.
B. Offer cervical dilatation and retry to take the smear.
C. Offer colposcopy examination.
D. Offer hysterectomy.
E. Offer withdrawal from the NHS cervical screening programme.

2.

A 30-year-old woman has had her cervical screening result reported as borderline.

What will be your plan of management?

A. Cervical biopsy.
B. Offer colposcopy.
C. Offer human papilloma virus (HPV) test.
D. Routine recall.
E. Repeat smear in six months.

3.

A woman has had her cervical smear. It shows moderate dyskaryosis. She subsequently had a colposcopy and a loop excision of transformation zone (LETZ) procedure. The histopathology shows negative margins.

What will be your further plan of management?

A. Cervical smear and colposcopy in six months.
B. Cervical smear with or without test-of-cure in six months.
C. Cervical smear in six months.
D. HPV test-of-cure in six months.
E. Six monthly smears for 18 months.

4.

Using high-risk HPV as the primary screening test is an attractive option for countries with existing cervical screening programmes.

Compared to liquid-based cytology for detection of borderline changes or worse, HPV primary screening is:

A. 10% more sensitive and 3% less specific.
B. 15% more sensitive and 4% less specific.
C. 20% more sensitive and 5% less specific.
D. 25% more sensitive and 6% less specific.
E. 30% more sensitive and 7% less specific.

5.

A 43-year-old woman has had her cervical smear taken on day 14 of her menstrual period. The result shows no abnormality but there were normal endometrial cells in the sample. She has a history of bilateral tubal ligation.

What will be your further management?

A. Cervical biopsy.
B. Reassure the woman.
C. Transvaginal scan and endometrial sampling.
D. Repeat smear in six months.
E. Urgent referral for colposcopy.

6.

A 32-year-old woman attends the colposcopy clinic after a high-grade smear result. After discussion, the woman accepts the LETZ procedure.

What is the minimum depth of excision that is accepted in the LETZ procedure?

A. 3 mm.
B. 5 mm.
C. 7 mm.
D. 9 mm.
E. 11 mm.

7.

A 45-year-old woman has had the LETZ procedure for high-grade dyskaryosis. The histopathology result shows CIN3 with positive margins.

What will be your further management?

A. Cervical smear with or without test-of-cure in six months.
B. Cervical smear in six months.
C. Colposcopy in six months.
D. Re-excision.
E. Test-of-cure in six months.

8.

A 36-year-old woman has had a LETZ procedure for cervical glandular intraepithelial neoplasia (CGIN). The histopathology result showed negative margins. Six months later the repeat cervical smear is negative but the HPV test-of-cure is positive.

What will be your next management?

A. Cervical biopsy.
B. Colposcopy.
C. Re-excision.
D. Smear and HPV test-of-cure in six months.
E. Smear and HPV test-of-cure in 12 months.

9.

A 45-year-old woman has had a total hysterectomy for abnormal uterine bleeding. The histopathology result shows positive margins for CIN1.

What will be your further management?

A. Vault cytology and HPV test-of-cure at six and 12 months.
B. Vault cytology and HPV test-of-cure at six, 12 and 18 months.
C. Vault cytology and HPV test-of-cure at six, 12 and 24 months.
D. Vault cytology and high-risk HPV test-of-cure at six, 12 and 24 months and then annually for nine years.
E. Vault cytology and HPV test-of-cure at six and 12 months and then annually for 10 years.

10.

A woman was found to be 10 weeks pregnant when she attended for her colposcopy appointment for high-grade dyskaryosis. The colposcopy examination suspected CIN1.

What will be your further management?

A. Repeat colposcopy at 20 weeks' gestation.
B. Repeat colposcopy at six weeks postpartum.
C. Repeat colposcopy at 12 weeks postpartum.
D. Repeat colposcopy at 16 weeks postpartum.
E. Repeat colposcopy at term.

11.

A 32-year-old nulliparous woman has suffered post-coital and intermenstrual bleeding for 10 weeks before being diagnosed with stage IB2 cervical cancer.

What is the most appropriate management?

A. Chemoradiation.
B. Radical hysterectomy and bilateral pelvic lymph node dissection.
C. Radical trachelectomy and bilateral pelvic lymph node dissection.
D. Radical trachelectomy.
E. Simple hysterectomy.

12.

A 35-year-old woman is found to be 15 weeks pregnant when she is diagnosed with stage IB1 cervical cancer.

What will be the most appropriate management?

A. Delay treatment until after fetal maturity.
B. Delay treatment until after delivery at term.
C. Immediate chemoradiation after termination of the pregnancy.
D. Immediate chemoradiation followed by surgery after delivery.
E. Immediate radical hysterectomy and bilateral pelvic lymphadenectomy.

13.

In the UK, HPV) vaccination of girls aged 12–13 years started in September, 2008. Almost 90% of girls eligible for the vaccine in 2010/2011 received all three doses.

What is the predicted impact that HPV vaccination may have, based on the current high uptake?

A. 30% decrease in high-grade CIN and 50% reduction in cervical cancer.
B. 40% decrease in high-grade CIN and 60% reduction in cervical cancer.
C. 50% decrease in high-grade CIN and 70% reduction in cervical cancer.
D. 50% of woman will no longer need routine cervical screening.
E. 90% reduction on mortalities from cervical cancer.

14.

A 32-year-old nulliparous woman is diagnosed with a cancer lesion at the anterior lip of the cervix with extension of 6 mm and stromal invasion of 8 mm. There is no parametrial invasion, neither is there any lesion elsewhere. Cystoscopy and sigmoid-oscopy are normal. She asks for fertility sparing treatment.

What is the most appropriate treatment in her case?

A. Chemoradiation.
B. Radical hysterectomy.
C. Radical trachelectomy and pelvic lymph node dissection.
D. Simple hysterectomy.
E. Simple hysterectomy and pelvic lymph node dissection.

15.

A 32-year-old woman is referred to the colposcopy clinic because of a suspicious looking cervix on speculum examination done because of heavy menstrual bleeding. She is diagnosed with cervical adenocarcinoma with depth of invasion of 2 mm and horizontal spread of 6 mm.

What is the risk of lymph node invasion in her case?

A. None.
B. 1%.
C. 3%.
D. 5%.
E. 7%.

16.

The incidence of endometrial cancer is rising in postmenopausal women, but in the same time the five-year survival rates have improved.

In terms of order, currently, endometrial cancer is:

A. The most common female cancer.
B. The second most common female cancer.
C. The third most common female cancer.
D. The fourth most common female cancer.
E. The fifth most common female cancer.

17.

Obesity is now affecting 25% of adults in the UK and predisposes women to endometrial as well as other cancers.

What type of endometrial cancer is obesity predominantly associated with?

A. Type 1 (endometroid) endometrial cancer rather than type 2 (non-endometroid).
B. Type 1 and type 2 endometrial cancers, equally.

C. Type 1 (endometroid) endometrial cancer.
D. Type 2 (non-endometroid) rather than type 1 (endometroid) endometrial cancers.
E. Type 2 (non-endometroid) endometrial cancer.

18.

A 55-year-old woman, with a BMI of 34, attends the gynaecology clinic as an urgent two-week referral with postmenopausal bleeding. She has had a transvaginal scan, which shows a thin endometrium apart from a focal area with a thickness of 8 mm.

What will be the most appropriate further management?

A. Offer dilatation and curettage.
B. Offer hysteroscopy and biopsy.
C. Offer magnetic resonant imaging.
D. Offer Pipelle biopsy.
E. Offer repeat scan in six months.

19.

A 51-year-old woman has had hysteroscopy and biopsy for postmenopausal bleeding. The biopsy result shows endometrial hyperplasia without atypia.

What is the risk that she may progress to have endometrial cancer?

A. <1% in 10 years.
B. <5% in 10 years.
C. <1% in 20 years.
D. <5% in 20 years.
E. <25% in 20 years.

20.

A 49-year-old woman has had a Pipelle biopsy done for abnormal heavy uterine bleeding. The result shows endometrial hyperplasia without atypia.

What is the most appropriate management for her condition?

A. Expectant management.
B. Levonorgestrel intrauterine system.
C. Hysterectomy.
D. Medroxyprogesterone 10–20 mg per day.
E. Northisterone 10–15 mg per day.

21.

A 46-year-old woman attends the gynaecology clinic six months after being diagnosed with endometrial hyperplasia without atypia; she is on northisterone 15 mg daily. She has had a surveillance Pipelle biopsy. The result shows a persistence of the same endometrial pathology.

What will be your further management?

A. Continue treatment for a further six months and then biopsy.
B. Continue the treatment for a further 12 months and then biopsy.
C. Levonorgestrel intrauterine system.
D. Offer hysterectomy.
E. Offer endometrial ablation.

22.

A 55-year-old woman attends the gynaecology clinic with postmenopausal bleeding. She had a transvaginal scan, which showed an endometrial thickness of 8 mm. She had a successful Pipelle biopsy in the clinic. The result shows endometrial hyperplasia with atypia.

What is the most appropriate management?

A. Laparotomy, total abdominal hysterectomy and bilateral salpingo-oophorectomy.
B. Laparoscopy, total hysterectomy and bilateral salpingo-oophorectomy.
C. Laparotomy and total abdominal hysterectomy.
D. Laparoscopic total hysterectomy.
E. Laparoscopy, total hysterectomy, bilateral salpingo-oophorectomy and pelvic nodes sampling.

23.

A 60-year-old woman, BMI 40, attends the outpatient hysteroscopy clinic as part of the investigation for her third episode of heavy postmenopausal bleeding. The endometrium looks suspicious and copious curettings are obtained. The result shows endometrial cancer. Stage I endometrial cancer is suspected after magnetic resonant imaging.

What is the most appropriate management?

A. Laparotomy, total abdominal hysterectomy and bilateral salpingo-oophorectomy.
B. Laparoscopy, total hysterectomy and bilateral salpingo-oophorectomy.
C. Laparotomy, total abdominal hysterectomy, bilateral salpingo-oophorectomy and omentectomy.
D. Laparoscopy, total hysterectomy, bilateral salpingo-oophorectomy, pelvic nodes dissection and radiotherapy.
E. Radiotherapy.

24.

A 65-year-old woman is diagnosed with stage IB endometrial cancer. She declines any surgical intervention and requests radiotherapy as an alternative.

What will be the risk of recurrence if she is treated using radiotherapy?

A. 6%.
B. 12%.
C. 18%.
D. 24%.
E. 30%.

25.

A 65-year-old woman is referred to the two-week-wait general gynaecology clinic because her general practitioner observed an irregular vulval ulcer with raised edges while he was performing a rectal examination for suspected haemorrhoids.

What will you do next?

A. Magnetic resonant imaging (MRI).
B. Take an excisional biopsy.
C. Urgent referral to cancer centre.

D. Urgent referral to gynaecology consultant.
E. Wide local excision.

26.

Vulval cancer spreads by direct extension to adjacent structures, by embolization to the regional inguinal and femoral lymph nodes, or by haematogenous spread.

What proportion of the women with vulval cancer who are operable have nodal spread?

A. 10%.
B. 20%.
C. 30%.
D. 40%.
E. 50%.

27.

A 70-year-old woman is diagnosed with vulval cancer. The tumour involves the vagina and the urethra. The pelvic nodes are negative.

What is the most likely stage of her disease?

A. Stage I.
B. Stage II.
C. Stage IIIA.
D. Stage IIIB.
E. Stage IV.

28.

A 68-year-old woman is diagnosed with vulval cancer. The lesion is 2 cm and lateral. The pathologist has phoned and informed you that the frozen section for the sentinel lymph node biopsies is positive.

How will you proceed with the surgery?

A. Proceed with bilateral lymphadenectomy.
B. Proceed with *en bloc* radical vulvectomy.
C. Proceed with contralateral lymphadenectomy.
D. Proceed with ipsilateral lymphadenectomy.
E. No further surgery.

29.

A 72-year-old woman is diagnosed with verrucous vulval cancer. The lesion is 3 cm in diameter and 2 cm lateral to the left labia majora.

What is the most appropriate management?

A. Radical vulvectomy with sentinel lymph node biopsies.
B. Wide local excision.
C. Wide local excision with ipsilateral lymphadenectomy.
D. Wide local excision with contralateral lymphadenectomy.
E. Wide local excision with bilateral lymphadenectomy.

30.

A 60-year-old woman is diagnosed with vulval basal cell carcinoma. The lesion is 3 cm in diameter and less than 10 mm above and lateral to the anus.

What is the most appropriate management?

A. Radical vulvectomy with sentinel lymph node biopsies.
B. Radiotherapy.
C. Wide local excision.
D. Wide local excision with ipsilateral lymphadenectomy.
E. Wide local excision with bilateral lymphadenectomy.

31.

A 54-year-old woman presents to you in the gynaecology outpatient clinic with vulval soreness and itching. On examination you find suspicious vulval lesions and you take a biopsy. Two weeks later you review her and the histology report shows irregular saw-toothed acanthosis, increased granular layer and basal cell liquefaction and a band-like dermal infiltrate that is mainly lymphocytic.

Which of the following conditions does this woman have?

A. Lichen planus.
B. Lichen sclerosis.
C. Lichen simplex.
D. Vulval intraepithelial neoplasia.
E. Vulval psoriasi.

32.

A 54-year-old woman presents to you in the gynaecology outpatient clinic with vulval soreness and itching. On examination you find suspicious vulval lesions and you take a biopsy. Two weeks later you review her and the histology report shows thinned epidermis with subepidermal hyalinization and deeper inflammatory infiltrate.

Which of the following conditions does this woman have?

A. Lichen planus.
B. Lichen sclerosis.
C. Lichen simplex.
D. Vulval intraepithelial neoplasia.
E. Vulval psoriasis.

33.

Your ST1 feels confused about vulval intraepethial neoplasia (VIN) and wishes to know which of these has the highest malignant potential.

Which of the following VINs has the highest risk to change into squamous cell carcinoma of the vulva?

A. VIN associated with HPV type 8.
B. VIN associated with HPV type 16.
C. VIN associated with HPV type 18.
D. VIN associated with HPV type 32.
E. VIN associated with lichen sclerosis.

ANSWERS

Q1: B. Offer cervical dilatation and retry to take the smear.[1]

- Cervical dilatation should be considered if it is difficult to obtain a cytology sample that represents the entire transformation zone from women who have severe cervical stenosis.

Q2: C. Offer human papilloma virus (HPV) test.[1]

- A reflex human papilloma virus (HPV) test (test-of-cure) tests for the high-risk HPV types 16, 18, 31, 33 and 45. They can induce malignancy even if they are at low levels.
- **Borderline or low-grade dyskaryosis** should have a reflex test. Those with a positive reflex test showing a high-risk HPV type should be referred for colposcopy. If the reflex test is negative, they are returned to the routine call–recall system.
- **Moderate, high-grade dyskaryosis or worse** are referred straight for colposcopy without a high-risk HPV test.

Q3: B. Cervical smear with or without test-of-cure in six months [evidence level 2+].[2]

- A high-risk HPV test-of-cure is to detect the persistence or clearance of high-risk types 16, 18, 31, 33 and 45.[1]
- A test-of-cure is an early valid prognostic evidence of failure or cure after treatment for cervical intraepithelial neoplasia (CIN) 2+ and is more accurate than cytology.
- The absence of high-risk HPV DNA has a 100% negative predictive value for cure after treatment of CIN2+.[1]

The UK National Health Service screening programme (NHSCSP)[1]
- First invitation at 25 years of age, then every three years until the age of 49 years.
- From ages 50 to 64, women are called every five years.
- For women older than 65, an invitation is required for women who have had recent abnormal tests.

Q4: D. 25% more sensitive and 6% less specific.[1]

- Primary screening with high-risk HPV testing generally detects more than 90% of all cases of CIN2, CIN3 and invasive cancer.[1]

Q5: D. Transvaginal scan and endometrial sampling.[1]

- In women aged over 40 years, who are beyond the 12th day of the menstrual cycle, the finding of normal endometrial cells in a cervical sample may indicate endometrial pathology ranging from benign polyps to carcinoma. Hence, endometrial biopsy is indicated.
- There is now a considerable body of evidence suggesting that endometrial cells in a sample from a woman <40 years do not indicate significant endometrial pathology.

Q6: C. 7 mm.[1]

- The goal of excision is to remove all the abnormal epithelium.
- **Type I cervical transformation zone**: depth of excision should be >7 mm and <10 mm.
- **Type II cervical transformation zone**: the depth of excision should be >10 mm and <15 mm.
- **Type III cervical transformation zone**: the depth of excision should be >15 mm and <25 mm.

Q7: A. Cervical smear with or without test-of-cure in six months. [1]

- **CIN3** extending to the lateral or deep margins of excision (or uncertain margin status) results in a higher incidence of recurrence but does not justify routine re-excision, provided there is no evidence of glandular abnormality or invasive disease and the woman is under 50 years of age.
- A cervical cytology sample should be taken six months after treatment. If the cytology sample is reported as high-grade dyskaryosis or suspected invasive squamous carcinoma, the woman must be referred for colposcopy without test-of-cure (absence of high-grade HPV type).
- **Cervical glandular intraepithelial neoplasia (CGIN)** has a risk of recurrence; if excision is not complete with a positive or unclear margin, re-excision should be done. Then repeat test-of-cure should be done after six months and 12 months. If both are negative, the woman should be recalled in three years.

Q8: B. Colposcopy.[1]

- In a woman who undergoes excision for CGIN, if she has a positive high-risk HPV test and no abnormality is detected at colposcopic examination, the woman should have a second test-of-cure sample 12 months later. If this sample is negative for cytology and high-risk for HPV, the woman can be discharged, for recall in three years.

Q9: D. Vault cytology and high-risk HPV test-of-cure at six, 12 and 24 months and then annually for nine years.[1]

- For women who undergo a hysterectomy and have incompletely excised CIN, the procedure is: **CIN1** vault cytology at six, 12 and 24 months; for **CIN2/3**, vault cytology at six and 12 months, followed by nine annual vault cytology samples until she is 65 years old or until ten years after surgery.[1]

Q10: C. Repeat colposcopy at 12 weeks postpartum.[1]

- The safety of delaying treatment of pregnant women has been demonstrated in a number of cohort and retrospective uncontrolled studies.
- The incidence of invasive cervical cancer in pregnancy is low, and pregnancy itself does not have an adverse effect on the prognosis.[1]

Q11: A. Chemoradiation.[2]

- For women diagnosed with cervical cancer stages IA1–IB1, the procedures are: surgery; stages IB2 or more, chemoradiation.
- Removal of pelvic lymph nodes is not recommended during treatment for International Federation of Gynaecology and Obstetrics (FIGO) stage IA1 disease.
- Pelvic lymph nodes should be removed if FIGO IA2 disease is present.
- Patients who have undergone surgery for cervical carcinoma and have positive nodes should be considered for adjuvant treatment with concurrent chemo-radiotherapy with platinum-based chemotherapy.
- Women requesting fertility conservation should be offered radical trachelect-omy and pelvic lymph node dissection, providing the tumour diameter is less than 2 cm and there is no lymphatic-vascular space invasion.

Q12: E. Immediate radical hysterectomy and bilateral pelvic lymphadenectomy.[2]

- For pregnant women with early stage disease (FIGO IA1, IA2, IB1) diagnosed after 16 weeks of gestation, treatment may be delayed to allow fetal maturity to occur.

- If gestational age is <20 weeks at diagnosis of advanced cervical cancer (FIGO 1B2 or greater), a systematic review supports immediate termination and treatment of the disease.

Q13: C. 50% decrease in high-grade CIN and 70% reduction in cervical cancer.[2]

- Since September 2012, the vaccine used in the national programme changed to the quadrivalent vaccine (HPV 6/11/16/18), which gives additional protection against genital warts.
- Despite vaccination, cervical screening will remain an essential component of the programme.

Q14: B. Radical trachelectomy and pelvic lymph node dissection.[2]

- She is Stage IB1 (clinically visible lesions limited to the cervix uteri).

Q15: B. 1%.[2]

- The risk of pelvic lymph node metastases is no more than 1% for stage FIGO IA1 and 3%–6% for FIGO IA2 cervical squamous cell cancer.
- The FIGO classification for early stage squamous cervical cancer (FIGO IA) is also applicable to early stage adenocarcinomas.
- The presence of lymphovascular invasion is an indicator of prognosis and should be considered when determining whether to perform pelvic lymphadenectomy in early stage cervical cancer.[2]

Q16: D. The fourth most common female cancer.[3]

- Endometrial cancer is the fourth most common cancer in women, accounting for around 5% of all female cancers.
- Five-year survival rates have improved to more than 77%, although women from deprived backgrounds have up to a 4% lower five-year survival rate.
- The incidence rates peak between the ages of 60 and 79 years.

Q17: A. Type 1 (endometroid) endometrial cancer rather than type 2 (non-endometroid).[3]

- Obesity is predominantly associated with type 1 (endometroid) endometrial cancer rather than type 2 (non-endometroid, such as serous or carcinosarcoma) endometrial cancer; however, both subtypes are increased with obesity.
- Risk of endometrial cancer is increased in women with a BMI >30 kg/m^2 and the risk increases linearly with increasing BMI.[3]
- In the UK, approximately 50% of endometrial cancers are attributable to obesity.

Q18: B. Offer hysteroscopy and biopsy.[3]

- Hysteroscopy can detect focal lesions such as polyps that may be missed by blind sampling.
- Up to 10% of endometrial pathology can be missed by blind sampling.

Q19: D. <5% in 20 years.[4]

Q20: B. Levonorgestrel intrauterine system.[4]

- Endometrial hyperplasia without atypia has a risk of <2% of progression to endometrial carcinoma during a period of 10 years.

- Simple or complex endometrial hyperplasia in the absence of cytological atypia poses an extremely low risk of progression to carcinoma and can be treated conservatively.
- Persistent or progressive disease will be found in approximately one-third of conservatively managed cases.
- Both continuous oral and local intrauterine progestogens (levonorgestrel-releasing intrauterine system (LNG-IUS)) are effective in achieving regression of endometrial hyperplasia without atypia.
- The LNG-IUS should be the first-line medical treatment because, compared with oral progestogens, it has a higher disease regression rate with a more favourable bleeding profile and it is associated with fewer adverse effects.
- Continuous progestogens (medroxyprogesterone 10–20 mg/day or norethisterone 10–15 mg/day) should be used for women who decline the LNG-IUS.
- Cyclical progestogens should not be used.

Q21: A. Continue treatment for further six months and then biopsy.[4]

- Treatment with oral progestogens or the LNG-IUS should be for a minimum of six months in order to induce histological regression of endometrial hyperplasia without atypia.
- Endometrial surveillance should be arranged at a minimum of six-monthly intervals. At least two consecutive six-monthly negative biopsies should be obtained prior to discharge.
- Hysterectomy is indicated in women not wanting to preserve their fertility when there is no histological regression of hyperplasia despite 12 months of treatment.
- Endometrial ablation is not recommended for the treatment of endometrial hyperplasia.

Q22: B. Laparoscopy, total hysterectomy and bilateral salpingo-oophorectomy.[4]

- Women with atypical hyperplasia should undergo a total hysterectomy because of the risk of underlying malignancy or progression to cancer.
- A laparoscopic approach to total hysterectomy is preferable to an abdominal approach as it is associated with a shorter hospital stay, less postoperative pain and quicker recovery.
- Lymphadenectomy should not be routinely performed in atypical hyperplasia because this would result in unnecessary surgical risk.

Q23: B. Laparoscopy, total hysterectomy and bilateral salpingo-oophorectomy.[4,5]

- Laparoscopic hysterectomy and bilateral salpingo-oophorectomy has been demonstrated to be the surgical technique of choice for women with endometrial cancer.[1]
- For stage I disease: simple hysterectomy and bilateral salpingo-oophorectomy.[2]
- For stage II disease: laparotomy/laparoscopy, bilateral salpingo-oophorectomy and lymphadenectomy.[4]
- Stage III disease: laparotomy/laparoscopy, bilateral salpingo-oophorectomy and adjuvant radiotherapy.[4,5]
- Stage IV disease: radiotherapy.[6]

Q24: C. 18%.[5]

- Primary radiotherapy has inferior survival rates compared with hysterectomy, with the risk of intrauterine recurrence of up to 18%. Hence, it should be considered only in exceptional cases.

Q25: C. Urgent referral to cancer centre.[6]

- In women where a vulval cancer is strongly suspicious on examination, urgent referral to a cancer centre should not await biopsy.
- Clinical features strongly indicating vulval cancer include an irregular fumigating mass, an irregular ulcer or enlarged groin nodes.

Q26: C. 30%.[6]

- Overall, about 30% of women with operable vulval cancer have nodal spread.[7]

Q27: B. Stage II.[7]

- Vulval cancer has been staged surgicopathologically using the FIGO staging system (stages I–IV).

Q28: A. Proceed with bilateral lymphadenectomy.[7]

- The purpose of sentinel lymph node biopsy (SLNB) is to determine if the cancer has spread to the first draining lymph node.
- If the sentinel lymph node does not contain cancer, then the cancer has not developed the ability to spread to nearby lymph nodes or other organs.
- If the sentinel lymph node biopsy (SLNB) is negative then no further surgery is necessary.
- If the SLNB is positive then consideration should be given to complete lymphadenectomy of both groins.
- The five-year survival in cases with no lymph node involvement is >80%. This falls to <50% if the inguinal nodes are involved. In cases with iliac of other pelvic nodes involved, five-year survival is 10%–15%.

Q29: B. Wide local excision.[7]

- Groin node dissection should be omitted in verrucous tumour.

Q30: B. Radiotherapy.[7]

- Basal cell carcinoma is rarely associated with lymph node metastases and can be managed by wide local excision.
- It is also amenable to treatment by radiotherapy, which should be the preferred treatment if resection would compromise function of adjacent organs, e.g. anal orifice.

Q31: A. Lichen planus.[8]

- The clinical presentation of lichen planus of the vulva spans a spectrum from subtle, fine, reticulate papules to severe erosive disease.
- Vulval lichen planus is an uncommon cutaneous disease. Vulvar pruritus and pain are common symptoms. Examination reveals an erythematous, friable vestibule, atrophy of the labia minora or scarring and loss of the normal vulvar architecture.
- Diagnosis is based on clinical findings and/or a vulvar biopsy.
- Topical ultrapotent corticosteroid is an effective treatment, with a 71% relief of symptoms.

Q32: B. Lichen sclerosis.[9]

- Lichen sclerosus is a chronic inflammatory dermatosis with white plaques, epidermal atrophy and scarring.

- Vulvar lichen sclerosus usually presents with progressive pruritus, dyspareunia, dysuria or genital bleeding.
- Diagnosis is usually by skin biopsy.
- There is a slightly increased risk of developing squamous cell skin cancer.
- Strong topical steroids seem to be the best treatment.

Q33: E. VIN associated with lichen sclerosis.[10]

- VIN is a vulval skin condition that may become cancerous if left untreated. It is confirmed by histological diagnosis.
- The most common aetiology is HPV type 16.
- A second non-HPV (known as differentiated type) occurs in conjunction with lichen sclerosus or lichen planus. The risk of progression to squamous cell carcinoma is much greater with the differentiated type of VIN and needs specialized management.

References

1. National Health Service Cervical Screening Programme. *Colposcopy and Programme Management.* March, 2016. [https://www.gov.uk/government/uploads]
2. Scottish Intercollegiate Guidelines Network. *Management of Cervical Cancer.* January, 2008. [www.sign.ac.uk/pdf/sign99.pdf]
3. The Royal College of Obstetricians and Gynaecologists. *Endometrial Cancer in Obese Women.* June, 2012. [https://www/rcog.org.uk/en/guidelines-research-services/guidelines/sip32]
4. The Royal College of Obstetricians and Gynaecologists. *Management of Endometrial Hyperplasia.* February, 2016. [https://www.rcog.org.uk/en/guidelines-research-services/guidelines/gtg67]
5. Cruilshank ME. Endometrial cancer. In: Cardozo L, Drife J, Kean L, et al. eds. *Obstetrics and Gynaecology: An Evidence-Based Text for MRCOG*, 2nd edn. London, UK: Edward Arnold, 2010; pp. 798–807.
6. The Royal College of Obstetricians and Gynaecologists. *Guidelines for the Diagnosis and Management of Vulval Carcinoma.* May, 2014. [https://www.rcog.org.uk]
7. FIGO Committee on Gynecologic Oncology. *Revised FIGO Staging for Carcinoma of the Vulva, Cervix, and Endometrium.* September, 2009. [www.csh.org.tw/dr.tcj/education/Cancer%20center/2009pdf]
8. Cooper SM, Wojnarowska F. Influence of treatment of erosive *Lichen planus* of the vulva on its prognosis. *Arch Dermatol* 2006;142(3):289–94.
9. Funaro D, Lovett A, Leroux N, Powell J. A double-blind, randomized prospective study evaluating topical clobetasol propionate 0.05% versus topical tacrolimus 0.1% in patients with vulvar lichen sclerosus. *J Am Acad Dermatol* 2014;71(1):84–91.
10. British Association for Sexual Health and HIV. *UK National Guidance on the Management of Vulval Conditions.* February, 2014. [https://www.bashh.org]

Chapter 16

Menstruation

Radwa Mansour

QUESTIONS

1.

A 36-year-old woman is complaining of having had heavy menstrual bleeding (HMB) for two years. Abdominal examination reveals a 20-week sized uterus and her pelvic scan shows multiple interstitial fibroids. Her haemoglobin level is 9 gm/dL. She is nulliparous and wishes to preserve her fertility.

What management option would you recommend?

- A. Gonadotropin-releasing hormone (GnRH) analogue for six months followed by myomectomy.
- B. MRI-focused ultrasonography.
- C. Open/laparoscopic myomectomy.
- D. Ulipristal acetate.
- E. Uterine artery embolization.

2.

A 24-year-old woman is counselled regarding surgical treatment of a 7-cm symptomatic fibroid. She is keen to know all the facts and particularly wants to hear about new techniques. She wants to know the effect of the procedures on her future fertility.

What information can you give her?

- A. Laparoscopic myomectomy is associated with a lower chance of conception.
- B. Hysteroscopic resection is feasible for almost all types of myomas.
- C. Laparoscopic myomectomy is her best option.
- D. Myolysis and cryomyolysis offer the best chance of conception.
- E. Pregnancy rates are higher after laparoscopic myomectomy when compared to the open approach.

3.

A 48-year-old woman is complaining of abnormal uterine bleeding, which has lasted for two years. She has tried the combined oral contraceptive, oral progestogens, tranexamic acid and mefenamic acid but without any improvement. She has three children and has been sterilized. Her last cervical smear was two years previously and was normal. She had surgery for breast cancer four years before. Her pelvic scan shows no uterine abnormalities. Her endometrial sampling is normal.

What would you offer her as a further step of treatment?

A. Endometrial ablation.
B. Expectant management awaiting the menopause.
C. Hysterectomy.
D. Injectable long-acting progestogens.
E. Levonorgestrel-releasing intrauterine system (LNG-IUS).

4.

A 50-year-old woman has had two previous episodes of abnormal uterine bleeding. She had a cervical smear a year previously, which was normal. Pelvic ultrasound scanning shows an endometrial thickness of 15 mm. She is on anticoagulation for recurrent thromboembolic events.

What is your next step in management?

A. Book for inpatient dilatation and curettage.
B. Inpatient hysteroscopy and biopsy.
C. LNG-IUS.
D. Outpatient office hysteroscopy and biopsy.
E. Pipelle biopsy in the clinic and offer LNG-IUS.

5.

An 18-year-old woman is referred to you because of her concerns about the irregularity of her menstrual cycle. She thinks she has very frequent cycles, which come every 25 days but may increase to every 38 days. She also thinks that she loses a lot of blood. Her general practitioner says she is not anaemic and a 2D ultrasound scan was normal. He tried to reassure her but she insists on referral.

How best can you handle the situation?

A. Ask her to measure her menstrual blood loss for the next two periods and report it if it is >120 mL.
B. Reassure her and explain that the average cycle length is between 24 days and 38 days.
C. Counsel her for an endometrial sample.
D. Repeat the haemoglobin after three months.
E. Request a 3D ultrasound.

6.

A 45-year-old woman complains of HMB. She has tried medical treatment without any improvement. All her investigations came back as normal. She is frustrated and keen to have an explanation for her problem.

What information should you give her to reassure her?

A. Between 40% and 60% of women with HMB have no uterine, endocrine, haematological or infective pathology on investigation.
B. Endometriosis is associated with >10% of HMB.
C. HMB affects around 20%–30% of premenopausal women.

D. The most common age that is presented to secondary care with this problem is 41–50 years.
E. Uterine fibroids represent 10% of pathological causes of HMB.

7.

A 20-year-old woman with learning difficulties comes with her caregiver who states that she has frequent irregular menstruation, which is also causing her problems with her hygienic care. Her pelvic scan is normal and her BMI is 22.

What will you advise when prescribing medical treatment for her?

A. A three-month continuous use of combined oral contraceptive pills (COCP) and restart a new three-cycle after the end of the withdrawal bleed.
B. Depot medroxyprogesterone acetate (DMPA).
C. LNG-IUS.
D. Surgical options, including endometrial ablation or hysterectomy.
E. The combined transdermal contraception patch.

8.

A 30-year-old woman comes to see you because of her symptomatic fibroid uterus. She has read about uterine artery embolization. She wants to know how it may compare to other methods of treatment.

Which is the best statement you can give her regarding the complications of this procedure?

A. Equal complication rates with that of surgical techniques.
B. Higher rates of need of re-intervention when compared to the MRI-guided focused ultrasonography.
C. Higher satisfaction rate than surgery (myomectomy or hysterectomy).
D. Less need for further intervention if compared to surgical options of treatment.
E. The most common side effects reported after the procedure are pain and vaginal discharge.

9.

One of your junior colleagues comes to ask you about the pharmacological treatments for fibroid uterus. He wants to know the mechanism of action for some of these medications.

What is your best explanation?

A. LNG-IUS acts by reduction of the fibroid size.
B. There is a specific histological appearance of the endometrium, which appears with the use of ulipristal acetate (UA) and persists for a year after stopping the treatment.
C. UA induces apoptosis in fibroid cells and inhibition of cellular proliferation.
D. When compared to GnRH analogues, UA controls menstrual blood loss less rapidly.
E. GnRH analogue long-term use may produce permanent reduction of fibroid size.

10.

A 26-year-old woman is complaining of HMB and dysmenorrhea for six months. She has used tranexamic acid and mefenamic acid without any improvement and now she has a LNG-IUS that was fitted one month previously. She is still having slight irregular bleeding, although the pain has improved.

How long should she expect to have this irregular bleeding?

A. This could last up to six weeks.
B. This could last up to eight weeks.
C. This could last up to 12 weeks.
D. This could last up to 18 weeks.
E. This could last up to 24 weeks.

11.

A 36-year-old woman is referred to the gynaecology clinic complaining of secondary amenorrhea for the last eight months since stopping COCP, which she has been taking for two years. She is a mother of two children. Her BMI is 24. Hormonal assessment five weeks previously showed her follicular stimulating hormone (FSH) of 26 IU/L and luteinizing hormone (LH) of 20 IU/L.

What will be your next step for diagnosis?

A. Anti-Mullerian hormone assay.
B. Auto-ovarian antibody assay.
C. Diagnostic of ovarian failure; no need for further tests.
D. Progesterone withdrawal test to confirm diagnosis.
E. Repeat FSH and LH.

12.

An 18-year-old national gymnastic champion is referred to you. She experiences long periods of secondary amenorrhea and she only has two to three periods each year. She is training for the coming Olympics but her general practitioner advised her to visit you because she is worried about her. She suffers from backache. Her BMI is 16.

What will you offer her?

A. Cyclic COCP.
B. Cyclic progesterone for withdrawal bleeding.
C. Depomedroxy progesterone acetate.
D. GnRH analogue.
E. Reassure and review her after the championship.

13.

An 18-year-old woman is referred to you by her general practitioner because of severe dysmenorrhea. She is experiencing severe pain with her periods such that she skips her academic classes for three days each month. She has tried mefenamic acid and other analgesics without improvement. She has also tried oral contraceptive pills but is still in pain. She is not a smoker and is not sexually active.

What is the most appropriate approach?

A. Carry out a full sexually transmitted infection screening.
B. Computerized tomography.
C. Refer for acupuncture.
D. Try other codeine tablets during the periods.
E. Laparoscopy.

14.

You are reviewing a 36-year-old woman with severe premenstrual tension syndrome (PMS). She is tearful and says she was about to lose her job after an argument with a work colleague just before her last menses. She has completed her family. She is exercising regularly. She has tried cognitive behavioral therapy. Her BMI is 35 and she is a smoker.

What will offer her as treatment?

A. Non-cyclical COCP.
B. GnRH analogue and add back therapy.
C. Hysterectomy and bilateral salpingo-oohorectomy.
D. Low-dose selective serotonin reuptake inhibitor (SSRI).
E. Vitamin B6.

15.

A 39-year-old Jehovah's Witness woman attends the gynaecology clinic complaining of HMB. She has used hormonal and non-hormonal medical treatments with no effect. Her haemoglobin dropped to 90 g/L during her last period. A transvaginal scan showed multiple uterine fibroids 3–12 cm in size. She wishes to start a family soon and wants to avoid surgery.

What is the most appropriate management option?

A. Blood transfusion to treat anaemia.
B. Non-cyclical oral contraception.
C. Mirena coil.
D. GnRH analogues.
E. UAE.

16.

A 26-year-old woman attends the clinic complaining of intermenstrual bleeding. On direct questioning she explains that her periods are regular and of normal amount and duration. She been with her current boyfriend for the last nine months. She has also experienced post-coital bleeding for the last three weeks. Her last smear report one year ago was normal with a normal cervix. She was not keen on an internal speculum examination.

What would you like to offer next?

A. A self-collected vaginal swab.
B. A repeat cervix smear.
C. A transvaginal scan.
D. Referral to the genitourinary clinic.
E. Urgent referral to colposcopy.

17.

A 20-year-old female student attends the gynaecology clinic complaining of HMB and dysmenorrhoea. She is otherwise healthy and well. Currently, she has no concerns about her fertility.

What is the first line of management for this patient according to the NICE guidelines?

A. COCP.
B. LNG-IUS.
C. Northisterone.
D. Non-steroidal anti-inflammatory drugs (NSAIDs).
E. Tranexamic acid.

ANSWERS

Q1: A. GnRH analogue for six months followed by myomectomy [evidence level 1+].[1]

- A Cochrane review suggested a 36% reduction in leiomyoma size and an improvement in symptoms after 12 weeks preoperative GnRH analogue treatment in women undergoing hysterectomy or myomectomy.[1]
- GnRH analogue treatment also allows for correction of haemoglobin level and reduces intraoperative blood loss.[1]
- GnRH analogue treatment induces a menopausal state, which may result in intolerable side effects and bone loss.
- The hypo-oestrogenic side effects could be minimized by adding low-dose oestrogen and progestin or tibolone after the initial phase of down regulation. GnRH analogue treatment is therefore limited to a maximum of six months.

Q2: C. Laparoscopic myomectomy is her best option [evidence level 1−].[2]

- Laparoscopic myomectomy is considered the best treatment option for symptomatic uterine fibroids in women who wish to retain childbearing capacity.
- Systematic reviews and one meta-analysis showed that the laparoscopic approach is associated with longer operating times but less blood loss, less postoperative pain and fewer complications than open conventional myomectomy.
- Myolysis (in which an electric current is passed through a needle to destroy the fibroid) or cryomyolysis (in which a freezing probe is used in a similar manner) can be used for all types of fibroids through laparoscopic or hysteroscopic routes. They are associated with less blood loss but have the disadvantages of providing no tissue for histology, an increased risk of postoperative adhesions and the need for reintervention.[2]

Q3: A. Endometrial ablation.[3]

- In women with heavy menstrual bleeding alone, who do not wish to preserve fertility, and with a uterus no bigger than a 10-week pregnancy, endometrial ablation should be considered preferable to hysterectomy.[3]
- For option (E), the Mirena intrauterine device is category 3 of the UK medical eligibility criteria where the risk outweighs the benefits.

Q4: D. Outpatient office hysteroscopy and biopsy [evidence level 2−].[4]

- Hysteroscopy and directed biopsy is generally accepted as the gold standard for evaluating the endometrial cavity. Historic dilation and curettage alone is no longer acceptable.
- Outpatient hysteroscopy with targeted biopsies has a sensitivity, specificity, positive predictive value and negative predictive value 98%, 95%, 96% and 98%, respectively, when compared with the histological findings at hysterectomy.[4]
- The positive predictive value of Pipelle endometrial samples in detecting endometrial polyps is higher in postmenopausal women (72.7%) compared to premenopausal women (53.7%).

Q5: B. Reassure her and explain that the average cycle length is between 24 days and 38 days.

- The mean frequency of menses (or length of the menstrual cycle) is 28 days.[5]
- Accepted variations are frequent (<24 days) to infrequent (>38 days). The mean duration of blood loss is 5–7 days.

- The mean monthly menstrual blood loss is 40–80 mL, heavy is >80 mL, light is <5 mL.
- Regular cycle-to-cycle variation is between 2–20 days, irregular variation is >20 days or absent.
- Bleeding is heavy if there is enough blood to soak a pad or tampon every hour for several consecutive hours, night-time bleeding that requires getting up to change pads or tampons, passing large blood clots during menstruation and/or a period that lasts longer than seven days.

Q6: A. Between 40% and 60% of women with HMB have no uterine, endocrine, haematological or infective pathology on investigation.[6]

- HMB due to ovulatory or endometrial dysfunction that does not require secondary referral and treatment can be managed in primary care.
- Pathological causes of HMB include uterine fibroids (20%–30%), uterine polyps (5%–10%), adenomyosis (5%). Endometriosis is associated with 5% of cases.
- Endometriosis rarely presents as abnormal uterine bleeding, but is identified in <5% of cases.
- Some prevalence studies have identified a gap in women's knowledge on HMB and suggested a possible need for community-based education to raise awareness of HMB.[6]

Q7: A. A three-month continuous use of combined oral contraceptive pills (COCP) and restart a new three-month cycle after the end of the withdrawal bleed.[7]

- COCP reduces the menstrual flow and dysmenorrhoea and allows control over the timing of menstruation. It may be used continuously for three months; then wait for withdrawal bleeding. A new cycle can then be started. This method is not suitable for those in a wheelchair because of an increased risk of deep vein thrombosis.
- The main concern with DMPA (which eliminates the need for daily compliance and swallowing) is reduction of bone mineral density due to the suppression of the hypothalamic–pituitary–ovarian axis, which causes low circulating levels of oestrogen. The Committee on Safety of Medicines in the UK have advised that in adolescents 'DMPA should only be used when other methods of contraception are inappropriate'.
- Compared to COCP users, combined transdermal contraception patch users experienced more breast discomfort, dysmenorrhoea, nausea and vomiting.[7]
- The insertion of the LNG-IUS in this group of patients may require general anaesthesia with its risks.
- Surgical options are not suitable because of her young age.

Q8: E. The most common side effects reported after the procedure are pain and vaginal discharge [evidence level 2+].[8]

- Uterine artery embolization (UAE) involves cannulating the femoral artery and identifying the uterine arteries before injecting an embolic agent to impair the blood supply to the uterus and fibroids.
- UAE was introduced in 1994 and is considered an effective alternative to hysterectomy.
- An updated Cochrane review in 2014 reporting on 793 women showed that patient satisfaction with UAE was similar to that with surgery (myomectomy and hysterectomy) with quicker recovery and early return to work.
- UAE was associated with more minor complications and an almost five-fold increase in the likelihood of further interventions within 2–5 years. The long-term follow-up showed no significant difference in ovarian failure rates.

- The Hopeful Study, which included a five-year follow-up after UAE or hysterectomy, showed that both treatments were safe. A meta-analysis including randomized and non-randomized clinical trials also suggested that UAE was associated with a lower rate of major complications compared with surgery.
- However, UAE had an increased risk of re-intervention (OR 10.45; 95% CI 2.65–41.14).

Q9: C. UA induces apoptosis in fibroid cells and inhibition of cellular proliferation [evidence level 1+].[9]

- UA is a selective progesterone receptor modulator with the trade names EllaOne in the European Union, Ella in the United States for contraception and Esmya for uterine fibroids).
- Treatment dosage: one 5-mg tablet to be taken orally once daily for treatment courses of up to three months each. Treatments should only be initiated when menstruation has occurred.
- The first treatment course should start during the first week of menstruation.
- Treatment usually leads to a significant reduction in menstrual blood loss or amenorrhea within the first 10 days.
- Menstrual periods generally return within four weeks after the end of each treatment course.
- The PEARL II trial was a double-blind 13-week comparison of UA with a GnRH analogue and showed that repeated three-month UA courses effectively control bleeding and shrink fibroids in patients with symptomatic fibroids.
- UA has minor side effects (cramps, vaginal discharge, dizziness), which usually improve with time.
- There is general agreement among several reviews that use of the LNG-IUS in women with fibroids is successful in reducing menstrual blood loss, increasing haemoglobin and relieving symptoms. There are conflicting results regarding its effect on fibroids or uterine volume and device expulsion rates.
- GnRH analogue treatment in women undergoing hysterectomy or myomectomy suggested a 36% reduction in leiomyoma size and an improvement in symptoms after 12 weeks. After discontinuation of treatment, menstruation returned in four to eight weeks and fibroid size returned to pretreatment levels within four to six months.
- GnRH can be used short term to allow for treatment of anaemia or in the preparation for surgery.

Q10: E. This could last up to 24 weeks.

- Women offered the LNG-IUS should be advised of anticipated changes in the bleeding pattern, particularly in the first few cycles and maybe lasting longer than six months. Therefore, they should be advised to persevere for at least six cycles to see the benefits of the treatment.
- Common side effects of LNG-IUS include irregular bleeding that may last for over six months; hormone-related problems such as breast tenderness, acne and headaches, which, if present, are generally minor and transient.
- Less common side effect is amenorrhoea.
- Rare complication is uterine perforation at the time of insertion.[3]

Q11: E. Repeat FSH and LH.[10]

- For the diagnosis of premature ovarian failure (POF), testing should be repeated after at least four weeks from the first test. A persistent increase confirms a diagnosis of POF. Although proper diagnostic accuracy in POF is lacking, NICE recommends the following diagnostic criteria: oligo-/amenorrhoea for four months and FSH of >25 IU/L on two occasions more than four weeks apart .

- One-third to one-half of POF cases are idiopathic, other causes include X-chromosome deletions, radiation or chemotherapy, and genetic defects of the gonadotropin hormone receptors.
- Ultrasound examination of the pelvis should be arranged for every woman with the symptoms described here to assess endometrial thickness (oestrogen status), ovarian volume and antral follicle count.
- Anti-Müllerian hormone estimation can assess ovarian reserve.
- Ovarian biopsy has unknown clinical value, is not cost effective and has surgical risks. Pregnancy has been reported even when a specimen has shown absence of follicles.
- A dual-emission X-ray absorptiometry scan should be considered for baseline assessment, as women with POF have a 50% risk for osteopenia.

Q12: A. Cyclic COCP.[11]

- The diagnosis of exercise-induced amenorrhea is primarily a diagnosis of exclusion.
- Menstrual irregularities are common in sportswomen (44%).
- Intense exercise in highly competitive athletes who train daily can suppress the pulsatile nature of GnRH.
- Exercise-induced amenorrhea has the potential to cause severe long-term morbidity, particularly with regard to osteoporosis.
- Oestrogen is also important in the formation of collagen and in healing of soft tissue injuries, which are common in amenorrhoeic female athletes. Young athletes may be placing themselves at risk when the attainment of peak bone mass is important for long-term skeletal strength.
- Diet and the use of a cyclical oestrogen/progestogen preparation should be considered in order to reinstate a normal menstrual cycle with the aim of preventing long-term morbidity.

Q13: E. Laparoscopy.[12]

- Primary dysmenorrhea is menstrual pain that is not associated with pelvic disease. It occurs in the first few years after menarche and affects as many as 50% of postpubertal girls.
- Secondary dysmenorrhea is defined as menstrual pain resulting from anatomical or macroscopic pelvic pathology, e.g. endometriosis or chronic pelvic inflammatory disease. It is most often observed in women aged 30–45 years.
- Laparoscopy is indicated when initial interventions fail to relieve symptoms to exclude any associated pelvic pathology. It is the single most useful procedure to offer a complete diagnostic survey of the pelvis and reproductive organs.
- Psychological support and lifestyle modifications (alcohol, smoking and obesity) may be of benefit.

Q14: D. Low-dose selective serotonin reuptake inhibitor (SSRI) [recommendation grade A; evidence level 1a & 1b].[13]

- First-line therapy includes exercise, cognitive behaviour therapy, vitamin B6, combined new generation pill, continuous or luteal phase low-dose SSRI (e.g. citalopram/escitalopram, 10 mg).
- Because of her BMI and being a smoker, low-dose SSRI is the more suitable. According to the UKMEC, where there are multiple risk factors (obesity and smoking), the use of combined hormonal contraception is category 3 (proven risks usually outweigh the advantages of using the method).

Q15: E. UAE.[14]

- UAE is recommended as an option for women with HMB associated with uterine fibroids and who want to retain their uterus and/or avoid surgery.
- 80%–90% will be asymptomatic or significantly improved within 12 months of UAE with a 40%–70 % reduction in fibroid volume. Mean volume reduction of the fibroid and uterus was 44% and 43%.
- If pregnancy occurs after UAE, patients can have a successful birth and delivery, but careful obstetric monitoring is advised.
- Obstetric risks after UAE for fibroids include prematurity, intrauterine growth restriction, abnormal placentation and increased likelihood of Caesarean delivery.

Q16: A. A self-collected vaginal swab.[15]

- Young sexually active women presenting with intermenstrual or postcoital bleeding should be tested for chlamydia.[15]
- Center for Disease Control recommends the nucleic acid amplification test (NAAT) of a self-collected vaginal swab, which does not require a speculum examination, to diagnose chlamydia.

Q17: B. LNG-IUS.[3]

- If pharmaceutical treatment is appropriate and either hormonal or non-hormonal treatments are acceptable, treatments should be considered in the following order: LNG-IUS provided long-term (at least 12 months) use is anticipated, tranexamic acid or non-steroidal anti-inflammatory drugs (NSAIDs) or COCP, norethisterone (15 mg) daily from days 5 to 26 of the menstrual cycle or injected long-acting progestogens.[3]

References

1. Lethaby A, Vollenhoven B, Sowter MC. Pre-operative GnRH analogue therapy before hysterectomy or myomectomy for uterine fibroids. *Cochrane Database Syst Rev* 2001;(2):CD000547.
2. Desai P, Patel P. Fibroids, infertility and laparoscopic myomectomy. *J Gynecol Endosc Surg* 2011;2(1):36–42.
3. National Institute of Clinical Excellence. *Heavy Menstrual Bleeding: Assessment and Management.* January, 2007. [nice.org.uk/guidance/cg44]
4. Seto MT, Ip PP, Ngu SF, Cheung AN2, Pun TC. Positive predictive value of endometrial polyps in Pipelle aspiration sampling: a histopathological study of 195 cases. *Eur J Obstet Gynecol Reprod Biol* 2016;203:12–15.
5. Fraser IS, Critchley HOD, Munro MG, Broder M. Can we achieve international agreement on terminologies and definitions used to describe abnormalities of menstrual bleeding? *Hum Reprod* 2007;22:635–43.
6. Marsh EE, Brocks ME, Ghant MS, Recht HS, Simonb M. Prevalence and knowledge of heavy menstrual bleeding among African American women. *Int J Gynaecol Obstet* 2014;125(1):56–9.
7. Jeffery E, Kayani S, Garden A. Management of menstrual problems in adolescents with learning and physical disabilities. *Obstet Gynaecol* 2013;15:106–12.
8. Gupta JK, Sinha A, Lumsden MA, Hickey M. Uterine artery embolization for symptomatic uterine fibroids. *Cochrane Database Syst Rev* 2014;(12):CD005073.15.
9. Donnez J, Vázquez F, Tomaszewski J, et al. Long-term treatment of uterine fibroids with ulipristal acetate. *Fertil Steril* 2014;101:1565–73.
10. Arora P, Polson DW. Diagnosis and management of premature ovarian failure. *Obstet Gynaecol* 2011;13:67–72.

11. Balen A. Amenorrhoea. In: Balen A, ed. *Reproductive Endocrinology for the MRCOG and Beyond*, 2nd edn. London, UK: RCOG Press, 2007; pp. 77–88.
12. Calis KA, Erogul M, Popat V, Kalantaridou SN, Dang DK. *Dysmenorrhea*. October, 2016. [http://emedicine.medscape.com/article/253812-overview#a6]
13. Royal College of Obstetricians and Gynaecologists. *Management of Premenstrual Syndrome*. December, 2016. [https://www.rcog.org.uk/en/guidelines-research-services/guidelines/gtg48]
14. Smeets AJ, Nijenhuis RJ, van Rooij WJ, et al. Uterine artery embolization in patients with a large fibroid burden: long-term clinical and MR follow-up. *Cardiovasc Intervent Radiol* 2010;33(5):943–8.
15. Centers for Diseases Control and Prevention. *2015 Sexually Transmitted Diseases Treatment Guidelines*. June, 2015. [https://www.cdc.gov/std/tg2015/chlamydia.htm]

Chapter 17

Pelvic Pathology

Akanksha Sood

QUESTIONS

1.

A 26-year-old woman has had two previous miscarriages and has a BMI of 24, has been in a stable relationship for three years and is keen to conceive. She presents with cyclical lower abdominal pain, menstrual dyschezia, unregulated bowel habits and bloating of the abdomen. The transvaginal ultrasound scan (TVS) findings are: uterus measuring 8 x 6 x 3 cm, normal appearance of ovaries.

What is your interpretation of these findings?

A. Adenomyosis.
B. Bicornuate uterus.
C. Impacted faeces.
D. Irritable bowel syndrome.
E. Rectal endometriosis.

2.

One of your year ST2 junior colleagues shows you a study indicating that in 60% of adult females, endometriosis symptoms started before the age of 20 years. He wants to know if there is a way to prevent the occurrence of this disease.

What would you tell him?

A. Combined contraceptive pills.
B. Danazol.
C. Exercise and increased physical activity.
D. Progestogen only pill.
E. No primary prevention strategies.

3.

A 35-year-old woman is having difficulty in getting pregnant. She also gives a history of dysmenorrhea and menstrual dyschezia. Her symptoms and examination are suggestive of rectal endometriosis.

What is the recommended investigation to make to exclude such a diagnosis?

A. Abdominal ultrasound.
B. Magnetic resonance imaging.
C. Laparoscopy.
D. Transvaginal ultrasound.
E. 3D ultrasound.

4.

A 38-year-old woman, who is a para 6, has come to the gynaecology clinic with complaints of dull pain in her lower abdomen and pelvis radiating to the thighs; it increases on standing and after menses. She also complains of dyspareunia. There are no bowel or urinary complaints. On clinical examination, there are no signs of infection. A transvaginal scan of the pelvis was normal. Diagnostic laparoscopy was negative.

What is the appropriate treatment option for her?

A. Botox injections into the levator ani.
B. Gabapentin 300 mg three times a day.
C. Medroxyprogesterone acetate 5 mg three times a day for 21 days, followed by withdrawal bleeding, and continued for three to six months.
D. Total abdominal hysterectomy and bilateral salpingo-oophorectomy.
E. Transvenous embolization of the ovarian vein.

5.

A 32-year-old woman, who is a para 2, has come to the gynaecology clinic with chronic pelvic pain for the past two years. Pain increases in the squatting position and is relieved on standing/straightening of legs. It is associated with dyspareunia. She also gives a history of generalized malaise and tiredness. There are no bowel/urinary symptoms. On clinical examination, there is a tight ropy band palpable along the levator ani muscle. The transvaginal ultrasound scan of the pelvis was normal.

What is the appropriate treatment option for her?

A. Botox injections into the levator ani.
B. Gabapentin 300 mg three times a day
C. Medroxyprogesterone acetate 5 mg three times a day for 21 days, followed by withdrawal bleeding, and continued for three to six months.
D. Total abdominal hysterectomy and bilateral salpingo-oophorectomy.
E. Transvenous embolization of the ovarian vein.

6.

A 35-year-old woman, who is a para 1, has come to the gynaecological clinic with chronic pain in her lower abdomen and pelvis for the past 10 years. The pain is non-cyclical, dull-aching and not associated with movement. There are no bowel or urinary symptoms. The abdominal and pelvic examination was unremarkable. The TVS of the pelvis is normal. Diagnostic laparoscopy done one year previously was negative.

What is the appropriate treatment option for her?

A. Botox injections into the levator ani.
B. Gabapentin 300 mg three times a day.
C. Medroxyprogesterone acetate 5 mg three times a day for 21 days, followed by withdrawal bleeding, and continued for three to six months.
D. Total abdominal hysterectomy and bilateral salpingo-oophorectomy.
E. Transvenous embolization of the ovarian vein.

7.

A 40-year-old female, who is a para 2+1, had firstly a vaginal delivery and secondly a Caesarean section for fetal distress. She has presented with chronic pelvic pain three months after her lower uterine segment Caesarian section (LSCS).

What is the incidence of nerve entrapment after LSCS?

A. 2.7%.
B. 3.7%.
C. 4.7%.
D. 5.7%.
E. 6.7%.

8.

Chronic pelvic pain should be seen as a symptom with a number of contributory factors rather than as a diagnosis in itself. A patient presenting with chronic pelvic pain wants to know what the incidence is of chronic pelvic pain in the adult female population.

A. 1 in 6.
B. 1 in 12.
C. 1 in 18.
D. 1 in 24.
E. 1 in 30.

9.

A 40-year-old woman, who is a para 2+1, presents with secondary amenorrhea for the past 10 months and complains of weight gain. She has increased two dress sizes over the last year. The pelvic examination was normal. A TVS shows an increased antral follicle count (AFC) and increased ovarian volume.

What is the most appropriate next investigation for her?

A. Fasting insulin levels.
B. Oral glucose tolerance test (OGTT).
C. Serum prolactin.
D. FSH/LH ratio.
E. Thyroid stimulating hormone.

10.

A 35-year-old woman, who is a para 2+1, has presented with secondary amenorrhea for the past 10 months and complains of weight gain. She has increased two dress sizes over the last year. The pelvic examination was normal. The TVS shows an increased AFC and increased ovarian volume.

What is the best treatment option for her?

A. Clomiphene for induction of ovulation.
B. Gonadotropin.
C. Ovarian drilling.
D. Metformin for regulation of insulin metabolism.
E. Withdrawal bleed every three to four months.

11.

A 28-year-old woman has presented with oligomenorrhoea, hirsutism and weight gain over the past two years. She has been diagnosed with polycystic ovarian syndrome (PCOS). Her BMI is 40 kg/m². She was advised about lifestyle measures to lose weight, which failed. She is currently not in a relationship but wishes to have children later.

What is the next best option that can be considered regarding her weight?

A. To be referred for in vitro fertilization (IVF).
B. To consider bariatric surgery.
C. To continue lifestyle measures with an expert dietician's advice.
D. To start extensive exercises.
E. To start metformin 500 mg three times a day for six months.

12.

A young 25-year-old woman is diagnosed with PCOS. Her BMI is 22. Her mother had type 2 diabetes and her elder sister developed gestational diabetes in her first pregnancy. She is concerned about her risk of developing diabetes. The OGTT fasting glucose level was 6.5 mmol/L.

What is the recommended next step for her?

A. Annual HbA1c.
B. Annual OGTT.
C. Lifestyle measures to keep fit.
D. No further investigation required as her BMI is normal.
E. Start metformin 500 mg twice a day.

13.

Hirsutism, characterized by excess facial and body hair and midline hair growth, is a common clinical presentation of PCOS. Although free and total testosterone is used in the diagnosis of PCOS, the recommended baseline biochemical test for hyperandrogenism is the free androgen index.

How is the free androgen index calculated?

A. Free testosterone/sex hormone-binding globulin x 100.
B. Free testosterone/total testosterone x 100.
C. Total testosterone/free testosterone x 100.
D. Total testosterone/sex hormone-binding globulin x 100.
E. Total testosterone − free testosterone/sex hormone-binding globulin x 100.

ANSWERS

Q1: E. Rectal endometriosis.[1]

- In endometriosis, leading symptoms are dysmenorrhea, chronic pelvic pain, deep dyspareunia, cyclical intestinal complaints, fatigue/weariness and infertility.[1,2]
- The symptoms depend on the location of the disease. Deep endometriosis of the posterior pelvis is associated with increased severity of dyschezia.
- Deep endometriosis of the rectovaginal septum is associated with the most severe forms of dyschezia and dyspareunia.[1]

Q2: E. No primary prevention strategies [grade C recommendation].[1]

- Because the cause of endometriosis is unknown, the potential for primary prevention is limited. The usefulness of oral contraception and physical exercise is uncertain for primary prevention of endometriosis.[1]

Q3: D. Transvaginal ultrasound [grade A recommendation].[1]

- In women with symptoms and signs of rectal endometriosis, transvaginal ultrasound scan (TVS) is useful for identifying or ruling out rectal endometriosis.
- TVS results are operator dependent; the scan should be performed by an experienced sonographer.[1]

Q4: E. Transvenous embolization of the ovarian vein [evidence level 1+].[2]

- **Pelvic congestion syndrome:** chronic pelvic pain arising from dilated and refluxing incompetent pelvic veins.[2]
  - Presentation: multiparous women of reproductive age, suggesting mechanical and hormonal mechanism.
  - The pain typically is described as dull pelvic pain that radiates to the upper thighs and is aggravated by prolonged standing and walking.[2]
  - The proportion of women found to have pelvic vein incompetence and who report chronic pelvic pain varies from 39% to 91%.[2]
  - Transvaginal Doppler and MR venography are useful screening tools but definitive diagnosis can be made by venography.
- **Treatment:** embolization of the refluxing vein has been highly successful. There has been subjective improvement in pelvic pain frequency, dysmenorrhoea and dyspareunia lasting for up to five years. Re-intervention rates were low. Common complications observed were transient pain after the procedure and a 2% risk of dye migration.

Q5: A. Botox injections into the levator ani [evidence level 1+].[3]

- **Myofascial chronic pelvic pain** usually arises from a trigger point formed due to a metabolic crisis within the muscle. It is palpable as a taut, ropy band. Pain is movement related, aggravated by specific movement or activity and relieved by certain positions.
  - Trigger points involve the levator ani muscle in levator ani syndrome, and other pelvic floor muscles can cause chronic pelvic pain.
- **Treatment:** current guidelines by the RCOG and Cochrane database suggest trigger point injections with local anaesthetic, corticosteroids and botulinum toxin A to treat chronic myofascial pelvic pain. This also provides long-term analgesia.
  - Studies have shown that botulinum toxin type A may be a useful agent in women with pelvic floor muscle spasm and chronic pelvic pain, who do not respond to conservative physiotherapy.
  - Self-limiting adverse effects like *de novo* urinary retention, faecal incontinence and constipation and/or rectal pain have been reported but not any long-term adverse effects.

Q6: B. Gabapentin 300 mg three times a day [evidence level 1+].[4]

- Gabapentin is a gamma-aminobutyric acid analogue, which is an inhibitory neurotransmitter.
- A recent double-blind, multi-centre, randomized controlled trial found that chronic pelvic pain can be suppressed by gabapentin.
- It is reasonable to consider antidepressant and anticonvulsant drugs (although the mechanisms of action are not completely understood). Both classes of drugs are well tolerated with relatively minor adverse effects.

Q7: B. 3.7%.[5]

- Nerve entrapment in scar tissue, fascia or a narrow foramen may result in pain and dysfunction in the distribution of that nerve.
- The incidence of nerve entrapment (defined as highly localized, sharp, stabbing or aching pain, exacerbated by particular movements, and persisting beyond five weeks or occurring after a pain-free interval) after one Pfannenstiel incision is 3.7%.

Q8: A. 1 in 6.[5]

Q9: B. Oral glucose tolerance test (OGTT) [grade B recommendation].[6]

- Women presenting with PCOS who are overweight (BMI$\geq$25 kg/m^2), and women with PCOS who are not overweight (BMI<25 kg/m^2) but who have additional risk factors such as advanced age (>40 years), personal history of gestational diabetes or family history of type 2 diabetes, should have a two-hour post-75 g OGTT performed anually.[6]

Q10: E. Withdrawal bleed every three to four months [good practice point].[6]

- Oligo- or amenorrhoea in women with PCOS may predispose to endometrial hyperplasia and later carcinoma (2.89-fold) because of hyperoestrogenism. It is good practice to recommend treatment with gestogens to induce a withdrawal bleed, at least every three to four months.[5]
- There does not appear to be an association with breast or ovarian cancer and no additional surveillance is required.

Q11: B. To consider bariatric surgery [grade C recommendation].[5]

- Bariatric surgery may be an option for morbidly obese women with PCOS (BMI of 40 kg/m^2 or more, or 35 kg/m^2 or more with a high-risk obesity-related condition), if standard weight loss strategies have failed.[5]
- Bariatric surgery may be indicated in selected women with PCOS and morbid obesity. Bariatric surgery may induce a significant weight loss (up to 60% of excess weight) and improve diabetes, hypertension and dyslipidaemia, reducing mortality from cardiovascular disease and cancer when compared with lifestyle modification. Long-term weight loss of 14%–25% may result.

Q12: B. Annual OGTT [Grade B recommendation].[5]

- In women with impaired fasting glucose (fasting plasma glucose level from 6.1 mmol/L to 6.9 mmol/L) or impaired glucose tolerance (plasma glucose of 7.8 mmol/L or more but less than 11.1 mmol/L after a two-hour OGTT), an OGTT should be performed annually.[5]
- It would be reasonable to carry out HbA1c measurements where women are unwilling to have an OGTT or where the resources are not readily available.

Q13: D. Total testosterone/sex hormone-binding globulin x 100.[7]

- The recommended baseline biochemical test for hyperandrogenism is the free androgen index.

References

1. European Society of Human Reproduction and Embryology. *Management of Women with Endometriosis*. September, 2013. [https://www.eshre.eu/guidelines]
2. Champaneria R, Shah L, Moss J, et al. The relationship between pelvic vein incompetence and chronic pelvic pain in women: systematic reviews of diagnosis

and treatment effectiveness. *Health Technol Assess (Winchester, England)* 2016;20 (5):1–108.

3. Adelowo A, Hacker MR, Shapiro A, Modest AM, Elkadry E. Botulinum toxin type A (BOTOX) for refractory myofascial pelvic pain. *Female Pelvic Med Reconstr Surg* 2013;19(5):288–92.

4. Royal College of Obstetricans and Gynaecologists. *Therapies Targeting the Nervous System for Chronic Pelvic Pain Relief.* January, 2015. [https://www.rcog.org.uk/en/guidelines-research-services/guidelines/sip46]

5. Royal College of Obstetricans and Gynaecologists. *The Initial Management of Chronic Pelvic Pain.* May, 2012. [https://www.rcog.org.uk/en/guidelines-research-services/guidelines/gtg41]

6. Royal College of Obstetricans and Gynaecologists. *Long-term Consequences of Polycystic Ovarian Syndrome.* November, 2014, [https://www.rcog.org.uk/en/guidelines-research-services/guidelines/gtg33]

7. Cho LW, Kilpatrick ES, Jayagopal V, Diver MJ, Atkin SL. Biological variation of total testosterone, free androgen index and bioavailable testosterone in polycystic ovarian syndrome: implications for identifying hyperandrogenaemia. *Clin Endocrinol* (Oxford) 2008;68:390–4.

Chapter 18

Urogynaecology

QUESTIONS

1.

You review a woman in the urogynaecology outpatient clinic. You decided to start her on anticholinergic therapy as she has symptoms of overactive bladder that has failed to respond to lifestyle modification and bladder retraining.

How long will it take before she can expect to see the full benefits of taking this medication?

A. Three weeks.
B. Four weeks.
C. Five weeks.
D. Six weeks.
E. Eight weeks.

2.

A 51-year-old woman with two previous vaginal deliveries is seen in the gynaecology outpatient clinic complaining of leaking urine on coughing and sneezing for the past three months. She has no other urinary symptoms and is not on any medications. Abdominal and pelvic examination is normal.

What would you tell her regarding the number of pelvic floor contractions to perform and the frequency of the exercise programme per day?

A. Pelvic floor muscle training programme: at least four contractions, three times per day.
B. Pelvic floor muscle training programme: at least six contractions, three times per day.
C. Pelvic floor muscle training programme: at least eight contractions, three times per day.
D. Pelvic floor muscle training programme: at least 10 contractions, three times per day.
E. Pelvic floor muscle training programme: at least 12 contractions, three times per day.

3.

A 65-year-old woman is prescribed mirabegron (Betmiga, Astellas Pharma) for detrusor overactivity.

What type of drug is mirabegron?

A. Anti-muscarinic.
B. B1-adrenoceptor agonist.
C. B2-adrenoceptor agonist.
D. B3-adrenoceptor agonist.
E. Serotonin–norepinephrine reuptake inhibitor.

4.

You see a woman in the gynaecology outpatient clinic. She has symptoms of frequency and urgency of micturition. You asked her to keep a bladder diary.

Over what length of time should a bladder diary be undertaken?

A. Two days.
B. Three days.
C. Four days.
D. Seven days.
E. 10 days.

5.

A 36-year-old patient presents to the clinic with a lower abdominal dragging feeling for the past 10 days. Her urine dipstick shows positive for nitrites but she has no other symptoms of urinary tract infection (UTI).

What is the management plan?

A. Advise her to increase her water intake.
B. Commence antibiotics.
C. Repeat urine dipstick.
D. Send midstream urine.
E. Send midstream urine and start antibiotics.

6.

You review a 49-year-old woman in the gynaecology outpatient clinic with symptoms of frequency and urgency of micturition. She is a para 1, delivered vaginally 15 years ago. Her BMI is 27 and she smokes 15 cigarettes a day. She drinks four cups of coffee daily.

Which of the following lifestyle interventions is the most important to improve her symptoms?

A. Lose weight.
B. Reduce caffeine intake.
C. Reduce fluid intake.
D. Stop smoking.
E. Walk more.

7.

A 67-year-old woman is seen in the gynaecology outpatient clinic. She has tried various medications for detrusor instability and all failed. She is keen to try the least invasive procedure.

Which of the following options would be most appropriate for her?

A. Bladder distention.
B. Botulinum toxin A.
C. Percutaneous posterior tibial nerve stimulation.
D. Percutaneous sacral nerve stimulation.
E. Transcutaneous sacral nerve stimulation.

8.

A 75-year-old woman presents to the gynaecology outpatient clinic complaining of continuous leaking of urine. She is known to have had multiple sclerosis for the past 10 years. She is chair-bound. On examination, there are pressure ulcers that are contaminated by the urine.

Which of the following initial management options would be most appropriate?

A. Book her for examination under anaesthesia and cystoscopy.
B. Clean intermittent self-catheterization.
C. In-dwelling suprapubic catheter.
D. In-dwelling urethral catheter.
E. Prescribe tolterodine tablets.

9.

An 82-year-old patient presents to the gynaecology outpatient clinic with symptoms of frequency and urgency. A post-void bladder scan shows 100 mL residual urine. Conservative management did not help and now you have decided to start her on medical treatment for overactive bladder (OAB).

Which of the following would you recommend?

A. Desmopressin.
B. Mirabegron.
C. Botulinum toxin.
D. Oxybutynin.
E. Tolterodine.

10.

A 72-year-old patient presents to the gynaecology outpatient clinic with symptoms of frequency and urgency. A post-void bladder scan shows 75 mL residual urine. Conservative management did not help and now you have decided to start her on medical treatment for OAB.

How soon after commencing medical treatment does she need a review?

A. Two weeks.
B. Four weeks.
C. Six weeks.
D. Eight weeks.
E. 12 weeks.

11.

A 53-year-old para 2 presents with a 12-month history of leaking on sneezing. She tried pelvic floor exercise for six months with no improvement. On examination, there was no evidence of uterovaginal prolapse.

What is the most appropriate surgical intervention?

A. Anterior colporrhaphy.
B. Burch abdominal colposuspension.
C. Intramural bulking agent.
D. Laparoscopic colposuspension.
E. Synthetic mid-urethral tape.

12.

You review a 61-year-old patient in the gynaecology outpatient clinic, who is complaining of leaking of urine on coughing or sneezing. Pelvic floor exercises have not helped. You counselled her and booked her for a mid-urethral tape surgery.

The theatre nurse asks you which type of tape do you prefer?

A. Type 1: macroporous polypropylene tape.
B. Type 2: microporous polypropylene tape.
C. Type 3: macroporous, multifilament polypropylene tape.
D. Type 4: submicronic polypropylene tape, coated biomaterials with pores of <1 mm.
E. Type 5: microporous monofilament polypropylene tape.

13.

A 62-year-old woman is referred to the gynaecology outpatient clinic because of hesitancy of micturition and dribbling of urine after micturition.

Which of the following initial investigations would you recommend?

A. Measure post-void residual urine volume by bladder ultrasound scan.
B. Measure post-void residual urine volume by catheterization.
C. Request urodynamic studies.
D. Send for pelvic ultrasound scan.
E. Send for urethral pressure studies.

14.

A 49-year-old woman who has multiple uterine fibroids is booked for total abdominal hysterectomy with conservation of the ovaries.

What is her risk of developing post-hysterectomy vault prolapse (PHVP)?

A. 1%–5%.
B. 6%–12%.
C. 15%–20%.
D. 21%–25%.
E. 26%–30%.

15.

A 63-year-old woman is booked for vaginal hysterectomy for pelvic organ prolapse stage 2, according to the Pelvic Organ Prolapse Quantification (POP-Q) classification.[1]

What is the best surgical procedure to perform to prevent vault prolapse in the future?

A. Approximating the round ligament and suturing it to the vaginal vault.

---

[1] N.B. For a review of the pelvic organ prolapse quantification (POP-Q), please refer to: Persu C, Chapple CR, Cauni V, Gutue S, Geavlete P. Pelvic organ prolapse quantification system (POP–Q) – A new era in pelvic prolapse staging. *J Med Life* 2011;4(1):75–81.

B. Closure of the peritoneum as high as possible.
C. McCall culdoplasty.
D. Vaginal Moskowitz operation.
E. Vaginal packing of the vagina for 24 hours postoperatively.

16.

You have obtained consent from a 67-year-old woman for a vaginal hysterectomy plus pelvic floor repair and a possible sacrospinous fixation. She is diagnosed with stage 2 uterovaginal prolapse. After you complete the hysterectomy and anterior vaginal wall repair, you pull on the vault and it comes down to 1 cm above the introitus.

Which of the following options would you perform next?

A. Attach the uterosacral and cardinal ligaments to the vaginal cuff and obliterate the peritoneum of the pouch of Douglas, before closing the posterior vaginal wall.
B. Continue and close the posterior vaginal wall.
C. High uterosacral ligament suspension.
D. Perform sacrospinous fixation before closing the posterior vaginal wall.
E. Perform posterior slingoplasty.

17.

A 55-year-old woman is seen in the clinic complaining of feeling a lump in the vagina. She has a history of vaginal hysterectomy six years previously. On examination, she has a complete vaginal vault prolapse, stage 4 POPQ.

Which of the following options would you recommend to her?

A. Abdominal sacrocolpopexy.
B. High uterosacral ligament suspension.
C. Laparoscopic sacrocolpopexy.
D. Sacrospinous fixation.
E. Transvaginal mesh.

18.

UTI is common in pregnancy and hence the regular check of urine in antenatal clinics.

What is the incidence of UTI during pregnancy?

A. Up to 3%.
B. Up to 8%.
C. Up to 13%.
D. Up to 18%.
E. Up to 23%.

19.

Asymptomatic bacteriuria (ASB) is most commonly seen in early pregnancy, which is the reason why it is standard antenatal practice to send a urine sample for microscopy and culture at the initial booking.

Which of the following organisms is the most common cause of ASB?

A. Enterococcus.
B. *Escherichia coli*.
C. Group B streptococcus.
D. *Klebsiella pneumoniae*.
E. *Proteus mirabilis*.

20.

A 26-year-old primigravida presented to the labour ward at 18 weeks' gestation with a fever of 38.6°C, rigors, abdominal and loin pain. She was diagnosed with pyelonephritis, and received intravenous antibiotics, antipyretics and fluid hydration

What is the risk of recurrence of pyelonephritis in the current pregnancy?

A. 1%–9%.
B. 10%–19%.
C. 20%–29%.
D. 30%–39%.
E. 40%–49%.

21.

A 32-year-old woman in her first pregnancy was admitted to hospital at 29 weeks' gestation because of colicky pain in the left loin, vomiting and a fever of 37.8°C. Investigations showed that she has a left ureteric stone. The patient is counselled and offered conservative management with pain killers, antibiotics and hydration.

What is the success rate of conservative management?

A. Up to 20% success rate.
B. Up to 40% success rate.
C. Up to 60% success rate.
D. Up to 80% success rate.
E. Up to 90% success rate.

22.

A 48-year-old woman presented to the gynaecology outpatient clinic complaining of hesitancy of and dribbling after micturition. Uroflometry was requested and you have the result.

What is the normal female maximum flow rate?

A. >10 mL/s.
B. >15 mL/s.
C. >20 mL/s.
D. >25 mL/s.
E. >30 mL/s.

23.

A 66-year-old woman is booked for a urodynamic study because of frequency, urgency and leaking of urine. The urodynamic study shows the maximum bladder capacity of 200 mL. The Pabd remained unchanged. The Pves and Pdet were consistently rising by 2cm H_2O for every 30 mL of infused fluid into the bladder. At the end of the infusion, the Pves and Pdet remained raised. There was no leak on coughing at the end of the filling phase.

What is the most likely diagnosis?

A. DOA.
B. Low-compliance bladder.
C. Mixed urodynamics stress and detrusor incontinence.
D. Normal urodynamics study results.
E. Urodynamic stress incontinence.

24.

You are teaching medical students about urodynamic studies; they are confused about Pdet.

How is Pdet calculated?

A. Urodynamic equipment calculates Pdet directly.
B. Urodynamic equipment calculates Pdet by subtracting Pabd from Pves.
C. Urodynamic equipment calculates Pdet by subtracting rectal from vesical pressure.
D. Urodynamic equipment calculates Pdet by subtracting Pves from Pabd.
E. Urodynamic equipment calculates Pdet by subtracting vaginal pressure from Pves.

25.

The renal plasma flow increases in pregnancy, leading to increased glomerular filtration rate, creatinine clearance and protein excretion.

By how much does the renal plasma flow increase in pregnancy?

A. 5%–20%.
B. 20%–30%.
C. 30%–40%.
D. 40%–50%.
E. 60%–80%.

26.

A 32-year-old woman in her first pregnancy was admitted to hospital at 29 weeks' gestation because of colicky pain in the left loin, vomiting and a fever of 37.8 degrees centigrade. Investigations showed that she has a left ureteric stone. The patient was counselled and offered conservative management with pain killers, antibiotics and hydration. Unfortunately, 48 hours later she was still spiking a temperature with deteriorating renal function.

Which of the following methods is the most frequently used to treat obstruction caused by calculi during pregnancy in this situation?

A. Continue conservative treatment for a further 48 hours.
B. Open through a renal incision and remove the calculi.
C. Percutaneous nephrostomy.
D. Ureteric stenting.
E. Ureteroscopy and stone removal.

27.

A 51-year-old woman has had urodynamic studies done because of multiple lower urinary tract symptoms. The result shows the following:

During the filling phase, maximum bladder capacity of 460 mL.

Pves and Pabd increased synchronously when the patient was asked to cough. Pdet fluctuated between +5 and –5 cm H_2O.

During the voiding phase, the patient leaked on coughing and Pdet was +5 cm H_2O.

Which of the following options is the most likely diagnosis?

A. DOA.
B. DOA incontinence.

C. Mixed urodynamics stress and detrusor incontinence.

D. Normal urodynamics study results.

E. Urodynamic stress incontinence.

28.

Your consultant examines a 65-year-old patient who presented with symptoms of pelvic organ prolapse. She had a hysterectomy 10 years previously. The prolapse is noticed. The most distal portion of the prolapse protrudes more than 1 cm below the hymen but no farther than 2 cm less than the total vaginal length.

What is the stage of this prolapse?

A. Stage 0.

B. Stage 1.

C. Stage 2.

D. Stage 3.

E. Stage 4.

ANSWERS

Q1: B. Four weeks.[1]

Q2: C. Pelvic floor muscle training programme: at least eight contractions, three times per day.[1]

- Offer a trial of supervised pelvic floor muscle training for at least three months' duration as first-line treatment to women with stress or mixed urinary incontinence (UI).
- Pelvic floor muscle training programmes should comprise at least eight contractions performed three times per day.[1]
- Do not use perineometry or pelvic floor electromyography as biofeedback as a routine part of pelvic floor muscle training.[1]
- Continue an exercise programme if pelvic floor muscle training is beneficial.[1]

Q3: D. B3-adrenoceptor agonist.[2]

- Mirabegron has a marketing authorization in the UK for the 'symptomatic treatment of urgency, increased micturition frequency, and/or urgency incontinence as may occur in patients with overactive bladder' (OAB).[2]
- It is an oral beta-3-adrenoceptor agonist, which activates beta-3-adrenoceptors causing the bladder to relax, which helps it to fill and store urine.
- Mirabegron is available as 25 mg and 50 mg tablets, with the recommended dose being 50 mg daily. The 25 mg is indicated if there is renal or hepatic impairment.

Q4: B. Three days.[1]

- Use bladder diaries for three days in the initial assessment of women with UI or OAB. It is also useful to assess treatment.

The voiding diary (or frequency–volume chart)

- Is a simple and effective way to assess women with UI or OAB.
- Most voiding dairies record the frequency of voids and voided volumes, leakage episodes, pad changes and type and volume of fluid intake.

Q5: D. Send midstream urine.[1]

In women who have symptoms of urinary tract infection (UTI)
- Send a midstream urine specimen for culture and antibiotic sensitivity regardless of the strip reagent result and consider prescribing a suitable antibiotic pending sensitivity results.
- In women who do not have symptoms of UTI, but their urine tests positive for both leucocytes and nitrites, do not offer antibiotics without the results of a midstream urine culture.
- UTI is diagnosed when there are bacterial counts >100 000 CFU/mL and a single strain of pathogen is identified on culture.

Q6: B. Reduce caffeine intake.[1]

- Recommend a trial of caffeine reduction to women with OAB.
- Consider advising modification of high or low fluid intake in women with UI or OAB.
- Advise women with UI or OAB who have a BMI greater than 30 to lose weight.[1]

Q7: C. Percutaneous posterior tibial nerve stimulation.[1]

- Do not offer percutaneous posterior tibial nerve stimulation for OAB unless there has been a multidisciplinary team review; conservative management including OAB drug treatment has not worked adequately nor does the woman want botulinum toxin A or percutaneous sacral nerve stimulation.
- Do not offer transcutaneous sacral nerve stimulation to treat OAB in women.[1]

Q8: D. In-dwelling urethral catheter.[3]

In-dwelling urethral catheters: long-term use for women with UI
- Indicated for long-term use in cases of: (1) chronic urinary retention in women who are unable to manage intermittent self-catheterization; (2) skin wounds, pressure ulcers or irritations that are contaminated by urine; (3) distress or disruption caused by bed and clothing changes; (4) if a woman expresses a preference for this form of management.
- An in-dwelling uretheral catheter is appropriate for women with cognitive impairment, lower-limb spasticity and loss of manual dexterity, together with increasing detrusor overactivity, as clean intermittent self-catheterization, even with the aid of a caregiver, is no longer feasible.

Suprapubic catheters: long-term use
- Indicated if there is urethral erosion or according to patient's preference.[1,3]
- Suprapubic catheters are comfortable and more convenient for catheter changes; may offer better self-image and sexual function.
- Disadvantages include risk of cellulitis, leakage and prolapse through the urethra; higher levels of expertise are required for insertion.

Q9: E. Tolterodine.[1]

- Do not use flavoxate, propantheline and imipramine for the treatment of UI or OAB in women.
- Do not offer oxybutynin (immediate-release) to frail older women.
- Offer one of the following choices first to women with OAB or mixed (UI): oxybutynin (immediate-release), tolterodine (immediate-release) or darifenacin (once-daily preparation).

- Desmopressin may be considered specifically to reduce nocturia. Use with particular caution in women with cystic fibrosis and avoid in those over 65 years with cardiovascular disease or hypertension.[1]

Q10: B. Four weeks.[1]

Q11: E. Synthetic mid-urethral tape.[4]

- The current evidence supports the retropubic synthetic sling with bottom-up approach as the primary procedure for stress urinary incontinence.
- Mid-urethral slings seem to have replaced colposuspension.

Q12: A. Type 1: macroporous polypropylene tape.[4]

- Use a device manufactured from type 1 macroporous polypropylene tape.
- Consider using a tape coloured for high visibility, for ease of insertion and revision.

Q13: A. Measure post-void residual urine volume by bladder ultrasound scan.[1]

- Use a bladder scan in preference to catheterization on the grounds of acceptability and lower incidence of adverse events (trauma and infection).[1]

Q14: B. 6%–12% [evidence level 3].[5]

- Post-hysterectomy vault prolapse (PHVP) has been reported to follow 11.6% of hysterectomies performed for prolapse and 1.8% for other benign diseases.
- A large study from Austria estimated the frequency of PHVP requiring surgical repair to be between 6% and 8%.

Q15: C. McCall culdoplasty.[5]

- McCall culdoplasty involves approximating the uterosacral ligaments using continuous sutures, to obliterate the peritoneum of the posterior cul-de-sac as high as possible. A similar approach has been described for abdominal hysterectomy.
- No comparative studies are available to assess the value of such a step at the time of abdominal hysterectomy, which is often carried out for indications other than prolapse.
- In a retrospective study evaluating the anatomical and functional results of the McCall culdoplasty in 185 patients undergoing vaginal hysterectomy for mild or moderate uterine prolapse, at 24 months' follow-up, the vaginal vault was well supported in 99.2%, with 89.2% showing stage 0 vaginal vault prolapse and 10% showing stage 1 prolapse that did not require revision surgery.

Q16: D. Perform sacrospinous fixation before closing the posterior vaginal wall [evidence level 2+].[5]

- Prophylactic sacrospinous fixation has been suggested at the time of vaginal hysterectomy for marked uterovaginal prolapse, when the vault (point C on the POP-Q system) could be pulled to the introitus at the end of anterior vaginal wall closure.
- A small retrospective study reported only one case of recurrent PHVP in 48 patients with a mean follow-up of two years. In this series, 20 women complained of right buttock pain; all resolved spontaneously by six weeks' follow-up, while five women subsequently developed de novo anterior vaginal wall prolapse. No information was provided about sexual dysfunction in this study.[5]

Q17: C. Laparoscopic sacrocolpopexy [evidence level 1–].[6]

- One relatively small multicentre randomized controlled trial compared abdominal sacrocolpopexy (ASC) with laparoscopic sacrocolpopexy (LSC) in women with PHVP, with or without other compartment prolapse. The results showed significant improvement in the objective outcome in both groups, with no significant difference between groups. At 12 months, 67% of the ASC group and 54% of the LSC group reported themselves to be 'very much better'.
- The potential advantages of LSC were ascertained with significantly less intraoperative blood loss (P<0.01) and shorter hospital stays (P = 0.02).

Q18: B. Up to 8%.[7]

Urinary tract infection (UTI) is common in pregnancy, with an overall incidence of up to 8%. It can be symptomatic or asymptomatic and is associated with an increased risk of preterm, prelabour rupture of membranes, preterm labour and fetal growth restriction.[7]

Q19: B. *Escherichia coli*.[7]

- The most common organism found in women with asymptomatic bacteruria (ASB) is *E. coli*, being responsible for up to 90% of all cases.
- The next most frequently observed pathogens are Gram-negative bacteria (*Proteus mirabilis*, *Klebsiella pneumoniae* and enterococcus).
- Gram-positive pathogens, such as *Staphylococcus aureus* and Group B streptococcus can also be found in ASB.[7]

Q20: B. 10%–19%.[7]

- The recurrence rate for pyelonephritis in the same pregnancy has been quoted to be as high as 10%–18%; therefore, there is an argument for commencing long-term suppressive antimicrobial prophylaxis for the remainder of the pregnancy.[7]

Q21: D. Up to 80% success rate [evidence level 2+].[7]

- The initial management of renal calculi in pregnancy is conservative, with up to 80% passing spontaneously with analgesia, hydration and antibiotics for any infective complications.
- If the symptoms are refractory to this treatment, or there is sepsis or a single obstructed kidney with deteriorating renal function, active management (percutaneous nephrostomy, ureteric stenting, ureteroscopy and stone removal) is indicated.[7]

Q22: B. >15 mL/s.[8]

- The normal female maximum flow rate should be more than 15 mL/s with a 'bell-shaped' curve and no residual urine, measured by ultrasound scanning after voiding.
- Ideally, more than one flow should be performed to diagnose voiding dysfunction, as the initial flow can be affected by anxiety about voiding into a flowmeter.
- In addition, the voided urine should be of reasonable volume, about 150 mL, similar to the voided volumes recorded in their bladder diaries.[8]

Urodynamics
- Urodynamics is a number of different physiological tests of bladder and urethral function to diagnose the pathology causing the woman's symptoms on which a management plan can be based and to predict problems that may follow treatment interventions, for example:

- A decreased flow rate may predict a higher incidence of retention after mid-urethral tape insertion.
- The presence of detrusor overactivity (DOA) in addition to urodynamic stress incontinence (USI) will predict a higher risk of worsening OAB symptoms after mid-urethral tape insertion.
- Urodynamics is not required before commencing non-invasive treatment for storage symptoms.
- Urodynamics consist of cystometry, uroflowmetry and more complex urodynamic investigations, e.g. videourodynamics, urethral pressure profilometry, ambulatory urodynamics.

Cystometry
- Cystometry studies both the filling and voiding phases of micturition. During the test, the patient has two catheters in the bladder, one for filling the bladder and the other for measuring pressure. Additionally, the patient has a pressure catheter in the rectum.
- Cystometry is an invasive test with a small risk of UTI and haematuria due to minor trauma from the catheters.

Filling cystometry phase of the study
- This part of the test diagnoses DOA and USI and records bladder sensations at different bladder volumes. The bladder is filled slowly with normal saline, usually at a rate of 50 mL/min. As it fills, the bladder pressure catheter measures intravesical pressure (Pves) while the rectal pressure catheter measures intra-abdominal pressure (Pabd). The detrusor pressure (Pdet) is calculated by subtracting Pabd from Pves.
- Pabd and Pdet are necessary in order to diagnose USI and DOA.

Urodynamic stress incontinence
- The woman is asked to cough vigorously. The sharp rises in Pves are due solely to rises in Pabd. There is no rise in the Pdet; any leakage has to be the result of USI. In this trace, leakage is recorded as the woman is sitting over a flowmeter. Leakage is confirmed visually by seeing urine escape from the urethra if she is not sitting over a flowmeter when she coughs.

Detrusor overactivity
- DOA is diagnosed if a pressure change is seen on Pves and Pdet but not on Pabd.
- **Uroflowmetry** is a simple non-invasive test to record the flow parameters.

Q23: B. Low-compliance bladder.[8]
- Bladder compliance is a mathematical calculation of the volume required for a unit rise of pressure measured during filling. It indicates how the bladder wall reacts on stretching.
- It is calculated by subtracting Pabd from Pves.
- A large rise in bladder pressure (>1 cm H_2O per 40 mL) in relation to bladder capacity is termed low compliance.
- It would, however, be unusual to see low compliance in a woman without underlying neurological or intrinsic bladder disease. It is usually seen in spinal cord injury, multiple sclerosis, following pelvic radiotherapy and recurrent urinary tract infection.
- Low compliance can be functional (treated with antimuscarinics and botulinum toxin A) or structural, which requires surgical management.

Q24: B. Urodynamic equipment calculates Pdet by subtracting Pabd from Pves.[8]

Q25: E. 60%–80%.

Q26: C. Percutaneous nephrostomy.[7]

- **Percutaneous nephrostomy** is entering the kidney through a small incision in the back. For the insertion of a nephroscope, the kidney stones are then remove under vision. It can be inserted under local anaesthetic and is a temporizing measure to prevent further deterioration in renal function until definitive treatment can be performed following delivery.
- **Urinary stents (double J-stents)** are also effective at relieving obstruction; however, they can become infected or encrusted and may need changing several times throughout the pregnancy.
- **Stone removal with ureteroscopy** (insertion of a ureteroscopy tube through the urethra) has been found to be safe during pregnancy and has good success rates. It is, therefore, a treatment option.
- The decision for which intervention is most appropriate is dependent on the case and will require multidisciplinary input from urology specialists.[8]

Q27: E. Urodynamic stress incontinence.[8]

- There is no rise in the Pdet, thus it is not an OAB. There is good bladder compliance because there is no large rise in Pves, the first red line in the graph. The spikes in the red line at the bottom of the chart show urine leakage corresponding with the spike in the Pabd, second line on the graph during coughing.

Q28: D. Stage 3.[9]

- **The Pelvic Organ Prolapse Quantification (POP-Q)** system is a standard system of terminology approved by the International Continence Society, the American Urogynecologic Society and the Society of Gynecologic Surgeons for the description of female pelvic organ prolapse and pelvic floor dysfunction.
  - **Stage 0:** No prolapse.
  - **Stage 1:** The most distal portion of the prolapse is more than 1 cm above the level of the hymen.
  - **Stage 2:** The most distal portion of the prolapse is 1 cm or less proximal or distal to the hymenal plane.
  - **Stage 3:** The most distal portion of the prolapse protrudes more than 1 cm below the hymen but no farther than 2 cm less the total vaginal length (for example, not all of the vagina has prolapsed).
  - **Stage 4:** Vaginal eversion is essentially complete.

References

1. National Institute for Health and Clinical Excellence. *Urinary Incontinence in Women: Management.* December, 2014. [https://www.nice.org.uk/guidance/cg190]
2. National Institute of Clinical Excellence. *Mirabegron for Treating Symptoms of Overactive Bladder. Technology Appraisal Guidance.* June, 2013. [https://www.nice.org.uk/guidance/ta290]
3. Barnes DG, Shaw PJ, Timoney AG, Tsokos N. Management of the neuropathic bladder by suprapubic catheterisation. *Br J Urol* 1993;72:169–72.
4. Hussain U, Kearney R. Surgical management of stress urinary incontinence. *Obstet Gynaecol Reprod Med* 2013;23(4):108–13.

5. The Royal College of Obstetricians and Gynaecologists. *Post-Hysterectomy Vaginal Vault Prolapse*. July, 2015. [https://www.rcog.org.uk/ guidelines-research-ser vices/guidelines/gtg46]
6. Freeman RM, Pantazis K, Thomson A, et al. A randomised controlled trial of abdominal versus laparoscopic sacrocolpopexy for the treatment of post-hysterectomy vaginal vault prolapse: LAS study. *Int Urogynecol J* 2013;24:377–84.
7. Cox S, Reid F. Urogynaecological complications in pregnancy: an overview. *Obstet Gynaecol Reprod Med* 2015;25(5):123–7.
8. Swithinbank LV, Watson A. Basic understanding of urodynamics. *Obstet Gynaecol Reprod Med* 2015;25(11):321–6.
9. Bump RC, Mattiasson A, Bø K, et al. The standardization of terminology of female pelvic organ prolapse and pelvic floor dysfunction. *Am J Obstet Gynecol* 1996;175:10–17.

Chapter 19

Conception and Assisted Reproduction

Magdy EL Sheikh

QUESTIONS

1.

A 31-year-old woman presents to the accident and emergency department three days following an oocyte retrieval procedure. The patient is complaining of abdominal pain, vomiting, dizziness and shortness of breath. You are on your way to assess the patient.

What would you want the emergency attendant to do while waiting for you to arrive?

A. Attach a pulse oximeter and electrocardiogram, administration of analgesics and an antiemetic.
B. Administer intravenous albumin.
C. Admit to the hospital and intravenous administration of 2–3 L fluids.
D. Arrange urgent abdominal and chest ultrasound evaluation.
E. Arrange a chest X-ray and electrocardiogram (ECG).

2.

Severe ovarian hyperstimulation syndrome (OHSS) is a recognized serious complication of fertility treatments.

What is the triggering factor for this condition?

A. Administration of human chorionic gonadotropins (hCG) for follicle maturation.
B. Embryo replacement.
C. Failure to monitor serum oestradiol and perform proper ultrasound folliculometry.
D. Inappropriate evaluation of the patient prior to treatment.
E. The use of large doses of gonadotrophins for ovarian stimulation.

3.

A 28-year-old female diagnosed with polycystic ovarian disease is undergoing an in vitro fertilization (IVF) cycle. The patient is counselled and informed that all possible measures will be taken to avoid the complication of OHSS.

Which protocol of ovarian stimulation would be advisable?

A. Clomiphene citrate in conjunction with a small dose of gonadotrophins.
B. Gonadotrophin releasing hormone (GnRH) antagonist protocol with GnRH agonist used for ovulation induction.
C. Recombinant follicular stimulating hormone (FSH) should be used in combination with recombinant hCG.
D. Soft stimulation with GnRH agonist and a step-up protocol and a minimal dose of hCG.
E. Soft stimulation with GnRH agonist and a step-down protocol followed by hCG.

4.

A 29-year-old woman with primary infertility due to tubal obstruction has undergone two trials of IVF with no success. Ovarian response and embryo cleavage had always been good. Previous ultrasonography and hysteroscopy were normal. Her partner's semen analysis is satisfactory. Karyotyping for the couple is normal.

What is the most probable cause of failure of implantation in this patient?

A. Aneuploidy of the embryos.
B. Antiphospholipid antibodies.
C. Toxic fluid, in a hydrosalpinx draining to the uterus.
D. Progesterone deficiency.
E. Thick or hard zona pellucida.

5.

A couple have been trying to achieve a spontaneous pregnancy for three years. The female partner is 37 years old and was diagnosed with endometriosis stage III.

Which of the following would be the most appropriate recommendation?

A. Laparoscopic surgery with ablation of endometriotic tissues.
B. Laparoscopic surgery followed by a six-month period of ovulation induction.
C. Laparoscopic laser surgery followed by three trials of artificial insemination.
D. Treatment with GnRH analogue for a period from three to six months.
E. The couple should proceed to IVF as soon as possible.

6.

A 35-year-old infertile patient is classified as having stage I endometriosis and was prepared for IVF treatment. After counselling regarding the treatment, she asks you some questions.

Which of the following statements regarding IVF is correct?

A. Clinical pregnancy rate for IVF is reduced in endometriosis.
B. Miscarriage rate is higher than average in patients with stage I endometriosis.
C. Ovarian stimulation could make the endometriosis condition worse.
D. Stage of endometriosis has no impact on the number of oocytes produced.
E. Studies have shown lower fertilization rates in stage I endometriosis; however, implantation and clinical pregnancy rates are not affected.

7.

An HIV-discordant couple desiring children are counselled regarding the risk of viral transmission.

Which of the following information is correct?

A. Only IVF should be performed if the infected male partner's sperm is to be used.
B. Semen washing and artificial insemination is a safe option for both female partner and offspring.

C. The couple should defer pregnancy in order to avoid the risks of viral transmission.
D. The only safe approach is to use the sperm of a healthy matched donor.
E. Viral suppression therapy is instituted prior to the use of the male partner semen.

8.

A 27-year-old woman fails to conceive for four years. She is a heavy smoker with oligomenorrhea. Her BMI is 37 kg/m^2.

What would be the first line of management?

A. Attempt IVF without any further delay.
B. Assessment laparoscopy.
C. Diet control for weight reduction and advice to stop smoking.
D. Induction of ovulation with a combination of insulin sensitizer and clomiphene citrate.
E. Pelvic ultrasonography and measurement of serum testosterone and prolactin hormones.

9.

A 33-year-old woman is contemplating IVF for the third time. The patient is worried about the risk of developing ovarian cancer in the future due to the repeated administration of fertility drugs.

Which of the following statements is correct?

A. Assisted reproduction medications increase the incidence of ovarian malignancies developing at a younger age.
B. Collective evidence denies any correlation between IVF drugs and an increased risk of ovarian cancer.
C. Only females with BRCA1 or BRCA2 mutations are at a significantly higher risk of developing ovarian cancer following the use of fertility treatments.
D. Recent evidence suggests an increase in benign ovarian lesions and a reduction in the incidence of ovarian malignancies following IVF treatment.
E. Studies confirmed the positive correlation between fertility medications and the incidence of ovarian cancer.

10.

The WHO criteria for values of semen analyses are reached on evaluation of 4500 men in 14 different countries. The lower limits defined as normal for various parameters are based on the fifth percentile obtained in 1900 men in whom the time to pregnancy did not exceed 12 months. The criteria suggested by WHO provide the current standardized reference to practitioners.

Which of the following statements about a semen sample correspond to the lowest normal WHO criteria?

	Volume mL/ejaculate	Number of sperm/mL	% progressive motility	% normal forms
A	1.5	5 million	60%	20%
B	1.5	40 million	40%	4%
C	2.0	20 million	40%	6%
D	1.5	15 million	32%	4%
E	2.0	40 million	40%	4%

11.

One of your junior colleagues wants to know what is meant by mild male factor infertility.

What will you tell him regarding the WHO criteria for mild male factor fertility?

A. A sperm count <40 million/mL with motility <40%.
B. A normal sperm count in the presence of >50% abnormal sperms.
C. A 30% reduction in any two of the semen parameters.
D. When two or more semen analyses have one or more variables below the fifth centile.
E. When two or more semen analyses have 30% reduction in two parameters.

12.

Spontaneous primary ovarian insufficiency (POI) affects 1:250 females at the age of 35 years.

What is the incidence of POI?

A. 0.5%.
B. 1%.
C. 2%.
D. 3%.
E. 5%.

13.

A couple with a child who has sickle cell anaemia are seeking pregnancy. The female partner is 39 years old. The couple request pregestational diagnosis in order to avoid a second affected child.

Which embryos can be transferred?

A. Both heterozygous and homozygous embryos can be transferred.
B. Both normal haemoglobin genotype (*HbAA*) and sickle cell trait (*HbAS*) embryos can be transferred.
C. Only heterozygous embryos will be transferred.
D. Only homozygous embryos will be transferred.
E. Only an *HbAC* embryo can be transferred.

14.

A couple come for preconceptional counselling. The woman is 29 years old, her partner is 32 years old. They both work in a pub. They wanted to know the safe limit of alcohol consumption that will not affect their fertility.

What is your advice?

A. They should abstain from drinking for a period of six months prior to conception.
B. They are only allowed one glass of wine a day.
C. The maximum permissible limit is three units per week.
D. They should not exceed the equivalent of 14 units of alcohol per week.
E. Three or four units of alcohol a day are unlikely to affect the quality of the semen.

15.

An overseas couple attends for consultation regarding pregnancy. She is 32 years old with four previous pregnancies and one living child. Their last pregnancy ended with an intrauterine fetal demise at 26 weeks due to severe rhesus isoimmunization.

What would be your management?

A. Advise amniocentesis at 24 weeks in any future pregnancy.
B. Advise spontaneous pregnancy and chorionic villous sampling with termination of any Rhesus (Rh)-positive fetus.
C. Advise the use of a donor sperm from an Rh-negative matched male.
D. Advise the couple to go for IVF and PGD of embryos.
E. Check the husband's genotype.

16.

A couple has come to consult you regarding NHS funding for IVF. They have been trying to conceive for three years. The female partner is 33 years old. The male partner has an adopted child because of failure to conceive in a previous relationship. They have not had any funded procedure previously.

What will you tell them?

A. They cannot be funded until they try for two more years.
B. They cannot be funded because they have a child in the house.
C. They cannot be funded until she reaches the age of 34 years old.
D. They can be funded if the anti-Müllerian hormone is more than 5.4 pmol/L.
E. They can be funded.

17.

A general practitioner requests your help. A man has just come back from a business visit to a region infected with the Zika virus (ZIKV). The man and his wife are wishing to try for pregnancy. The couple are free of any symptoms.

What would be your recommendation?

A. The man is advised to have a blood test for the ZIKV before any decision is made.
B. The man is advised to have a course of antiviral therapy.
C. The couple is advised to use contraception for a period of eight weeks.
D. The couple is assured that ZIKV is not transmitted via semen.
E. The couple can try artificial insemination with washed sperms.

18.

You had a panel discussion with colleagues from the oncology department about a 29-year-old patient diagnosed with cervical cancer. The lesion occupied the lower part of the cervix and appeared to be of 1–2 cm in diameter. The patient is requesting preservation of her future fertility.

You suggested radical vaginal trachelectomy (RVT) with lymph node dissection.

Which of the following statements is correct?

A. Radical abdominal hysterectomy (RAH) with lymph node dissection carries a significantly better five-year survival rate.
B. RVT with lymph node dissection is performed only in cervical adenocarcinomas.
C. Recurrences and five-year survival rates are not significantly different between RAH and RVT.
D. Radiotherapy is used in an attempt to maintain fertility.
E. Ovarian tissues cryopreservation should be offered.

19.

A boy of 15 years old has Hodgkin's lymphoma. His parents come to see you requesting counselling about preservation of fertility.

How will you counsel them?

A. He is too young for producing fertile semen.
B. He will be allowed to store semen for a maximum of five years according to law.
C. Semen viability is lost after five years.
D. It is not possible because there are no legal rules in relation to consent in this group.
E. It is possible if he can produce good quality semen before treatment.

20.

A couple has been booked for IUI. While reviewing their notes, you find they have not been screened for chlamydia.

How will you proceed?

A. Carry on with the procedure if their history does not indicate sexually transmitted infections.
B. Carry on with the procedure if the history of the male partner does indicate sexually transmitted infection.
C. Carry on with the scheduled procedure but offer prophylactic antibiotics.
D. Cancel the procedure and refer them to the genitourinary medicine clinic.
E. Delay the procedure until they are screened.

21.

A couple comes to see you, as they want to start a family. They tried unprotected intercourse for three months but the male partner complains of a lifelong problem with premature ejaculation.

What is your first-line management?

A. Advise pharmacotherapy of selective serotonin reuptake inhibitors.
B. Advise psychotherapy.
C. Advise consultation with a sex therapist.
D. Advise intrauterine insemination.
E. Offer different options to treat erectile dysfunction.

22.

A young 32-year-old woman is diagnosed with cancer of the ovary stage IA, grade 2 mucinous cancer. She does not have a steady partner. She was not keen on oocyte preservation as she wishes to achieve spontaneous pregnancy, if possible.

Which of the following is the most appropriate management option?

A. It is not possible to preserve any fertility organs for fear of recurrence.
B. She can have fertility-sparing surgery.
C. She can have pelvic radiotherapy without surgery.
D. She can have chemotherapy without surgery.
E. She can try sperm donation and embryo preservation.

23.

While counselling a couple about IVF, they voiced worries about the possibility of any increase in the rate of congenital anomalies if they achieve pregnancy.

What will you tell them?

A. There is an increased risk of 10%–20%.
B. There is an increased risk of 20%–25%.

C. There is an increased risk of 30%–40%.
D. There is no increased risk of congenital anomalies.
E. There is no increased risk if they have intracytoplasmic sperm injection.

24.

A couple comes to see you because they want to achieve a pregnancy. They have tried unprotected intercourse for the last 12 months. On history taking, you find that the male partner had a short trip abroad four months ago and had a ZIKV infection. He has been on condom contraception for the last four months.

What is your advice?

A. Continue contraception for four months to see if he develops any symptoms of reinfection.
B. Continue contraception for six more months to make sure he is completely cured.
C. He can stop contraception and wait for spontaneous pregnancy.
D. He can stop contraception and proceed with fertility treatment.
E. He should wait for two more months before they can start fertility treatment.

ANSWERS

Q1: A. Attachment of a pulse oximeter and electrocardiogram, administration of analgesics and an antiemetic [evidence level 3].[1]

- Patients complaining of abdominal pain and intolerance to oral fluids following oocyte collection are suspected to be suffering from ovarian hyperstimulation syndrome (OHSS). A normal electrocardiogram (ECG) and good oxygen saturation are reassuring in the initial stage.[1]
- The patient should be evaluated by a physician experienced in such conditions.[1] The treating fertility specialist will perform several blood tests including complete blood count and serum electrolytes. Other tests will be requested depending on the initial evaluation of the attending physician.[1]
- Dizziness and shortness of breath observed could be due to the accumulation of a large amount of ascetic fluid and hypovolaemia in conjunction with low osmolality and hyponatraemia.
- Pleural effusion, pericardial effusion and even pulmonary embolism are possible complications and should be ruled out.[1]
- Initial administration of analgesia in the form of paracetamol or oral opiates in conjunction with antiemetic drugs is recommended.[1]
- Following confirmation of the diagnosis, fluid therapy is commenced.[1]

Q2: A. Administration of human chorionic gonadotropins (hCG) for follicle maturation [evidence level 3].[2]

- All the factors mentioned help in the prevention of OHSS.
- However, the triggering factor in ovarian hyperstimulation cascade of events is the administration of hCG.[2] The syndrome is not likely to occur if the administration of hCG is avoided [evidence level 3].[2]

Q3: B. Gonadotrophin releasing hormone (GnRH) antagonist protocol with GnRH agonist used for ovulation induction [evidence level 2].[3]

- It has been shown, recently by meta-analysis and Cochran reviews, that the use of GnRH antagonists in the stimulation programme and the utilization of GnRH agonist to complete the oocyte maturation instead of hCG markedly reduces the incidence of severe OHSS.[3]

- Native GnRH stimulates gonadotrophins of the anterior pituitary.
- The GnRH agonists, have greater potency and a longer half-life than native GnRH, and produce an initial stimulation of pituitary gonadotrophs with secretion of follicle-stimulating hormone and luteinizing hormone. This response is followed by down regulation and inhibition of the pituitary–gonadal axis.
- The GnRH antagonists suppress pituitary gonadotropin by GnRH-receptor competition, thus avoiding the initial stimulatory phase of the agonists.

Q4: A. Aneuploidy of the embryos [evidence level 3].[4]

- Even in normal euploid couples, chromosomal aberrations of human embryos are common.
- Aneuploidy is recognized as the most common cause behind repeated implantation failure and early pregnancy loss.[4]
- Her tubal factor fertility is not likely to be the cause of the implantation failure. Hydrosalpinx was excluded by previous hysteroscopy and ultrasonography.

Q5: E. The couple should proceed to IVF as soon as possible [evidence level 3].[5]

- The patient has been diagnosed as endometriosis stage III.
- Diagnosis of endometriosis is made via laparoscopy.
- She is 37 years old and has been trying for pregnancy for three years.
- The patient should resort to IVF as the age factor is extremely important.[5]

Q6: E. Studies have shown lower fertilization rates in stage I endometriosis; however, implantation and clinical pregnancy rates are not affected [evidence level 3].[6]

- Several studies have shown similar results for IVF treatment in patients with stage I endometriosis compared to other groups with no endometriosis.
- There has been no indication that miscarriage rate is increased in endometriosis.
- A recent meta-analysis of 27 observational studies included 8984 cases and showed lower fertilization rates for IVF in endometriosis stage I; however, implantation and pregnancy rates were normal.[6]

Q7: B. Semen washing and artificial insemination is a safe option for both female partner and offspring [evidence level 1+].[7]

- A recent systemic review and meta-analysis including 40 studies confirmed that semen washing as performed in artificial intrauterine insemination (IUI) treatments prevents HIV transmission. Therefore, IVF is not the only possible option.
- The female partner does not need to receive antiviral therapy prior to IUI.

Q8: E. Pelvic ultrasonography and measurement of serum testosterone and prolactin hormones [evidence level 3].[8]

- The patient has not been diagnosed fully yet but has a strong possibility of polycystic ovarian syndrome.
- An ultrasound examination and measurement of serum androgen and serum prolactin is essential to confirm the diagnosis.
- Following diagnosis confirmation, advice regarding cessation of smoking and weight reduction measures are mandatory.

Q9: B. Collective evidence denies any correlation between IVF drugs and an increased risk of ovarian cancer [evidence level 1+].[9]

- Recent Cochrane reviews of related studies have failed to demonstrate 'any significant' treatment-related impact on the incidence of ovarian cancer in assisted reproduction patients.

Q10:[10]

	Volume mL/ejaculate	Number of sperm/mL	% progressive motility	% normal forms
D	1.5	15 million	32%	4%

These are the lower limits of normal as suggested by WHO.[10]

Q11: D. When two or more semen analyses have one or more variables below the fifth centile [evidence level 2].[10]

- According to the WHO criteria, the diagnosis of mild male infertility problem is made when two or more semen analysis results show one or more variables below the fifth centile.[10]

Q12: B. 1%.[11]

- The definition of primary ovarian insufficiency is cessation of menstruation before the age of 40 years.[11]

Q13: B. Both normal haemoglobin genotype (*HbAA*) and sickle cell type (*HbAS*) embryos can be transferred.[12]

- Haemoglobinopathies are the most frequent indications for preimplantation genetic diagnosis (PGD).
- A normal or a carrier embryo can be transferred.
- Sickle cell disease is caused by mutation in the haemoglobin gene (*Hb*) on chromosome 11.
- A normal copy of the gene is expressed as A, an abnormal is expressed as S or C.
- Normal individuals have two copies of the normal gene (*HbAA*); affected individuals with sickle cell disease have two abnormal copies of the gene and are either *HbSS* or *HbSC*.
- Carriers of the disease or sickle cell trait (SCT) have one normal copy *HbA* and one abnormal copy of the gene (*HbAS* or *HbAC*).
- If both parents have SCT, there is a 50% (or 1 in 2) chance that any child of theirs will also have SCT if the child inherits the sickle cell gene from one of the parents. Such children will not have symptoms of SCD, but they can pass SCT on to their children.
- If both parents have SCT, there is a 25% (or 1 in 4) chance that any child of theirs will have SCD. There is also a 25% (or 1 in 4) chance that the child will not have sickle cell disease (SCD) or SCT.
- In PGD, IVF with embryo blastomere biopsy and identification of affected embryos will follow. Healthy embryos are then transferred. In this case a chromosomal examination of embryos for aneuploidy is also carried out in order to avoid trisomies as the mother is 39 years old.[12]

Q14: D. They should not exceed the equivalent of 14 units of alcohol per week.[13]

- According to guidelines of the UK chief medical officer, women seeking pregnancy or who are pregnant should not drink alcohol at all to avoid risks of fetal alcohol syndrome (e.g. restricted growth, facial abnormalities, long-term learning and behavioural disorders). They should not exceed one to two units a day.

- One unit of alcohol is equivalent to 25 mL of spirits (whisky, gin, vodka), 76 mL (half a pint) of average 4% strength lager, or 76 mL (two-thirds of a 125-mL glass) of average-strength (12%) wine.

Q15: E. Check the husband's genotypye.[14]

- About 40% of Rh (D)-positive individuals are homozygous for the D antigen (DD); the remainder is heterozygous (Dd).
- The husband should be checked for genotype (zygosity). A homozygous male (DD) will always cause an affected pregnancy. In this case, an Rh-negative donor sperm option is possible.
- A heterozygous male (heterozygous (Dd), 50% chance that the child would be Rh-positive) might be offered IVF and PGD where Rh-negative embryos are selected for transfer.[14]

Q16: B. They cannot be funded because they have a child in the house.[15]

- NHS does not supply any funding if there is a child in the house, from this relationship, from a previous relationship, or even if the child is adopted (for full information regarding NHS funding criteria, please review: [www.nhs.uk/Conditions/IVF/Pages/Availability/aspx])

Q17: C. The couple is advised to use contraception for a period of eight weeks.[16]

- Zika virus (ZIKV) disease is transmitted by mosquitoes in endemic areas. The virus is isolated from an infected person's blood and semen [evidence level 3].
- WHO recommends safe sex or contraceptive measures to be taken if an individual is visiting an infected country.
- A male partner returning from such areas should use contraception for at least eight weeks.[16]

Q18: C. Recurrences and five-year survival rates are not significantly different between RAH and RVT [evidence level 3].[17]

- Five-year recurrence rate is not significantly different between patients who received RAH and RVT. RVT could be implemented in the early stages of cervical carcinomas in an attempt to preserve fertility.

Q19: E. It is possible if he can produce good quality semen before treatment [evidence level 3].[18]

- Advances in assisted reproductive technologies have led to adult cancer patients being offered sperm cryopreservation routinely, and this has only recently started to be offered to adolescent and younger cancer patients.[18]
- Any strict policy of age-related referral to a sperm bank would have denied significant numbers of adolescent cancer patients the chance to store their sperm.
- For instance, if the threshold age of 16 years were applied, this would have amounted to 28.8% (59/205) of the successful group being denied the chance to store sperm.
- If the child understood the issues, it seems unreasonable to deny him this potential just because of age alone.
- Available studies for the outcome of pregnancy and offspring born after childhood cancer fertility preservation do not provide evidence of germ cell

mutagenesis, increased congenital malformations, neonatal mortality or cancers in offspring.
- Fertility preservation techniques improve the reproductive potential in adolescent and young adult patients receiving cancer therapies.

Q20: C. Carry on with the scheduled procedure but offer prophylactic antibiotics.[19]

- NICE recommends screening for *Chlamydia trachomatis*. If screening is not done, then prophylactic antibiotics should be offered.

Q21: A. Advise pharmacotherapy of selective serotonin reuptake inhibitors (SSRI) [evidence level 1+].[20]

- Lifelong premature ejaculation is best managed with pharmacotherapy (SSRIs).
- Acquired premature ejaculation may be due to erectile dysfunction and is managed by pharmacotherapy and basic psychosexual education in an integrated treatment programme.

Q22: B. She can have fertility-sparing surgery.[17]

- In 507 women with early ovarian cancer, who had fertility-sparing surgery (conserving the uterus and the contralateral ovary), there was a 10.3% chance of recurrence and 5.5% chance of death from disease, which is comparable to historical controls. A total of 186 (36.68%) full-term deliveries were achieved in that population.
- The European Society of Gynaecologic Oncology concluded that Stage IA grade 1 and possibly grade 2 tumours of mucinous endometrioid or serous types were suitable for fertility-sparing surgery.

Q23: C. There is an increased risk of 30%–40% [evidence level 1+].[21,22]

- The background risk for congenital anomalies lies between 3% and 5% of all infants. IVF is associated with a 30%–40% increased risk of major congenital anomalies.
- This excess risk is not only related to multiple pregnancies, because it is observed even in singleton pregnancies.
- This increased risk is partly attributable to the underlying infertility or its determinants as couples who take longer than 12 months to conceive also exhibit an increased risk of anomalies.
- The main anomalies that occur in IVF pregnancies include gastrointestinal, cardiovascular (specifically septal heart defects), musculoskeletal defects and cleft lip, esophageal atresia and anorectal atresia.
- Nevertheless, the absolute risk is low as the background risk per se is low.

Q24: E. He should wait for two more months before they can start fertility treatment.[23]

- Zika virus (ZIKV) is transmitted through the bite of an infected *Aedes* mosquito.
- ZIKV can pass to the fetus during pregnancy and is a cause of microcephaly and other severe fetal brain defects.
- ZIKV can be transmitted through sex, even if the infected person does not have symptoms at the time.
- History taking for fertile couples seeking conception should specifically include recent travel.
- A person who has had a known ZIKV infection should not try to conceive naturally, donate gametes or proceed with fertility treatment for six months or until the semen tests negative for ZIKV RNA by nucleic acid testing.

References

1. Royal College of Obstetricians and Gynaecologists. *The Management of Ovarian Hyperstimulation Syndrome*. February, 2016. [https://www.rcog.org.uk/en/guide lines-research-services/guidelines/gtg5]

2. Al-Inany HG, Abou-Setta AM, Aboulghar M. Gonadotrophin-releasing hormone antagonists for assisted conception: a Cochrane review. *Reprod Biomed Online* 2007;14:640.

3. Griesinger G, Diedrich K, Devroey P, Kolibianakis EM. GnRH agonist for triggering final oocyte maturation in the GnRH antagonist ovarian hyperstimulation protocol: a systematic review and meta-analysis. *Hum Reprod Update* 2006;12:159.

4. Sugiura-Ogasawara M, Ozaki Y, Katano K, et al. Abnormal embryonic karyotype is the most frequent cause of recurrent miscarriage. *Hum Reprod* 2012:27:2297–303.

5. European Society for Human Reproduction and Embryology. *Guideline on the Management of Women with Endometriosis*. September, 2013. [https://www.eshre/eu]

6. Harb HM, Gallos ID, Chu J, Harb M, Coomarasamy A. The effect of endometriosis on in vitro fertilisation outcome: a systematic review and meta-analysis. *Brit J Obstet Gynaecol* 2013;120(11):1308.

7. Zafer M, Horvath H, Mmeje O, et al. Effectiveness of semen washing to prevent human immunodeficiency virus (HIV) transmission and assist pregnancy in HIV-discordant couples: a systemic review and meta-analysis. *Fertil Steril* 2016:105 (3):645–55.

8. The Rotterdam ESHRE/ASRM-Sponsored PCOS Consensus Workshop Group. Revised 2003 consensus on diagnostic criteria and long-term health risks related to polycystic ovary syndrome. *Fertil Steril* 2004;81(1):19–25.

9. Rizzuto I, Behrens RF, Smith LA. Risk of ovarian cancer in women treated with ovarian stimulating drugs for infertility. *Cochrane Database Syst Rev* 2013;(8): CD008215.

10. New World Health Semen Analysis Parameters. February, 2016. [http://ivfmd .net/]

11. Nelson LM. Clinical practice. Primary ovarian insufficiency. *N Engl J Med* 2009;360(6):606.

12. Kuliev A, Pakhalchuk T, Verlinsky O, Rechitsky S. Preimplantation genetic diagnosis for hemoglobinopathies. *Hemoglobin* 2011;35(5–6):547–55.

13. Department of Health. *UK Chief Medical Officers' Low Risk Drinking Guidelines*. August, 2016. [https://www.gov.uk/government/uploads]

14. Zipursky A, Paul VK. The global burden of Rh disease. *Arch Dis Child Fetal Neonatal Ed* 2011;96(2):F84–5.

15. National Health Service. *Template Criteria for NHS Funded Assisted Reproductive Technologies*. October, 2013. [www.medwayccg.nhs.uk/app/uploads/2015/05/MED-14-57-Attachment]

16. World Health Organization. *Information for travelers visiting Zika-affected countries*. [www.who.int/csr/disease/zika/information-for-travelers/en]

17. Royal College of Obstetricians and Gynaecologists. *Fertility Sparing Treatment in Gynaecological Cancer*. February, 2013. [https://www.rcog.org.uk/en/guidelines-research-services/guidelines/sip35]

18. Bahadur G, Ling KLE, Hart R, et al. Semen quality and cryopreservation in adolescent cancer patients. *Hum Reprod* 2002;17(12):3157–61.

19. National Institute for Health and Care Excellence. *Fertility Problems: Assessment and Treatment*. February, 2013. [https://www.nice.org.uk/guidance/cg156]

20. McMahon CG, Porst H. Oral agents for the treatment of premature ejaculation: review of efficacy and safety in the context of the recent International Society for Sexual Medicine criteria for lifelong premature ejaculation. *J Sex Med* 2011;8 (10):2707–25.

21. Hansen M, Bower C, Milne E, de Klerk N, Kurinczuk JJ. Assisted reproductive technologies and the risk of birth defects – a systematic review. *Hum Reprod* 2005;20:328–38.
22. Royal College of Obstetricians & Gynaecologists and British Fertility Society. *In Vitro Fertilisation: Perinatal Risks and Early Childhood Outcomes.* May, 2012. [https://www.rcog.org.uk/en/guidelines-research-services/guidelines/sip8]
23. British Fertility Society. *Zika Virus, Fertility Treatment and Gamete Donation.* June, 2016. (https://britishfertilitysociety.org.uk/2016/02/01/zika-virus-fertility-treatment-and-gamete-donation/#sthash.tDHYNPxr.dpuf)

Chapter 20

Medical Statistics

QUESTIONS

1.

A drug company is undergoing a trial for a new medication for the treatment of heavy menstrual bleeding. One thousand women are recruited; 550 women are given the new medication and the rest are given a placebo. The mean age is 32 (SD=5) and 36 (SD=7) years for the former and the latter group, respectively. The women's ages are normally distributed.

What is the percentage of the women whose ages range between 29 and 43 years in the placebo group?

A. 38%.
B. 58%.
C. 68%.
D. 78%.
E. 86%.

2.

A drug company ran a trial for the effect of a new medication on the prevention of pregnancy-induced hypertension (PIH). Following the appropriate approval from the Regional ethics committee and the women's consent, 1000 pregnant women were randomly allocated to one of two different groups. The women were considered to be at low risk for PIH. The treatment group received a regular single low dose of the new drug and the control group did not. The following table shows the number of women in each group who did and who did not develop PIH.

	Developed PIH	Did not develop PIH
Treatment group	250	250
Control group	200	300

What is the relative risk for the treatment group?

A. 0.25.
B. 0.50.
C. 0.75.
D. 1.00.
E. 1.25.

3.

A researcher has developed a new prenatal screening test for Down syndrome. Following the appropriate approval from the Regional ethics committee and the women's consent, 2000 pregnant women were randomly allocated to one of two different groups. The women were considered to be at low risk for pregnancy affected by Down syndrome. The following table shows the number of women in each group who did and who did not have babies affected by Down syndrome.

	Screen positive	Screen negative
Baby affected by Down syndrome	800	200
Baby not affected by Down syndrome	400	600

What is the positive predictive value of this test?

A. 20%.
B. 40%.
C. 60%.
D. 80%.
E. 100%.

4.

A drug company ran a trial for the effect of a new medication on the treatment of PIH. Following the appropriate approval from the Regional ethics committee and consent from the women, 1000 pregnant women were randomly allocated to one of two different groups. The treatment group received a regular single low dose of the new drug and the control group did not. The number needed to treat (NNT) is calculated as 10.

What is meant by the number needed to treat (NNT)?

A. It is the inverse of the absolute risk.
B. It is the inverse of the attributed risk.
C. It is the difference in the relative risk between the exposed and the non-exposed groups.
D. It is the number of patients needed to be exposed to the risk factor to cause harm in one patient.
E. It is the number of patients needed to treat during a specific period.

5.

A researcher has done a comparative study between two populations with regard to the intelligence quotient (IQ). The mean IQ for the first group is 75 and it is 80 for the second ($P<0.1$).

What would be the conclusion of this study?

A. Null hypothesis can be accepted.
B. Null hypothesis cannot be accepted.

C. Type I error.
D. Type II error.
E. Significant difference is detected.

6.

The forest plot diagram here illustrates a study that has been done to identify a common genetic variant associated with the risk of endometrial cancer.

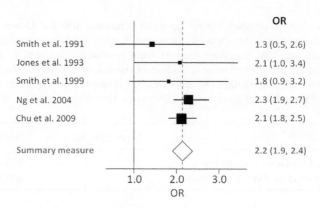

	OR
Smith et al. 1991	1.3 (0.5, 2.6)
Jones et al. 1993	2.1 (1.0, 3.4)
Smith et al. 1999	1.8 (0.9, 3.2)
Ng et al. 2004	2.3 (1.9, 2.7)
Chu et al. 2009	2.1 (1.8, 2.5)
Summary measure	2.2 (1.9, 2.4)

What is the overall conclusion of the study?

A. P-value is most probably <0.001.
B. P-value is most probably <0.05.
C. P-value is most probably <0.1.
D. P-value is most probably <0.1%.
E. P-value is most probably <5%.

7.

A researcher is studying the relationship between high beta-human chorionic gonadotropin (BhCG), low pregnancy-associated plasma protein A (PAPP-A), increased nuchal translucency and the risk of Down syndrome.

Which of the following tests can the researcher use to analyze the results?

A. ANOVA test.
B. Chi-squire (X^2) test.
C. Multiple linear regression test.
D. Simple linear regression test.
E. Student (t)-test.

8.

A researcher is studying the side effects of a new antihypertensive medication in two groups of pregnant women (100 women in each group) with PIH. The first group receives the new medication while the other receives a conventional one.

Which type of the epidemiological studies will suit this study?

A. Case-controlled study.
B. Cohort study.
C. Cross-sectional study.
D. Double-blind randomized case-controlled study.
E. Survey.

ANSWERS

Q1: C. 68%.[1]

- When data follow a normal (Gaussian) distribution:
  - Mean, median and mode are equal.
  - 68% of the variables will be within one standard deviation (SD) from the mean (M) (i.e. M±SD).
  - 95% of the variables will be within two SDs from the mean (M±2SD).
  - 99.7% of the variables will be within three SDs from the mean (M±3SD).

Q2: E. 1.25.[1]

- Relative risk = 250 in 500 divided by 200 in 500 or 250/200 = 1.25.
- **Relative risk or risk ratio** (RR) is the ratio of the probability of an event occurring (e.g. developing a lung disease) in an exposed group (smokers) compared to the probability of the event (developing lung disease) occurring in a matched, non-exposed group (non-smokers). Another example is the probability of the occurrence of side effects in people exposed to a medication compared to those not exposed.
- An RR=1 means there is neither an increased nor a decreased risk
- An RR>1 means there is a risk of developing the condition; an RR of 2 means the risk is doubled. An RR of 7.0 means that the affected group has seven times the risk of a non-affected group.
- If the RR<1, it means that the chance of a bad outcome is twice as likely to occur without the intervention.

Q3: D. 80%.[1,2]

- **Positive and negative predictive values (PPV)** are used for diagnostic tests to indicate the probability that, in case of a positive test, the patient really has the specified disease.
- **Sensitivity** is the probability that a test will indicate 'disease' among those with the disease.
- **Specificity** is the fraction of those without disease who will have a negative test result.

Q4: A. It is the inverse of the absolute risk.[1]

- The number needed to treat (NNT) is an epidemiological measure used in communicating the effectiveness of a healthcare intervention, typically a treatment with medication or an intervention (e.g. Caesarian section for breech presentation).
- NNT is the number of patients needed to be treated to prevent one additional bad outcome.
- It is the inverse of the absolute risk reduction.
- The lower the NNT, the more effective the intervention.

Q5: A. Null hypothesis can be accepted.[1]

- Null hypothesis states that there is no difference between the samples being compared, and any difference observed is simply the result of random variation.
- The conventional values for the critical level of significance (P-value) are equal to 0.05 (5%), 0.01 (1%) and 0.001 (0.1%).
- Where the level of significance (P-value) is more than these critical levels, the difference between the two compared groups will be insignificant and the null hypothesis will be accepted.

Q6: C. P-value is most probably <0.1.[2]

- A forest plot is a graphical representation of a meta-analysis.
- It is usually accompanied by a table listing references (author and date) of the studies included in the meta-analysis.
- It has one line representing each study in the meta-analysis, plotted according to the standardized mean difference (SMD approximates the difference between the average score of participants in the intervention group and the average score of participants in the control group). The box on each line shows the standardized mean difference (SMD) for each study.
- The diamond shape (usually black) at the bottom of the graph shows the average and the overall effect size of the studies included.
- The dotted line is called the line of action.
- If the diamond shape crosses the line of action, it means the study has not found any significant difference or association, i.e. $P<0.5$ or $P<0.1$.
- If the diamond shape finds a significant difference in favour of any side of the study, then the diamond shape will be on that side of the line of action, and the P-value will be significant at <0.05 (5%), <0.01 (1%) or <0.001 (0.1%).

Q7: C. Multiple linear regression test.[2,3]

Tests of significance include:

- Parametric tests: students (t)-test and ANOVA test.
- Non-parametric tests: X^2-test, Fisher's exact test, Man–Whitney U test, Wilcoxon test.
- **Linear regression** is an approach for modelling the relationship between a position on a scale (scalar) of the dependent variable Y against and an independent variable denoted X.
- **A dependent variable** is a variable that may change and is dependent on other factors, e.g. weather.
- **An independent factor** is a factor that does not depend on other conditions or variables and will not change, e.g. one's age at a certain time.
- In another example in an experiment to test the theory that a vitamin could extend a person's life-expectancy, the independent variable is the amount of vitamin that is given to the subjects within the experiment; the dependent variable is lifespan.
  - The case of one explanatory variable is called simple linear regression analysis.
  - For more than one explanatory variable, as in this question, the process is called multiple linear regression.
- **Student test (t)** is a statistical hypothesis test in which the test statistic follows a Student's-t distribution (or t-distribution) if the null hypothesis is true.
- **Chi-square test (X^2-test)** is used to determine whether there is a significant difference between the expected frequencies and the observed frequencies in one or more categories. An example is a researcher expects that women of low social class will have a higher percentage rate of suicide. The X^2-test will show the difference between the actual figures of those who commit suicide versus the expected figures assumed by the researcher. A large difference between collected numbers and expected numbers means rejecting the null hypothesis, i.e. there is no interaction between the variables.

Q8: B. Cohort study.[2,3]

Cohort studies

- These involve a group of people with defined characteristics who are followed-up to determine the incidence of, or mortality from, some specific exposure.[2,3]

- A well-designed cohort study can provide powerful results.
- Cohort studies are an example of longitudinal analysis. They can be prospective or retrospective.
- They are more suitable for common diseases and can determine incidence.
- Attrition bias (loss of follow-up) is the most common drawback of prospective cohort studies.

Case-control studies

- Compare patients who have a disease or outcome of interest (cases) with patients who do not have the disease or outcome (controls).
- They identify subjects by outcome status at the outset of the investigation. For example, the outcomes of interest may be whether the subject has undergone a specific type of surgery or experienced a complication.[2,3]
- In comparison to cohort studies, case-control studies are quick, relatively inexpensive to implement, require comparatively fewer subjects and allow for multiple exposures or risk factors to be assessed for one outcome.
- They are more suitable for rare diseases.
- In a case-control study, it is imperative that the investigator has explicitly defined inclusion and exclusion criteria prior to the selection of cases or randomization.

References

1. Harris M, Taylor G. *Medical Statistics Made Easy*. London, UK: Martin Dunitz, Taylor and Francis, 2004.
2. Easterbrook PJ. *Basic Medical Sciences for MRCP Part 1*. London, UK: Churchill Livingstone, 2005.
3. Sharp VF. *Statistics for the Social Sciences*. Boston, MA: Little, Brown, 1979.

Chapter 21

Professional Dilemmas, Consent and Good Medical Practice

Irene Gafson

QUESTIONS

1.

You have just finished your night shift as the registrar on call. There was a very difficult vaginal breech delivery. You struggled to deliver the after-coming head.

While checking your Facebook account, you note that the foundation year 2 doctor (FY2) who was on call with you has posted a message: 'What an awful night. Saw a horrendous vaginal breech. Why would anyone opt for a vaginal breech delivery?'

What is the most appropriate next step?

A. Fill in an incident form when you return to work.
B. Immediately call the FY2 colleague and advise removal of this Facebook post.
C. Inform the General Medical Council (GMC).
D. Leave a comment on Facebook saying this was an exception.
E. Telephone the consultant who was on call and ask him/her to investigate.

2.

You have recently started working at a new Trust as an ST3 grade. A woman with threatened preterm labour arrives at 29 weeks' gestation. In the hospital guideline for the management of preterm labour, you notice that the first-line drug choice is nifedipine. You have not previously used this drug for tocolysis. When you consult the British National formulary, you note that nifedipine is not licensed for this use.

What is the most appropriate course of action?

A. Contact the on-call pharmacist for advice.
B. Omit the tocolysis and just prescribe steroids.
C. Prescribe atosiban instead as you are more familiar with it.
D. Prescribe the nifedipine but explain to the patient it is unlicensed and document this.
E. Refuse to prescribe nifedipine as it is unlicensed.

3.

You are an ST4 in the obstetrics department. Your good friend contacts you for some medical advice. She is three weeks postpartum and breasteeding her child. She says that, over the last 24 hours, her right breast has become very painful and red and it really hurts to feed. She has also been feeling very feverish. She has looked up her symptoms online and thinks she has mastitis. She is wondering if you could prescribe her antibiotics as she does not feel well enough to leave the house.

What is the single most appropriate course of action?

A. Check if she has any allergies and prescribe her appropriate antibiotics and take them to her house.
B. Give her a box of antibiotics you happen to have at home that is appropriate for mastitis.
C. Take a box of antibiotics from the day assessment unit cupboard at work and drop them off at her house.
D. Tell her to book an urgent appointment with her general practitioner to fully assess and treat her.
E. Reassure her that this is probably just engorgement and nothing to worry about.

4.

You are supervising an ST2 performing an elective Caesarean section for breech presentation. He makes a small laceration on the baby's right buttock when incising the uterus. It is not actively bleeding and is approximately 1.5 cm in length and superficial. The ST2 is extremely upset about this complication.

What is the single most appropriate next step?

A. Ask the ST2 to go and explain it to the parents in recovery as it was their complication.
B. Fill in an incident form and notify the delivery suite manager.
C. Go to the parents with the junior doctor, explain and apologize about the complication and document it in the notes.
D. Reassure your colleague that it is a non-significant complication and it happens to everyone.
E. Tell the paediatrician and ask them to highlight it to the parents at the baby check.

5.

You are the ST3 performing an elective Caesarean section. The anaesthetic registrar on call seems to be unwell. You notice that he smells of alcohol and is sweating profusely. When he draws up the local anaesthetic you notice that he is trembling. You ask to speak to him in private and ask if he is unwell. You explain your concerns and he storms off and continues with preparing his spinal anaesthetic equipment.

What is the most appropriate next step?

A. Contact your defence union for urgent advice.
B. Escalate to the consultant on call urgently.
C. Fill in an incident report form.
D. Make an urgent call referring him to the GMC.
E. Refuse to operate with him because of the altercation.

6.

You are an ST4 in the obstetrics department and sitting in the doctor's office. Your colleague sitting next to you is in the process of submitting an article for publication.

She asks for your help with the submission as she is having difficulty with the system. You note that she has checked the box stating 'no conflicts of interest'. You know that her project revolves around the use of a new drug for managing menorrhagia. She received sponsorship for the last hospital social event. The drug representative has been involved heavily in this project. When you ask your colleague about this, she states that as she has not received money directly; this does not count as a conflict of interest.

What is the single most appropriate next step?

A. Accept your colleague's explanation; there is nothing further to do.
B. Await publication and then submit a comment online.
C. Contact the journal to highlight your concerns.
D. Highlight your concerns to the consultant involved in the research.
E. Notify the GMC as this is a probity issue relating to research.

7.

You are an ST4 doing night duty with a new foundation year 2 doctor (FY2). He has been working fairly independently when seeing patients in maternity triage. The midwife tells you she has concerns about the FY2 as he does not examine the patients before discharging them. As the labour ward is fairly quiet, you suggest seeing the next patient together as an opportunity for a work place-based assessment. The FY2 dismisses the patient's complaint and does not examine her appropriately. You notice he is clearly unable to perform a speculum examination. After completing the consultation yourself, you ask the doctor about his confidence with speculum examination and he states that he does not need any help and walks away.

What is the single most appropriate course of action?

A. Complete a clinical incident form for the inability to perform a speculum.
B. Complete the FY2s case discussion highlighting your concerns.
C. Establish who the FY2's educational supervisor is and meet with him/her at the end of your shift.
D. Liaise with the GMC emergency hotline for advice.
E. Tell the consultant on call about your concerns as s/he would officially be the clinical supervisor.

8.

You have recently joined a new Trust and worked several shifts as the gynaecology registrar on call. You notice some recurring issues in the organization of the emergency gynaecology services. At your previous Trust, you carried out a quality improvement project in emergency gynaecology and feel that your experience could be invaluable in trying to improve things at this hospital.

Who is the most appropriate person to arrange a meeting with to discuss this?

A. Clinical director for gynaecology.
B. Clinical supervisor.
C. Educational supervisor.
D. Medical director.
E. Risk management lead.

9.

You have a keen interest in medical education. You have been an ST5 grade at the Trust for six months and have noticed that there is a lack of departmental teaching on up-to-date RCOG and NICE guidance. You have some ideas about trying to institute changes to the departmental teaching sessions.

Who is the single most appropriate person to speak to about your ideas?

A. Clinical director.
B. College tutor.
C. Educational supervisor.
D. Training programme director.
E. Undergraduate lead for education.

10.

You are assisting your consultant in performing a laparoscopic bilateral salpingo-oophorectomy. You have assisted this same consultant several times and have significant experience in laparoscopic surgery yourself. The consultant is the clinical director for gynaecology within your unit. Whenever he operates, he tends to get quite frustrated and aggressive towards the scrub nurse and his assistant. You have previously seen the scrub nurse cry after a theatre list with him. On this particular occasion, the surgery is complicated by significant adhesions. The consultant keeps blaming the equipment for the difficulties he is having, although it appears to be working well from your perspective. You offer a suggestion of swapping the equipment in the ports and he tells you to 'Shut up. What do you know dear?' After only partially removing one of the ovaries, he decides to abandon the surgery. You offer to contact another consultant to assist and he states 'I warned you once already, you stupid girl'.

What is the most appropriate next course of action?

A. Arrange a meeting with your educational supervisor.
B. Ask to never be rostered to work with him again.
C. Fill in an incident report form.
D. Liaise with the other registrars to find out if he behaves similarly with them.
E. Refer him to the GMC.

ANSWERS

Q1: B. Immediately call the foundation year 2 (FY2) colleague and advise removal of this post.[1]

- It is thoroughly unprofessional to write posts like this on social media. Even if there is no identifiable information about the patient, this is not an appropriate thing to post openly on Facebook.
- In the first instance, you would want to protect the profession and encourage your colleague to remove the post. You may wish to fill in an incident form or inform the consultant afterwards.
- British Medical Association (BMA) guidance states: 'Although the way medical professionals use social media in their private lives is a matter for their own personal judgement, doctors and medical students should consider whether the content they upload onto the internet could compromise public confidence in the medical profession.[1]

Q2: D. Prescribe the nifedipine but explain to the patient it is unlicensed and document this.[2,3]

- Nifedipine is mentioned in the RCOG Green Top guideline for tocolysis. It is also recommended in the hospital guideline as the first-line drug choice. It is therefore appropriate to prescribe it.

- The GMC guidance on the prescribing of unlicensed medications states that when prescribing an unlicensed medicine you must:
  - Be satisfied that there is sufficient evidence or experience of using the medicine to demonstrate its safety and efficacy.
  - Take responsibility for prescribing the medicine and for overseeing the patient's care, monitoring and any follow-up treatment or ensure that arrangements are made for another suitable doctor to do so.
  - Make a clear, accurate and legible record of all medicines prescribed and, where you are not following common practice, your reasons for prescribing an unlicensed medicine.

Q3: D. Tell her to book an urgent appointment with her general practitioner to fully assess and treat her.[4]

- Although it is very tempting to help your friends and family when they have a medical condition you are experienced in dealing with, this is not appropriate.
- The GMC has very strict guidance about self-prescribing and prescribing for friends and family.
- While her symptoms are very suggestive of mastitis, she needs a proper medical assessment.

Q4: C. Go to the parents with the junior doctor, explain and apologize about the complication and document it in the notes.[5,6]

- All doctors have a professional responsibility to be open with the patients. This duty of candour was highlighted after the Francis report. As the ST2 is very upset, it would be appropriate for you as the senior to liaise with the parents but invite the ST2 to see how you have this conversation.
- It is vital that you document the complication in the operation note including your explanation to the parents.
- As a doctor, you should not be afraid of saying sorry.[5,6]

Q5: B. Escalate to the consultant on call urgently.[7]

- According to the GMC guidance on raising concerns,
  'If you have concerns that a colleague may not be fit to practice and may be putting patients at risk, you must ask for advice from a colleague, your defense body or us. If you are still concerned you must report this, in line with our guidance and your workplace policy, and make a record of the steps you have taken.'
- As you have tried to approach your colleague without success, you need to take further action as there is a clear patient safety issue here. Something needs to be done as soon as possible as this anaesthetist does not seem fit to carry out his job in his current state. Escalating it to your senior could allow for senior anaesthetic input.
- This issue will obviously require further investigation but, in the first instance, the immediate patient safety issue needs to be addressed.[8]

Q6: D. Highlight your concerns to the consultant involved in the research.[8]

- The GMC has very explicit guidance about declaring conflicts of interest in research.
  - You must be open and honest in all financial and commercial matters relating to your research and its funding.

- You must not allow your judgement about a research project to be influenced, or be seen to be influenced, at any stage, by financial, personal, political or other external interests.
- You must identify and notify any actual or potential conflicts of interest as soon as possible to the research ethics committee, other appropriate bodies and the participants, in line with the policy of your employing or contracting body.
- You have a duty to raise your concern. Liaising with the lead consultant for the research in the first instance would be most sensible. If they too deny any concerns and fail to offer you enough evidence of this, it would be appropriate to then escalate your concern and seek guidance from the GMC about your next steps.[8]

Q7: C. Establish who the FY2's educational supervisor is and meet with him/her at the end of your shift.[9]

- You have already tried to address your concerns and they have not been accepted. The midwife has raised concerns about the FY2 to you as well.
- There is a potentially serious patient safety issue as this doctor appears to lack basic skills required and, more importantly, seems to lack insight.
- Liaising with ther educational supervisor for further investigation is the most appropriate course of action. The educational supervisor needs to know about your concerns and investigate them.
- As an educational supervisor, s/he can try to find out if there have been previous concerns with this trainee and escalate things accordingly.[9]

Q8: A. Clinical director of gynaecology.[10,11]

- While many of the people listed would have some role to play in discussing your ideas, the most appropriate is the clinical director. S/he is directly responsible for making decisions regarding the services in the gynaecology department and would be most aware of the way the service is run and why.
- The medical director takes a more macro view of the way in which the hospital is run, which is not going to be specific to the gynaecology department.

Q9: B. College tutor.[12,13]

- The person responsible for ensuring that those within a department are appropriately trained is the college tutor. S/he would be the most appropriate first port of call.
- The clinical director has more say regarding organisational issues within a department and resources allocation.
- While your educational supervisor might be interested in your educational aspirations, s/he is less likely to have a pivotal role in department educational activities.
- The training programme director would be more appropriate if you have thoughts or suggestions related to regional teaching.
- The undergraduate lead for education would be relevant if it was an educational initiative for medical students but, in this case, this sounds more like postgraduate departmental teaching.[12,13]

Q10: E. Refer him to the GMC.[7]

- The consultant has been verbally aggressive and sexist towards you. He is the clinical director of the gynaecology department and there is nobody above to refer to locally for advice. You have tried to approach him directly, unsuccessfully.
- His surgical skills seem below par and might be putting patients at risk. He does not show insight or ask for help from someone else. The GMC

recommends that 'If you cannot raise the issue with the responsible person or body locally because you believe them to be part of the problem', it is appropriate to refer to the GMC.

- While asking to not work together might benefit you, it does nothing to address the issues with this individual.
- Your educational supervisor might be able to offer advice but it might delay an investigation.
- Incident report forms will be sent directly to the clinical director for investigation and this would be the individual you are reporting.
- Liaising with colleagues is often the most tempting first course of action but does not serve to address the problem directly.

References

1. British Medical Association. *Using Social Media: Practical and Ethical Guidance for Doctors and Medical Students*. [www.bma.org.uk/-/media/files/pdfs/practical%20advice]%20].
2. Royal College of Obstetricians and Gynaecologists. *Developing New Pharmaceutical Treatments for Obstetric Conditions*. May, 2015. [https://www.rcog.org.uk/global assets/documents/guidelines/scientific-impact-papers/sip-50.pdf]
3. General Medical Council. *Hot Topic: Prescribing Unlicensed Medicines*. November, 2015. [www.gmc-uk.org/guidance/28349.asp]
4. General Medical Council. *Hot Topic: Prescribing for Friends and Family*. August, 2015. [www.gmc-uk.org/guidance/27549.asp]
5. General Medical Council. *Hot Topic: Duty of Candour*. July, 2015. [www.gmc-uk.org].
6. General Medical Council. *Openness and Honesty when Things go Wrong: The Professional Duty of Candour*. June, 2015. [www.gmc-uk.org/DoC_guidance_english.pdf_61618688.pdf]
7. General Medical Council. *Raising and Acting on Concerns about Patient Safety*. January, 2012. [www.gmc.uk.org/Raising_and_acting_on_concerns_about_patient_safety]
8. General Medical Council. *Good Practice in Research and Consent to Research*. March, 2013. [www.gmc.uk.org/static/documents/content/Good_practice_in_research_and_consent]
9. General Medical Council and NACT UK. *Roles and Responsibilities of an Educational Supervisor*. [www.gmc-uk.org/Final_Appendix_2___Roles_of_Supervisors.pdf_53817452.pdf]
10. Supporting the Role of the Medical Director. May, 2014. [https://www.gov.uk/government/uploads]
11. The King's Fund. *Leadership Needs of Medical Directors and Clinical Directors*. August, 2010. [https://www.kingsfund.org.uk/sites/files/kf/Leadership-needs-clinical-directors-August2010.pdf]
12. Royal College of Obstetricians and Gynaecologists. *College Tutor: Job Description*. October, 2014. https://www.rcog.org.uk/globalassets/documents/careers-and-training/resources/college]
13. Royal College of Obstetricians and Gynaecologists. *Undergraduate Academic Education and Training*. [https://www.rcog.org.uk/en/careers-training/academic-og/ undergraduate-academic].

Chapter 22

Ethics

Wafaa Basta

QUESTIONS

1.

The four pillars of medical ethics principles as described by Beauchamp and Childress include the following principles except:

A. Autonomy.
B. Beneficence.
C. Justice.
D. Non-maleficence.
E. Veracity.

2.

A 32-year-old recent immigrant woman in labour is attended by your ST2 colleague because of fetal distress. He decided to do vacuum delivery. The woman is stressed and anxious. Although communication is difficult, she expressed her request to stop the procedure. The doctor proceeds with the vacuum delivery for the sake of the baby.

Which of the following principles better describes this action?

A. Autonomy.
B. Battery.
C. Beneficence.
D. Non-maleficence.
E. Paternalism.

3.

A Jehovah's Witness has an elective Caesarean section for a placenta praevia. Despite being counselled about the risks, she wishes not to have a blood transfusion under any circumstance. Despite timely management, the patient dies on the table during a Caesarean hysterectomy.

Which of the following principles better describes this situation?

A. Autonomy.
B. Beneficence.
C. Equality.
D. Non-maleficence.
E. Veracity.

4.

An 18-year-old woman was coming alone to the early pregnancy assessment unit. Suddenly she collapsed and became unconscious, having a suspected ruptured ectopic pregnancy. After immediate resuscitation, an emergency laparotomy with right salpingectomy was done and the patient survived.

Which of the following principles better describes this action?

A. Battery.
B. Beneficence.
C. Negligence.
D. Non-maleficence.
E. Paternalism.

5.

An 83-year-old lady undergoes a laparotomy for suspected ovarian cancer. The family asks if you would disclose the results to them so they can explain better to her.

What ethical principle should guide you to take your decision?

A. Autonomy.
B. Beneficence.
C. Paternalism.
D. Confidentiality.
E. Fidelity.

6.

A 32-year-old lady in her fifth pregnancy is asking for termination of pregnancy. She had four previous Caesarean deliveries resulting in four male children. She is 12 weeks pregnant with another male. She asks for termination to be able to have a female baby later.

This decision is consistent with which Clause of the Abortion Act 1967?

A. Clause A.
B. Clause B.
C. Clause C.
D. Clause D.
E. Clause E.

ANSWERS

Q1: E. Veracity.[1]

The framework used in the analysis of medical ethics is the "four principles" approach postulated by Tom Beauchamp and James Childress in their textbook *Principles of Biomedical Ethics*.

- Respect for autonomy – the patient has the right to refuse or choose his/her treatment.

- Beneficence – a practitioner should act in the best interest of the patient.
- Non-maleficence – 'first, do no harm'.
- Justice – concerns the distribution of scarce health resources, and the decision of who gets what treatment (fairness and equality).[1]

Q2: B. Battery.[2,3]

- Touching/treating someone without permission could be considered assault or battery under criminal and civil laws, even if the person was helped by your actions.[2,3]

Q3: A. Autonomy.[4]

- Autonomy is based on the Principle of Respect for Persons; individual persons have the right to make their own choices and develop their own life plan.[4]
- Physicians should take care to avoid coercion and deception that can deny a patient's autonomy and can result in charges of battery.[4]

Q4: C. Beneficence.[5]

- The term beneficence in the medical context means actions that serve the best interests of patients.[5]
- When an emergency arises in a clinical setting and it is not possible to find out a patient's wishes, you can treat them without their consent, provided the treatment is immediately necessary to save her life or to prevent a serious deterioration of her condition.
- The treatment you provide must be the least restrictive of the patient's future choices.
- If the patient regains capacity while in your care, you should tell her what has been done, and why, as soon as she is sufficiently recovered to understand.[5]

Q5: D. Confidentiality.[6]

- Confidentiality is 'the protection of a patient's personal information or personal informed decision from unauthorised parties'. This includes a patient's name and address, not just medical information.[6]
- A patient's right to confidentiality has, for centuries, been an integral part of ethics in healthcare and is highlighted in the Hippocratic oath.

Q6: C. Clause C.[7]

- The fact that fetal sex is not specifically included in the Act does not necessarily mean that abortion on the grounds of fetal sex would be unlawful, just as is the case with rape.[7]
- All that needs to be established is that, in good faith, two doctors believe that continuing the pregnancy would involve a risk, greater than if the pregnancy were terminated, of injury to the woman's physical or mental health. A doctor could conclude that the prospect of giving birth to a fifth son, or yet another son, would pose a risk to the woman's mental health, greater than termination.[7]
- It is simply wrong to say that abortion on the grounds of fetal sex is unlawful in the UK. That is not what the law says.[7]

References

1. Beauchamp TL, Childress JF. *The Principles of Biomedical Ethics.* Oxford, UK: Oxford University Press, 1979.
2. Ministry of Ethics: *Main Principles of Consent.* [www.ministryofethics.co.uk/]

3. *Offences against the Person Act.* 1861.
4. American College of Physicians Ethics Manual, 6th edn. *Ann Intern Med* 2012;156:73–104.
5. General Medical Council Consent Guidance: *The Scope of Treatment in Emergencies.* [www.gmc-uk.org/guidance/ethical_guidance/consent_guidance_scope_of_treatment_in_emergencies.asp]
6. General Medical Council (UK). *Confidentiality: Protecting and Providing Information.* September, 2000. [www.gmc-uk.org/standards/secret.htm]
7. Jackson E. *The Legality of Abortion for Fetal Sex.* [www.reproductivereview.org/images/uploads/Britains_abortion_law.pdf]

Chapter 23

Breast Disorders

Youssef Abo Elwan

QUESTIONS

1.

A 23-year-old woman has asked her general practitioner if it is appropriate for her to breastfeed.

Which of the following maternal infections is a contraindication to breastfeeding?

A. Hepatitis B virus.
B. Hepatitis C virus.
C. HIV in a developed country.
D. HIV in a developing country.
E. Zika virus.

2.

You are explaining to your ST1 colleague the physiology of lactation.

What will you tell him?

A. A rise in oestrogen levels stimulates lactation.
B. Dopamine receptor agonist bromocriptine stimulates lactation.
C. Rise in progesterone levels stimulates lactation.
D. Removal of the placenta is necessary for the initiation of milk secretion.
E. Sucking initiates breastmilk secretion.

3.

You review a 24-year-old woman with epilepsy controlled by lamotrigine who delivered spontaneously. She is keen to breastfeed her baby. Her last fitting episode was two months prior to pregnancy.

What advice would you give her?

A. Avoid breastfeeding if possible.
B. Administer 1 mg intravenous vitamin K to the neonate.

C. Consider breastfeeding prior to taking the lamotrigine dose.
D. Stop her antiepileptic medication.
E. Stop lamotrigine and commence carbamazepine.

4.

While on call on the labour ward, the midwife asks you to see a primigravida who has just delivered by a vacuum-assisted delivery after a long painful 16 hours' labour. The woman feels exhausted and is reluctant to breastfeed. She seemed to understand the benefits of breastfeeding.

When is the most appropriate time to start breastfeeding if she wishes to exclusively breastfeed?

A. Breastfeeding within 20 minutes of delivery is the best way to sustain exclusive breastfeeding.
B. Breastfeeding within one hour of delivery is the best way to sustain exclusive breastfeeding.
C. Breastfeeding within two hours of delivery is the best way to sustain exclusive breastfeeding.
D. Breastfeeding within three hours of delivery is the best way to sustain exclusive breastfeeding.
E. Breastfeeding within five hours of delivery is the best way to sustain exclusive breastfeeding.

5.

Breastfeeding immediately after delivery of a baby can reduce the risk of bleeding by causing uterine contraction.

Which hormone is released to cause this?

A. Adrenocorticotropic hormone.
B. Oxytocin.
C. Prostacyclin.
D. Prostaglandin F2α.
E. Vascular endothelial growth factor (VEGF).

6.

A healthy multiparous woman has just delivered. She suffered from mastitis with her previous child.

What is your advice if she develops mastitis?

A. Antibiotics are contraindicated as they are secreted in breastmilk and harm the baby.
B. Cabergoline to stop lactation to prevent the occurrence of breast abscess.
C. If a breast abscess develops, treat it conservatively.
D. Reassurance and encourage breastfeeding or expressing milk.
E. The milk from the affected breast will harm the baby.

7.

A 35-year-old woman has an unplanned pregnancy. She is considering termination of this pregnancy. She has a family history of breast cancer. She has read some information about the relationship between pregnancy and breast cancer and wanted to know if termination of pregnancy would increase her risk of breast cancer.

What will you tell her?

A. Abortion will increase the risk if her mother had breast cancer.
B. If she has a normal mammography, termination will not increase the risk.
C. Induced abortion increases the risk.
D. Spontaneous, medical or surgical termination will not increase the risk.
E. Spontaneous miscarriage increases the risk.

8.

A 31-year-old nulliparous woman with breast cancer underwent a radical mastectomy of her right breast last year. She wishes to achieve pregnancy in the near future. She is worried that pregnancy may precipitate recurrence of the cancer.

What advice you will you give her?

A. Delay pregnancy for at least four years to improve the chance of survival.
B. Nulliparity increases the risk of breast cancer.
C. Pregnancy confers no increased risk of breast cancer in *BRCA1* and *BRCA2* gene mutation carriers.
D. Subsequent pregnancy improves the chance of survival.
E. Subsequent pregnancy may precipitate recurrence of cancer.

9.

A 28-year-old woman is diagnosed with early stage breast cancer at 19 weeks of gestation.

How would you counsel her regarding her management options?

A. Combination chemotherapy is contraindicated.
B. Radiotherapy is absolutely contraindicated.
C. Surgery (mastectomy or lumpectomy with axillary clearance) is the last-resort line of treatment.
D. Surgery should be performed as soon as possible with termination of pregnancy to improve survival.
E. Surgery should be performed as soon as possible without termination of pregnancy.

10.

A 35-year-old woman attends the preconception clinic for counselling after the treatment for breast cancer. She is planning a pregnancy.

How long after completion of the treatment, should she wait before attempting to conceive?

A. Three months.
B. Six months.
C. One year.
D. Two years.
E. Three years.

11.

A 32-year-old woman is diagnosed with breast cancer. She is 10 weeks pregnant with a 3 cm tumour in her breast. You are part of the multidisciplinary team at the gynaecology oncology department.

What is your recommendation for her treatment?

A. Surgical excision as soon as possible.
B. Surgical excision and chemotherapy as soon as possible, within the first trimester.
C. Surgical excision as soon as possible, and administering of chemotherapy in the second trimester.
D. Surgical excision and administering chemotherapy six weeks post-delivery.
E. Surgical excision in the second trimester.

12.

Which of the following maternal therapies is neither absolutely nor relatively contra-indicated while breastfeeding?

A. Bromocriptine.
B. Cabergolin.
C. Cyclosporine.
D. Digoxin.
E. Radioactive iodine.

13.

A 35-year-old parous woman who is 35 weeks pregnant has just completed her adjuvant chemotherapy for breast cancer after surgical treatment.

What advice would you give about the timing of delivery?

A. Await spontaneous labour.
B. Immediate induction after a course of corticosteroids.
C. Induction at 38 weeks.
D. Induction one week after a course of corticosteroids.
E. Induction two weeks after completion of chemotherapy.

14.

A 38-year-old woman has just delivered after completion of both surgical and adjuvant chemotherapy for breast cancer during the current pregnancy. She is now healthy and disease free. She is breastfeeding and asks your advice regarding a safe form of contraception.

What will you recommend?

A. Condoms.
B. Safe period method.
C. The combined oral contraceptive pill.
D. The copper intrauterine device.
E. The Mirena coil.

15.

A 37-year-old woman has just delivered. She had completed surgical and adjuvant chemotherapy treatment for breast cancer during this pregnancy.

What is your breastfeeding advice?

A. She should not breastfeed for six months until she is sure there is no recurrence.
B. She can breastfeed safely.
C. She can only use formula-feeding.
D. She cannot breastfeed if she has had chemotherapy.
E. She can only breastfeed if she had radical mastectomy of the affected breast.

ANSWERS

Q1: C. HIV in a developed country [evidence level 4].[1]

- UNICEF states that 'Without preventive interventions, approximately one-third of infants born to HIV-positive mothers contract HIV during pregnancy, childbirth or breastfeeding'.
- In developing countries with low resources, the risk of HIV-infection has to be compared with the risk of morbidity and mortality due to not breastfeeding.
- Breastfeeding is protective against death from diarrhoea, respiratory and other infections, particularly in the first months of life. It is for this reason that breastfeeding is recommended in developing countries despite maternal HIV infection.
- Transmission of hepatitis B and C is not increased through breastfeeding.[1]
- The World Health Organization (WHO), February 2016 states that breastfeeding is not contraindicated to maternal infection of Zika virus.[1]
- WHO recommends that infants start breastfeeding within one hour of birth, and are exclusively breastfed for six months.

Q2: D. Removal of the placenta is necessary for the initiation of milk secretion.[2]

- High levels of progesterone inhibit lactation before birth. Cessation of placental progesterone synthesis at delivery triggers lactation.
- Prolactin stimulates milk production and oxytocin stimulates its ejection.
- Prolactin is a polypeptide hormone synthesized by lactotrophic cells in the anterior pituitary. Oxytocin contracts the smooth muscle layer of band-like cells surrounding the alveoli to squeeze the newly produced milk into the duct system.[2]
- The breast parenchyma contains the functional secretory and ductal tissue. The stroma constitutes the supportive tissue (connective tissue, fibroblasts, adipose tissue, nerve tissue and endothelial cells associated with blood vessels and lymph vessels).
- The breast alveoli comprise secretory epithelial cells surrounding a central lumen, and basal myoepithelial cells which contract to allow milk expression.

Q3: C. Consider breastfeeding prior to taking lamotrigine dose.[3,4]

- Woman with epilepsy should be encouraged to breastfeed as most antiepileptic drugs cross into the breastmilk in only minimal amounts (3%–5% of maternal levels).
- Women taking lamotrigine should be advised to breastfeed prior to taking their medication in order to minimize neonatal exposure as it crosses into breastmilk in much larger doses (30%–50%).
- Many infants have been breastfed without adverse reactions.
- However, infants should be observed for side effects (apnoea, rash, drowsiness or poor sucking).
- Measurement of serum levels may be indicated to rule out toxicity if there is a concern.
- Monitoring of the platelet count and liver function may also be advisable. If an infant rash occurs, breastfeeding should be discontinued until the cause can be established.[3,4]

Q4: B. Breastfeeding within one hour of delivery is the best way to sustain exclusive breastfeeding.[5,6]

- If every child was breastfed within an hour of birth, and given only breastmilk for their first six months of life, about 800 000 children's lives would be saved every year.

- Breastmilk gives infants all the nutrients they need for healthy development.
- It contains antibodies that help protect infants from common childhood illnesses (diarrhoea and pneumonia, the two primary causes of child mortality worldwide).[6]
- Breastmilk is readily available and affordable, which helps to ensure that infants get adequate nutrition.

Q5: B. Oxytocin.[6]

- Oxytocin produced by the posterior pituitary gland stimulates milk secretion and prevents uterine bleeding because of contractions of the breast myoepithelial alveoli and the uterine muscles.

Q6: E. Reassurance and encourage breastfeeding or expressing milk [evidence level 2+].[7,8]

- Supportive counselling and reassurance are important.
- Effective milk removal by continuing breastfeeding or expressing milk is essential.
- The milk from the affected breast will not harm the baby.[1]
- Using warmth to the sore area sparingly and just before a feed (for up to five minutes) can trigger the let-down reflex to help clear the blockage, which may relieve the pain.
- Ice packs and cold compresses after feeding will help reduce congestion and pain. Published studies and anecdotal reports seem to support the value of chilled or even room-temperature cabbage leaves in reducing breast engorgement.[8]
- Women should be advised to start breastfeeding from the painful breast where the child sucking is stronger, to help in emptying the breast.
- Antibiotics are indicated if leucocyte counts in the milk and culture indicate infection.
- If a breast abscess develops, ultrasound-guided aspiration or incision and drainage should be performed; complete cure can be expected.[8]

Q7: D. Spontaneous, medical or surgical termination will not increase the risk [evidence level 2+].[9]

- Rigorous prospective studies consistently showed no association between induced abortion or spontaneous abortion and breast cancer risk.

Q8: D. Subsequent pregnancy improves the chance of survival [evidence level 2+].[10]

- Several studies show better survival in women who conceive after treatment for breast cancer.[10]
- There are no adverse effects of a subsequent pregnancy after breast cancer.
- There are several studies to demonstrate that there may be improved prognosis if she has another pregnancy.
- She is advised not to conceive for at least two years following completion of treatment.[11]
- Nulliparity increases the risk of developing breast cancer.[10]

Q9: E. Surgery should be performed as soon as possible without termination of pregnancy.[10]

- The woman should understand that delay in therapy has serious consequences.
- Treatment can be started during pregnancy, as soon as possible.

- Therapeutic termination of pregnancy does not improve survival.[10]
- Surgery is the first-line treatment.
- Combination chemotherapy is not contraindicated [evidence level 3].[10,11]
- Radiation is better delayed until after delivery unless it is lifesaving.
- The abdomen must be properly shielded and radiation dose is limited to 500 µGy.

Q10: D. Two years [evidence level 3].[10,11]

- Women are advised to wait for at least two years after treatment for breast cancer before conception because of the risk of early relapse.
- The rate of disease recurrence is highest in the first three years and then declines, although late relapses do occur up to 10 years and more from the time of diagnosis.[11]

Q11: C. Surgical excision as soon as possible, and administering of chemotherapy in the second trimester [evidence level 3].[10,12]

- Breast surgery can be performed safely at any time during gestation with little risk to the fetus.
- Chemotherapy is safe in the second and third trimester. It should be avoided in the first trimester because of the risk of fetal malformation and miscarriage.[12]

Q12: D. Digoxin.[13]

- Dopamine receptor agonist bromocriptine and cabergoline both suppress milk production.
- Case reports have described acute myocardial infarction in women treated with bromocriptine for suppressing lactation.[13]
- Radioactive iodine therapy will cause fetal goiter and is contraindicated during pregnancy and breastfeeding.
- Only few drugs are absolutely contraindicated, e.g. radiopharmaceuticals, cytotoxic and immunosuppressants such as cyclosporine.[13]

Q13: A. Await spontaneous labour.[10]

- Most women can be allowed to go to term and have a normal or induced delivery after successful treatment of breast cancer during pregnancy.
- Birth should be more than two to three weeks after the last chemotherapy session to allow maternal bone marrow recovery and to minimize problems with neutropenia.
- Most of the available data do not show any increase in congenital malformations or stillbirth among the offspring of women who have completed treatment for breast cancer.[10]

Q14: D. The copper intrauterine device.[14]

- Hormonal contraception is contraindicated in women with current or recent breast cancer.[14]
- There is insufficient evidence to support the use of combined or progestogen-only hormonal contraceptives when alternative non-hormonal methods are suitable and acceptable.

Q15: B. She can breastfeed safely [evidence level 2+].[10]

- There is no evidence that breastfeeding increases the risk of recurrence in women who have completed treatment for breast cancer.[10]

References

1. World Health Organization. *Breastfeeding in the Context of Zika Virus*. February, 2016. [www.who.int/csr/resources/publications/zika/breastfeeding/en/]
2. Mohrbacher N, Stock J, Newton E. *The Breastfeeding Answer Book*, 3rd edn. (revised). La Leche League International (Open Library), 2003.
3. Nelson-Piercy C. *Handbook of Obstetric Medicine*, 4th edn. New York, NY: Informa Healthcare, 2010.
4. Drugs.com. *Lamotrigine Use while Breastfeeding*. [https://www.drugs.com/breastfeeding]
5. World Health Organization. *10 Facts on Breastfeeding*. February, 2012. [www.who.int/features/files/breastfeeding]
6. Collins S, Arulkumaran S, Hayes K, Jackson S, Impey L, eds. *Oxford Handbook of Obstetrics and Gynaecology*. Oxford, UK: Oxford University Press, 2008; Ch. 9.
7. Roberts K. A comparison of chilled cabbage leaves and chilled gel packs in reducing breast engorgement. *J Hum Reprod* 1995;11:17–20.
8. World Health Organization. Department of Child and Adolescent Health and Development. *Mastitis Causes and Management*. 2000. [www.apps.who.int/iris/bitstream/10665/66230/1/WHO_FCH_CAH_00.13_eng.pdf]
9. Michels KB, Xue F, Colditz GA, Willett WC. Induced and spontaneous abortion and incidence of breast cancer among young women: a prospective cohort study. *Arch Int Med* 2007;167(8):814–20.
10. Royal College of Obstetrician and Gynecologists. *Pregnancy and Breast Cancer*. April, 2011. [https://www.rcog.org.uk/guidelines/gtg_12.pdf]
11. Society of Obstetricians and Gynaecologists of Canada. *Breast Cancer, Pregnancy, and Breastfeeding*. February, 2002. [https://sogc.org/wp-content/uploads/2013/01/111E-CPG-February2002.pdf]
12. Padmagirison R, Gajjar K, Spencer C. Management of breast cancer during pregnancy. *Obstet Gynaecol* 2010;12:186–92.
13. Hopp L, Weisse AB, Iffy L. Acute myocardial infarction in a healthy mother using bromocriptine for milk suppression. *Can J Cardiol* 1996;12:415–18.
14. World Health Organization. *New Recommendations on the Safety of Contraceptive Methods for Women with Medical Conditions*. March, 2015. [http://who.int/reproductivehealth/publications/family_planning/MEC-5/en/]

Chapter 24

Neonatology

QUESTIONS

1.

During your postnatal ward round you are asked to review a baby with clinical jaundice. He was delivered two days ago and his unconjugated bilirubin blood levels are 320 mmol/L.

What is your first-line management?

A. ABO compatible blood transfusion.
B. Exchange transfusion.
C. Only observation.
D. Rh-negative blood transfusion.
E. Phototherapy.

2.

The community midwife called you to ask about one of her nursing mothers. Her baby has developed jaundice at three weeks of life and his bilirubin level is 210 mmol/L. The baby is exclusively breastfed. The baby seems in good health. She asks your advice for breastfeeding.

What will you tell her?

A. Combine breastfeeding with formula-feeding.
B. Continue breastfeeding at a three-hourly interval.
C. Continue breastfeeding but increase the frequency to 10–12 times a day.
D. Stop breastfeeding completely.
E. Stop breastfeeding until the bilirubin drops to 216 mmol/L.

3.

You performed a forceps delivery because of delayed second stage labour. The neonatologist assessed the Apgar score as 3 at one minute.

What does this score imply?

A. It is a process to indicate the condition of the baby at birth.
B. The baby is hypoxic.
C. The baby is hypoxaemic.
D. The baby will develop long-term neurological problems.
E. The baby has suffered antenatal hypoxia.

4.

Your ST2 delivered a male full-term baby by Caesarean section for failure to progress and has a suspicious cardiotocography (CTG) result. The baby was born with an Apgar score of 4 at one minute. The pediatrician informed you that the baby was asphyxiated.

What does this term indicate?

A. It is an accurate reflection of intrapartum events.
B. It is a description of a varying degree of severity and not an end point.
C. It indicates fetal hypoxia.
D. It indicates fetal hypoxemia.
E. It indicates the baby will develop long-term neurological sequela.

5.

You are called to the labour ward urgently because a newborn has not started breathing after 55 seconds. The heart rate was 100/min. It was a normal vertex vaginal delivery with no risk factors.

What are your first-line resuscitation methods?

A. Drying and/or blowing oxygen over the face.
B. Immediate intubation.
C. Immediate admission to the neonatal intensive care unit.
D. Start cardiac compression.
E. Start mouth-to-mouth breathing.

6.

You have just delivered a 32-week baby. He was breathing and did not seem to require positive pressure ventilation.

When should you clamp the cord in order to reduce the need for blood transfusions and increase iron stores.

A. After three minutes.
B. After four minutes.
C. After five minutes.
D. After six minutes.
E. Immediately.

7.

You have just carried out a Caesarian section on a baby because of failure to progress and a low fetal pH. The baby did not breathe after initial drying and gentle stimulation.

How soon should positive pressure ventilation be started?

A. After failed external cardiac massage.
B. After failed mouth-to-mouth breathing.

C. Only if the pulse is below 60 bpm.
D. Within one minute.
E. Within five minutes.

8.

You delivered a full-term baby who failed to breathe despite drying and gentle stimulation. The neonatologist decided to start positive pressure ventilation.

Which is the best method to use?

A. Chest compression.
B. Endotracheal intubation.
C. Face–mask interface.
D. Mouth-to-mouth breathing.
E. Nasal cannula.

ANSWERS

Q1: C. Only observation.[1]

- Jaundice appearing after 24 hours and fading before 14 days of age can be physiological.
- Jaundice that appears during the first 24 hours of life is likely to be non-physiologic; further evaluation is indicated.[1]
- Over 60% of term newborns develop jaundice by 48 to 72 hours of age with 5%–10% needing intervention for management (phototherapy) of hyperbilirubinaemia.
- Bilirubin levels up to 324 mmol/L may be accepted as normal in healthy term newborns.[2]
- In physiological jaundice with no rising bilirubin levels, mothers should be assured about the benign nature of the condition. Frequent exclusive breast-feeding with no glucose water is advisable.
- The mother should bring the baby to the clinic if the colour of the legs looks as yellow as that of the face.
- Any newborn discharged prior to 48 hours of life should be evaluated again in the next 48 hours for adequacy of breastfeeding and any jaundice.[1]
- Treatment for jaundice is only necessary if the bilirubin levels exceeds 360 mmol/L.
- Phototherapy can make the baby irritable. It is associated with loose stools.

Q2: C. Continue breastfeeding but increase the frequency to 10–12 times a day [evidence level 2+].[2]

- This condition is due to 'breastmilk jaundice'. It should be considered if the serum bilirubin is predominantly unconjugated, if other causes of prolonged jaundice have been excluded and if the infant is in good health, vigorously active, feeding well and has adequate weight gain.[2]
- It is not recommended to stop breastfeeding until bilirubin levels have reached an excess of 360 mmol/L.
- Decreased frequency of breastfeeding leads to exaggeration of physiological jaundice. Encouraging a mother to breastfeed at least 10–12 times per day would be helpful in the management of physiological jaundice in healthy term babies.
- For healthy term infants with breastmilk or breastfeeding jaundice and with bilirubin levels of 12 mg/dL (170 μmol/L) to 17 mg/dL, it is acceptable to increase the frequency of breastfeeding to 10–12 times per day.

Q3: A. It is a process to indicate the condition of the baby at birth.[3]

- The Apgar score conveys the condition of the newborn and its response to resuscitation. It is not intended to use as a means for when or how to resuscitate.[3]
- The Apgar score should be reported at one and five minutes after birth for all infants but thereafter every 20 minutes in babies with an initial Apgar score of <7.
- Apgar scores can be low because of other factors (anaesthesia and prematurity) that are not due to hypoxia.
- Low scores are not evidence of birth asphyxia nor a guide to neurological prognoses.

Hypoxemia is an abnormally low arterial oxygen tension (PaO_2) in the blood due to insufficient arterial oxygen content.
Hypoxia is a condition in which the oxygen is at an inadequate level for tissue oxygenation, e.g. in hypoventilation or high altitude, it is usually due to respiratory causes.

Q4: B. It is a description of a varying degree of severity and not an end point.[3]

- The term asphyxia does not indicate any specific condition. An impaired fetal oxygenation either in the antenatal period or due to intrapartum events can only be indicated according to the umbilical artery pH and any additional neurological manifestations, e.g. seizures, hypotonia or evidence of multi-organ dysfunction.[3]

Q5: A. Drying and/or blowing oxygen over the face.[4,5]

- Seventy-five percent of normal term infants breathe within one minute of delivery. Most of the rest will do so within three minutes.[7]
- Initially drying the baby to keep him warm and blowing air or oxygen over the face may stimulate breathing.[7]
- Newborn infants who are born at term and are breathing or crying and have good tone must be dried and kept warm. These actions can be provided with the baby lying on the mother's chest and should not require separation of mother and baby.
- Approximately 10% of newborns require some assistance to begin breathing at birth, and <1% require extensive resuscitation.

Q6: A. After three minutes [high quality evidence level 1–].[6,7]

- There is moderate- to high-quality evidence that late clamping of the umbilical cord is associated with a lower risk of anaemia requiring transfusion in preterm infants and with higher serum ferritin levels at follow-up in term neonates.

Q7: D. Within one minute [evidence level 4].[7]

- A prompt increase in heart rate remains the most sensitive indicator of resuscitation efficacy.
- There are no adequate human studies to define the optimum time to start positive pressure ventilation (PPV).
- Evidence from animal studies indicates that blood pressure and cerebral blood flow reductions occur within seven to 10 minutes and cardiac arrest occurs within 15 minutes after cord occlusion.
- In animal studies, initiation of PPV is associated with a significant improvement in myocardial function and cerebral oxygenation.
- Within the limitations of the current studies, the WHO recommends starting PPV if the baby does not start breathing within one minute after birth.[7]

Q8: C. Face–mask interface [evidence level 4].[8,9]

- Initial inflation pressure of 20 cmH$_2$O may be required for preterm babies. For some term babies, the pressure may be increased to 30–40 cmH$_2$O.
- International consensus and guidelines on neonatal resuscitation recommend that infants with inadequate respiration and/or bradycardia at birth be given positive pressure ventilation (PPV) with a manual ventilation device with a face mask or endotracheal tube (ETT).
- Endotracheal tube (ETT) ventilation requires extensive training and experience, without which infants frequently deteriorate during intubation attempts.
- Because of the limited experience of using nasal cannula, most healthcare providers still prefer the face–mask interface.
- In a randomized trial of 363 preterm infants at <30 weeks' gestation receiving PPV in the delivery room, there were no differences in short-term outcomes using the nasal tube compared with the face mask [evidence level 1−].
- Measurement of the heart rate with visible chest movements after 60 seconds of ventilation should be used to assess the adequacy of ventilation.
- Consider the addition of chest compression if the neonate continues to have a heart rate of less than 60 bpm after one minute or does not have visible chest movements after one minute of PPV.
- Injury to the neonate's lungs has been known to occur with over-zealous cardiopulmonary resuscitation (CPR).

To carry out chest compression:
- Place one hand on the forehead and gently tilt the head back and lift the chin to open the infant's airway. Remove any visible obstructions from the mouth and nose.
- Start with five initial rescue breathes; place your mouth over the mouth and nose of the infant and blow steadily but gently, checking that the chest rises.
- Place two fingers or the heel of the hand in the middle of the chest and push down gently by 4 cm (about 1.5 inches), which is approximately one-third of the chest diameter.
- After 30 chest compressions at a rate of 100–120/minute, give two rescue breaths.
- Continue with cycles of 30 chest compressions and two rescue breaths until the baby begins to recover or emergency help arrives.

References

1. World Health Organisation. *Jaundice in the Newborn*. [www.newbornwhocc.org/jaundice.pdf]
2. American Academy of Pediatrics Subcommittee on Hyperbilirubinemia. Management of hyperbilirubinemia in the newborn infant 35 or more weeks of gestation. *Pediatrics* 2004;114(1):297–316.
3. American College of Obstetricians and Gynaecologists, the American Academy of Pediatrics. *The Apgar Score*. November, 2015. [www.acog.org/Resources-And-Publications/Committee-Opinions/Committee-on-Obstetric-Practice/The-Apgar-Score]
4. Elkady A, Verhigen E, Fogarty P. Mastering Short Answer Questions for the Part 2 MRCOG with Evidence Based Answers. In: Fogarty PP, ed. *Neonatology*, 2009; 26, p. 188–193. [https://issuu.com/cambridge.org.uk/docs/27833_mktg_kit_rcog_issuu_web]
5. Perlman JM, Wyllie J, Kattwinkel J, et al. Part 11: Neonatal resuscitation. 2010 International Consensus on Cardiopulmonary Resuscitation and Emergency Cardiovascular Care Science with Treatment Recommendations. *Circulation* 2010;122(16,S2):S516–38. [circ.ahajournals.org/content/122/16_suppl_2/S516]

6. Strauss RG, Mock DM, Johnson KJ, et al. A randomized clinical trial comparing immediate versus delayed clamping of the umbilical cord in preterm infants: short-term clinical and laboratory endpoints. *Transfusion* 2008;48:658–65.

7. World Health Organization. *Guidelines on Basic Newborn Resuscitation*. July, 2012. [www.who.int/maternal_child_adolescent/documents/basic_newborn_resuscitation/en/]

8. Omar C, Kamlin F, Schilleman K, et al. Mask versus nasal tube for stabilization of preterm infants at birth: A randomized controlled trial. *Pediatrics* 2013;132(2): e381–8.

9. NHS choices. *First Aid – CPR*. [www.nhs.uk/conditions/Accidents-and-first-aid]

Chapter 25

Operative Gynaecological and Surgical Complications

QUESTIONS

1.

You are a year ST5 performing a total abdominal hysterectomy. It was a difficult case with adhesions and a right broad ligament fibroid. While doing the dissection of the right side and before clamping the uterine artery, you suspected ureteric injury.

What is your first reaction?

A. Continue with your surgery and leave a drain to see if urine comes out of the drain.
B. Call for help from a urologist.
C. Dissect the ureter to inspect any site of possible injury.
D. Inject indigo carmine dye to observe for any urine leak.
E. Request intraoperative intravenous urography (IVU).

2.

During a difficult hysterectomy, you call the urologist because you suspected ureteric injury. He diagnosed a transection injury distally, below the pelvic brim, 5 cm from the ureterovesicular junction.

What is the best management for this injury?

A. Boari flap.
B. End-to-end anastomosis of the two cut edges.
C. Ureteral stenting with ureterotomy.
D. Ureteral stenting without ureterotomy.
E. Ureteral substitution with gastrointestinal segments.

3.

You have performed a vaginal hysterectomy for a 60-year-old woman because of vaginal vault prolapse. There was some difficulty dissecting the bladder and opening the vesicovaginal pouch. At the end of the surgery, there was clear urine in the drainage catheter. Two weeks later, the patient came complaining of continuous leaking of urine vaginally. On examination and the methylene blue test, you noticed a vesicovaginal fistula of <5 mm diameter.

What is your first-line management?

A. Advise her to use vaginal tampons and come back for surgical repair after three months.
B. Check if she has a urinary infection.
C. Insert a suprapubic catheter to see if the patient remains dry.
D. Insert a Foley catheter for three to four weeks and review in four weeks.
E. Insert a Foley catheter for one to two weeks and review in four weeks.

Q4.

While reviewing the next operative list, you noticed that one of the women who was booked for abdominal hysterectomy has previously developed a surgical site infection from appendectomy surgery.

What is the overall incidence of this complication?

A. 3%.
B. 5%.
C. 10%.
D. 12%.
E. 15%.

5.

A patient who had a total hysterectomy is referred to the accident and emergency department because of a surgical site wound infection (SSI). She was threatening to sue the hospital because she thinks it is due to acquired hospital infection.

What will you tell her about the most common cause of SSI?

A. Contamination by micro-organisms from the patient's own body.
B. Contamination from the operating theatre environment.
C. Contamination from the surgeon's gloves.
D. Contamination from the swabs.
E. Contamination from surgical sutures.

6.

After operating on a morbidly obese patient, she complains of deep tissue pain in the buttocks with dark urine.

What is your provisional diagnosis?

A. Hypokalemia.
B. Hyperkalemia.
C. Surgical site infection.
D. Rhabdomyolysis.
E. Renal failure.

7.

At the preoperative assessment clinic, an obese 42-year-old woman (BMI 40) was booked for a total abdominal hysterectomy. She is healthy with no medical disorders or other comorbidity.

What is the most important specific risk-screening question you should ask?

A. Family history of ischemic heart disease.
B. Family history of uterine or ovarian malignancy.
C. If she had ever smoked.
D. Nocturnal orthopnea.
E. Sleep-disordered breathing.

8.

Your ST2 junior colleague asks you if he can arrange a day-surgery booking for a patient with a BMI of 45. She is booked for laparoscopic sterilization. She was keen on going home the same day.

What is your advice?

A. Advise her that she needs at least two adults to look after her when she is discharged.
B. Arrange for a day-surgery admission but ask her to sign a high-risk consent.
C. Obesity alone is not a contraindication for day surgery.
D. She cannot be booked for day surgery because of the perioperative risks associated with her obesity.
E. She can have the surgery at the day surgery but admit as an inpatient after completion of her surgery.

9.

Readmission because of postoperative adhesions costs the UK NHS £24.2 million/year.

What is the incidence of readmission because of adhesion-related disease?

A. 1%.
B. 3%.
C. 4.5%.
D. 7%.
E. 10%.

10.

Your ST3 colleague calls you during a surgical termination of pregnancy because he thinks he may have perforated the uterus before completion of emptying the uterus.

How will you handle the situation?

A. Ask him to abandon the technique and use misoprostol to complete emptying the uterus.
B. Complete the surgery to empty the uterus under ultrasound guidance.
C. Immediate laparoscopy and complete the surgery under laparoscopic guidance.
D. Immediate laparotomy.
E. Start a syntocinon infusion.

11.

A 42-year-old mother of four children is booked for abdominal hysterectomy because of an enlarged uterus and heavy menstrual bleeding resistant to other first-line managements. During counselling, she has expressed that she has completed her family and does not wish to have any more children. At the beginning of surgery, you discover she is pregnant.

How will you manage the situation?

A. Ask a colleague to endorse the decision to carry on with hysterectomy and document his view in the operative note.
B. Carry on with the procedure as she has already completed her family, but remove the uterus with the pregnancy inside.
C. Evacuate the pregnancy to show her the fetus, carry on with the evacuation of the uterus and proceed with the hysterectomy.
D. Seek legal advice.
E. Stop the procedure and explain that you could not have terminated the pregnancy because there was no prior consent.

12.

During a laparoscopic sterilization procedure, you discover a suspicious right ovarian cyst.

How will you proceed?

A. Ask for a frozen section and perform a total abdominal hysterectomy and bilateral salpingo-oophorectomy if malignancy is confirmed.
B. Carry on with the scheduled procedure but do not remove the suspicious ovarian cyst.
C. Carry on with the scheduled procedure and take a sample for histopathology.
D. Remove the right ovary.
E. Remove the suspicious ovarian cyst after seeking a second opinion.

13.

You were asked to perform a total abdominal hysterectomy because of a large right broad ligament fibroid.

How best should you avoid ureteric injury?

A. Ask a urological surgeon to assist you to help prevent injury.
B. Dissection and visualization of the ureter.
C. Intraoperative insertion of a ureteric catheter to identify the ureter.
D. Intraoperative insertion of illuminating ureteric catheters.
E. Preoperative intravenous urography to identify the course of the ureter.

ANSWERS

Q1: B. Call for help from a urologist.[1]

• Ureteral injury is a serious complication of gynaecological surgery, which may be complicated by ureterovaginal fistulae, urinary peritonitis or loss of kidney function.
• The frequency of ureteric injury in gynaecological surgery is approximately 1%, with a higher percentage during abdominal hysterectomies.[1]
• Ureteric injury may be due to crushing, transection, angulation ischaemia or resection.

Q2: A. Boari flap.[1]

• If the ureteric injury is mid-ureteral or proximal ureteral, and the distal ureteral segment is not suitable for anastomosis, a Boari tubularized bladder flap is a viable alternative. The bladder is opened on its anterior surface, and a full thickness bladder flap is swung cranially and tubularized for anastomosis to the proximal ureteral segment. It is a technically challenging procedure and should be carried out by an experienced urologist.

Q3: D. Insert a Foley catheter for three to four weeks and review in four weeks.

- This procedure may lead to spontaneous cure in 15%–20% of cases.[1]

Q4: B. 5%.[2]

Q5: A. Contamination by micro-organisms from the patient's own body.[2]

Q6: D. Rhabdomyolysis.[3]

- Rhabdomyolysis is a rare but serious complication in obese patients.
- The triad of muscle weakness, myalgia and dark urine characterizes rhabdomyolysis.
- To prevent further acute kidney injury, any rise in serum creatinine kinase concentration should be treated aggressively with intravenous fluids and diuretics. Alkalinization of urine may be required.

Q7: E. Sleep-disordered breathing.[3]

- Most obese patients presenting for surgery are relatively healthy with a similar perioperative/operative risk to that of patients of normal weight.
- The obese patients at high perioperative risk are those with central obesity and metabolic syndrome.
- **Metabolic syndrome** is a clustering of at least three of the following five factors: abdominal (central) obesity, elevated BP, elevated fasting plasma glucose, high serum triglycerides, low high-density lipoprotein (HDL) levels. It is associated with the risk of developing cardiovascular disease and type 2 diabetes.
- The perioperative assessment of obese patients should include screening patients for sleep-disordered breathing with a clear pathway for referral for specialist sleep studies if indicated.[3]
- All other options are risk factors for all patients but are not specific to obese patients.

Q8: C. Obesity alone is not a contraindication for day surgery.[4]

- Obese patients should not be denied the advantages offered by day surgery.
- Suitability for day surgery should relate to the patient's health as determined at the preoperative assessment and not limited by arbitrary limits of age or BMI.[4]

Q9: C. 4.5%.[5]

- Postoperative adhesions have serious consequences, e.g. subfertility, pain, intestinal obstruction and/or complications during future surgical procedures.
- Even if adhesions are surgically removed, they often reform.
- Adhesions are associated with clinical burden and extra cost to the NHS.[5]

Q10: C. Immediate laparoscopy and complete the surgery under laparoscopic guidance.[6]

- If perforation is suspected during a termination of pregnancy, immediate laparoscopy is mandatory.[6] It allows proper diagnosis and management of any bleeding, continuation of the process under visual guidance, and exploration of the peritoneal cavity and the gastrointestinal tract for any possible injury.
- If there is massive bleeding or suspected gastrointestinal tract injury, laparotomy should be started without delay.

Q11: E. Stop the procedure and explain that you could not have terminated the pregnancy because there was no prior consent.[7]

Q12: B. Carry on with the scheduled procedure but do not remove the suspicious ovarian cyst.[8]

- Removal of any organ should not be carried out without prior consent, even if this means a second surgery.[7]
- You cannot take a biopsy of the ovarian mass as this may help spread the disease if it is cancer or may precipitate bleeding. The case is best referred to a gynaecology oncology centre.[8]

Q13: B. Dissection and visualization of the ureter.[9]

- Even in the hands of an experienced surgeon, ureteral injuries may occur due to anatomical distortions or in cases of endometriosis, pelvic adhesions or pelvic tumours.
- The reported incidence of ureteric injuries is 0.03%–2.0% for abdominal hysterectomy, 0.02%–0.5% for vaginal hysterectomy and 0.2%–6.0% for laparoscopy-assisted vaginal hysterectomy
- Direct visualization of the ureter should be an initial necessary prevention in all pelvic surgery in conditions that may increase the risk of ureteric injury.

References

1. Abboudi H, Ahmed K, Royle J, et al. Ureteric injury: a challenging condition to diagnose and manage. *Nat Rev Urol* 2013;10(2):108–15.
2. National Institute of Clinical Excellence. *Surgical Site Infections: Prevention and Treatment*. October, 2008. [https://www.nice.org.uk/guidance/cg74]
3. Association of Anaesthetists of Great Britain and Ireland Society for Obesity and Bariatric Anaesthesia. *Peri-operative Management of the Obese Surgical Patient*. March, 2015. [onlinelibrary.wiley.com]
4. Association of Anaesthetists of Great Britain and Ireland and the British Association of Day Surgery. Day case and short stay surgery: 2. *Anaesthesia* 2011;66:417–34.
5. Lower AM, Hawthorn RJ, Ellis H, et al. The impact of adhesions on hospital readmissions over ten years after 8849 open gynaecological operations: an assessment from the Surgical and Clinical Adhesions Research Study. *Brit J Obstet Gynaecol* 2000;107:855–62.
6. Society of Obstetricians and Gynaecologists of Canada. *Induced Abortion Guidelines*. November, 2006. [www.sogc.org/wp-content/uploads/2013/01/gui184E0611.pdf]
7. Royal College of Obstetricians and Gynaecologists. *Obtaining Valid Consent*. January, 2015. [https://www.rcog.org.uk/globalassets/documents/guidelines.pdf]
8. Chen L-M, Bere JS. *Patient Education: Ovarian Cancer Diagnosis and Staging (Beyond the Basics)*. [www.uptodate.com/contents/ovarian-cancer-diagnosis-and-staging]
9. Messaoudi F, Ben Jemaa S, Yazidi M, et al. Lower urinary trauma complication in gyneacologic and obstetrical surgery. *Tunis Med* 2008;86(8):740–4.

Chapter 26

Training and Clinical Governance in Obstetrics and Gynaecology

Bismeen Jadoon

QUESTIONS

1.

You are the consultant instructing the new specialist training staff who recently joined your department.

Which of the following training modalities has shown improvement in the clinical outcome?

A. Computer-based courses.
B. Inhouse multidisciplinary training courses.
C. Mnemonics.
D. Pocket algorithms.
E. Weekly clinical departmental meeting.

2.

You are working at the ST6 level in a District General Hospital. You are asked to help with finding an effective obstetric emergencies training programme.

Which of the following do you recommend?

A. One-to-one training.
B. Practical, multi-professional, obstetric emergency training at your hospital.
C. Single one-day course at your hospital.
D. Single one-day course at a simulation centre.
E. Single 2-day course at your hospital.

3.

Patient feedback is an essential component of revalidation.

What is the proposed role of patient feedback in revalidation?

A. It helps your esteem and personal ego.
B. It is used as an essential prerequisite for a consultant appointment.

C. It is a prerequisite for applying for new jobs.

D. It is a prerequisite to continue with your current contract.

E. It reassures patients, employers and other professionals and contributes to improving patient care and safety.

4.

You are asked to design an audit within your department to review the use of prophylactic antibiotics prior to the instrumentation of the uterus in patients undergoing procedures for fertility treatment.

Which of the following would you recommend, regarding conducting an audit?

A. Choose a nationally agreed standard.

B. Choose an audit topic at random.

C. Choose an evidence-based topic.

D. Choose a topic where you expect the results to show a statistical significance.

E. Choose a topic that meets the auditable standards of the College guidelines.

5.

A 50-year-old woman with the likely diagnosis of cervical cancer is admitted to the emergency unit with abdominal pain and vaginal bleeding. She has experienced postmenopausal bleeding for the last four months and has not had cervical smears in the past. Her condition deteriorated rapidly the day after admission. She collapsed and could not be resuscitated. You were the doctor on duty. You were asked to join the risk management team to participate in the root cause analysis of the case.

What is your understanding of root cause analyses?

A. A process of structured investigations to identify the root causes of faults or problems.

B. A process to identify what went wrong with a problem.

C. A process to identify the responsible persons for an unwanted event.

D. A process to start legal proceedings.

E. A process of self-learning.

6.

You are working at the ST5 level. You have conducted a trial of forceps delivery in theatre on a 28-year-old primigravida. She had successful epidural analgesia. The procedure went well. The estimated blood loss was 700 mL. The woman is haemodyanamically stable and the episiotomy is repaired appropriately. While counting swabs at the end of the procedure, the midwife has found that one swab is missing.

An X-ray located the swab, buried under one of the sutures. You called the consultant who removed the swab.

What is the most appropriate clinical governance action you should take?

A. Class this as an adverse event and inform your consultant.

B. Class this as a never event.

C. Class this as a near miss and inform the midwife in charge.

D. Fill the incident form on Datix and initiate the root cause analysis.

E. Inform the patient and offer a follow-up appointment.

7.

You are working at the ST5 level as part of the gynaecology team. One of your patients had a hysterectomy for heavy menstrual bleeding. As a part of trust policy you are advised to find out about the patient's experience through the patient-reported outcome measure.

What is the purpose of the patient-reported outcome measures?

A. It is used for research purposes.
B. It is used to assess the effectiveness of care.
C. It reduces the inequalities in clinical care.
D. It is used to analyse a patient's behaviour.
E. It helps tailor treatment plans to meet the patient's preferences and needs.

8.

There has been an increased incidence of perineal tears in the month of July within your department. You are part of the risk management team and needed to review risk assessment regarding this issue.

How do you calculate the risk score?

A. By calculating the frequency of the incident.
B. By calculating the severity of the incident.
C. By calculating the likelihood of harm.
D. By the serious concern to the practice.
E. The risk is calculated by multiplying the severity of harm with the likelihood of harm.

9.

A 29-year-old girl is brought for an examination after being assaulted by her husband. You are the registrar on call. The police have been involved and requested access to the patient's information.

According to the Caldicott principles and the Data Protection Act of 1998, when may you allow access to confidential patient information?

A. Access to personal data should be on a strict need-to-know basis.
B. According to orders from your consultant.
C. According to orders from the hospital manager.
D. If it is for criminal proceedings.
E. The patient's information can only be shared after their written permission.

10.

As an ST5, you are going to have your appraisal with your educational supervisor.

What is the purpose of this process?

A. For policy making.
B. It is mainly for research purposes.
C. To review a doctor's performance.
D. To rate clinical services based on a doctor's performance.
E. To set out personal and professional development needs, career paths and goals.

ANSWERS

Q1: B. In-house multidisciplinary training courses [evidence level 3][1]

- Introduction of a mandatory one-day inhouse training course, which included an intensive cardiotocography training session, resulted in a significant reduction in five-minute Apgar scores <7 and the incidence of severe hypoxic ischaemic encephalopathy.
- However, currently there are no randomized controlled trials to support this.

Q2: B. Practical, multi-professional, obstetric emergency training at your hospital [evidence level 1][2]

- Training is the systematic acquisition of knowledge (what we think), skills (what we do) and attitudes (what we feel). It should lead to improved performance in a particular environment.
- The Simulation and Fire-drill Evaluation study is a large randomized controlled trial recently completed in the southwest of England. It evaluated the effect of training in local hospitals versus training at a central simulation centre and the effect of an additional day of specific teamwork training.
- The study concluded that practical, multiprofessional, obstetric emergency training increased midwives' and doctors' knowledge of obstetric emergency management regardless of the location of training, in a simulation centre or in local hospitals.
- The Clinical Negligence Scheme for Trusts recommends annual training for all staff.

Q3: E. It reassures patients, employers and other professionals and contributes to improving patient care and safety [evidence level 2].[3]

- Medical revalidation is the process by which the General Medical Council confirms the continuation of a doctor's license to practise in the UK.
- Revalidation is intended to reassure patients, employers and other professionals and to contribute to improving patient care and safety.
- The patient feedback questionnaires form an essential part of the assessment process along with multi-source feedback collected from colleagues.
- For the purpose of revalidation, it only needs to be collected five-yearly.
- Revalidation is mandatory and applies to all the clinical staff working in the NHS.

Q4: E. Choose a topic that meets the auditable standards of the College guidelines.[4]

- NICE defines clinical audit as 'a quality improvement process that seeks to improve patient care and outcomes through systematic review of care against explicit criteria and the implementation of change'.
- The lack of an existing standard does not preclude audit. A standard can be defined during the audit design.
- Ideally, a standard should be evidence-based but audit is still important in areas that are lacking clear evidence.
- Staff working in the area being audited should be involved from the planning stage. They may well need to collect the data initially, and for re-audit, and will be essential in implementing change if needed.
- A statistical significance need not be reached for useful audit.

Q5: A. A process of structured investigations to identify the root causes of faults or problems [evidence level 3].[5]

- Root cause analysis is a collective term to describe a wide range of approaches, tools and techniques used to uncover the root causes of problems.
- It is usually conducted for high-level incidents.

Q6: B. Class this as a never event.[6]

- A retained swab is classed as a never event.[6]
- Never events are serious, largely preventable patient safety incidents that should not occur if the available preventative measures have been implemented.

- They may act as a marker for a fundamental problem about patient safety within an organization.
- All missing items must be documented in the perioperative care plan, theatre register and patient's notes.
- The scrub practitioner must report the missing item to the nurse/midwife in charge and a clinical incident must be completed on Datix.

Q7: E. It helps tailor treatment plans to meet the patient's preferences and needs.[7]

- Patient-reported outcome measures can be used to assess quality and effectiveness of care from the patient's perspective.
- This can lead to reduction of inequalities of care and improved referral patterns to secondary care.

Q8: E. The risk is calculated by multiplying the severity of harm with the likelihood of harm [evidence level 3].[8]

- The multiplication of severity with the likelihood of occurrence gives the composite risk index.
- A risk score of 20 or more is considered unacceptable.

Q9: A. Access to personal data should be on a strict need-to-know basis [evidence level 3].[9]

- The Caldicott principles for obtaining, recording, holding, using or disposing of personal data are: (1) Justify the reason. (2) Do not use personal confidential data unless it is absolutely necessary. (3) Use the minimum amount of personal confidential data necessary. (4) Access to personal confidential data should be on a strict need-to-know basis. (5) Everyone with access to personal confidential data should be aware of their responsibilities. (6) Comply with the law. (7) The duty to share information can be as important as the duty to protect patient confidentiality.

10: E. To set out personal and professional development needs, career paths and goals [evidence level 3].[10]

- Appraisal is a part of clinical governance.
- It is arranged annually to set out personal and professional development needs, career paths and goals and to agree a plan for the following year.

References

1. Draycott T, Sibanda T, Owen L, et al. Does training in obstetric emergencies improve neonatal outcome? *Br J Obstet Gynaecol* 2006;113:177–82.
2. Crofts JF, Ellis D, Draycott TJ, et al. Change in knowledge of midwives and obstetricians following obstetric emergency training: a randomised controlled trial of local hospital, simulation center and teamwork training. *Br J Obstet Gynaecol* 2007;114:1534–41.
3. General Medical Council. *Colleague and Patient Feedback for Revalidation.* [www.gmc-uk.org]
4. National Institute for Health and Clinical Excellence. *Principles for Best Practice in Clinical Audit.* [https://www.nice.org.uk/about/what-we-do/into-practice/audit-and-service-improvement]
5. National Health Service. *Root Cause Analysis (RCA) Investigation.* [www.nrls.npsa.nhs.uk/resources/collection]

6. Government Publications. *The Never Events List*, 2012–13. January, 2012. [https://www.gov.uk/government/publications/the-never-events-list-for-2012-13]
7. Department of Health. *Guidance on the Routine Collection of Patient Reported Outcome Measures (PROMS)*. July, 2011. [https://www.gov.uk/government/publications/tliers–2]
8. Royal College of Obstetricians and Gynaecologists. *Improving Patient Safety: Risk Management for Maternity and Gynaecology*., September, 2009. [https://www.rcog.org.uk/en/guidelines-research-services/guidelines/clinical-governance-advice-2]
9. Department of Health. *Information to Share or not to Share? Government Response to the Caldicott Review*. September, 2013. [https://www.gov.ukgovernment/publications/caldicott-information-governance-review-department-of-health-response]
10. General Medical Council. *Good Medical Practice Framework for Appraisal and Revalidation*. March, 2013. [www.gmc.uk.org/doctors/revalidation/revalidation_gmp_framework.asp]

Index